Health Culture in the Heartland,
1880–1980

Health Culture in the Heartland, 1880–1980

An Oral History

LUCINDA McCRAY BEIER

University of Illinois Press

URBANA AND CHICAGO

Library of Congress Cataloging-in-Publication Data
Beier, Lucinda McCray.
Health culture in the heartland, 1880-1980 : an oral history /
Lucinda McCray Beier.
p. ; cm.
Includes bibliographical references and index.
ISBN-13 978-0-252-03348-3 (cloth : alk. paper)
ISBN-10 0-252-03348-5 (cloth : alk. paper)
ISBN-13 978-0-252-07554-4 (pbk. : alk. paper)
ISBN-10 0-252-07554-4 (pbk. : alk. paper)
1. Medicine—Illinois—McLean County—History.
2. Medical care—Illinois—McLean County—History.
3. Public health—Illinois—McLean County—History.
I. Title.
[DNLM: 1. Community Health Services—history—Illinois.
2. Delivery of Health Care—history—Illinois. 3. History,
19th Century—Illinois. 4. History, 20th Century—Illinois.
5. Public Health—history—Illinois. WA 11 A13 B422h 2009]
R210.M35B43   2009
610.9773'59—dc22   2008029715

Dedicated to the memory of my mother,
Janet Hough McCray (1927–2004),
Whose strength, wisdom,
creativity, love, and laughter
made my world.

Contents

Acknowledgments   viii

Introduction: A Matter of Life and Death   ix

1. Living and Dying in Nineteenth-Century McLean County   1

2. No Place Like Home: Hospitals and the Development of
   Institutional Care   22

3. Nursing, Gender, and Modern Medicine   44

4. Doctors and Organized Medicine   73

5. An Ounce of Prevention: Public Health Services   117

6. Matters of Life and Death: Experience and Expectations of
   Health, Illness, and Medical Care in the Twentieth Century   136

   Conclusion: Health Culture in Transition   179

   Appendix: Oral History Informants   191

   Notes   195

   Bibliography   223

   Index   233

Illustrations follow page 116

Acknowledgments

No book is truly written alone. However, few have enjoyed as much collective attention as this one. First of all, it is my pleasure and honor to thank the community volunteers who explored McLean County's experience of health, illness, and medicine with me: Ruth Carpenter, Margaret Esposito, Corlin Ferguson, Deborah Finfgeld, Christine Kibler, John Krueger, Nadine Reining, Michael Robak, and Madge Williams. I also want to thank the oral history informants whose memories compose the heart of this book.

I am very grateful to staff members at the McLean County Museum of History in Bloomington, Illinois, including Susan Hartzold, Preston Hawks, Bill Kemp, and Greg Koos. Thanks are also due to the Illinois Wesleyan University's College of Nursing, the McLean County Health Department, the McLean County Medical Society, the Mennonite College of Nursing (now of Illinois State University), and the Sisters of the Third Order of St. Francis for providing access to their records. Many thanks to the Bloomington-Normal Black History Project and Cynthia Baer for sharing their oral history transcripts with me. I wish to acknowledge the financial support provided to the original museum exhibit and book project by the Illinois Humanities Council. I am also grateful to the subject and interlibrary loan librarians at Milner Library, Illinois State University. In addition, I wish to acknowledge the suggestions of Laurie Matheson, of the University of Illinois Press, and three anonymous reviewers, whose comments made all the difference.

Finally, I must thank my family. My parents, Robert and Janet McCray, and wonderful siblings, Gary, Hollis, Bob, Leslie, Janet, and David, contested and nurtured the arguments contained in this book—many of which emerged during a half-century of dinner-table conversations. And my husband, Lee, and sons, Joe, Jesse, Jake, and Zach, tolerated and cheered the long revision process: thanks, guys.

A Matter of Life and Death

Suffering and Healing in
McLean County, Illinois

In 1879 two German nuns drove a horse-drawn wagon forty-five miles on dirt roads from Peoria to Bloomington, Illinois, to explore the possibility of opening a new hospital. Members of the Third Order of the Sisters of St. Francis, Reverend Mother Frances and Sister Augustina, had been in the United States for only five years, refugees from Otto von Bismarck's persecution of the Roman Catholic clergy.[1] The Sister nurses, fresh from setting up Peoria's St. Francis Hospital in 1876, discussed their ideas with two local physicians who agreed to assemble a medical staff for the proposed facility. In March 1880 St. Joseph's Hospital—McLean County's first—opened in an "old brick mansion" on the outskirts of town, purchased by the Order for $7,000.[2]

This event occurred at the end of a decade that had witnessed increasing attention to health issues in Bloomington. In 1871 an ordinance was passed stopping residents from letting livestock run at large in the streets.[3] In 1874 the city started construction of a sewerage system and a public water supply.[4] In 1877 it began paving streets with brick.[5] Thus, with hindsight, 1880 can be viewed as a watershed, marking significant changes in the ways urban McLean County residents thought about and dealt with health and illness. The year 1880 marked the beginning of a trend away from traditional, individualized, home-based, dominantly lay management of birth, ill-health, and death in the county, and toward collective professional and institutional management of these matters—a trend that would not be completed until the middle of the twentieth century, but was heralded by unlikely harbingers of change, two German Sister nurses in a horse-drawn wagon. Although Reverend Mother Frances and Sister Augustina would have seen themselves more as traditional religious providers of residential care than as trailblazers, by establishing the area's first hospital they helped spearhead a health-care revolution. Thus, 1880 is the point at which my account of health, illness, and medicine in McLean County begins.

It ends in about 1980, when McLean County's health-care delivery system began another major transition. Influenced by the opportunities and stresses of a changing business and regulatory climate, the county's medical organizations took new forms—collaborating, diversifying, and contending with new types of competition. The heyday of fee-for-service medicine was ending, but the shape of the future was not yet clear. Although the conclusion of this book provides a glimpse of the years between 1980 and 2000, that complicated period deserves its own study and a different research design.

Approach

This book is a history of community health culture.[6] That history subsumes the beliefs, behaviors, expectations, and experiences of sufferers and healers; women and men; and members of diverse social class, ethnic, and racial groups. It presumes that the theories, practices, and roles associated with "biomedicine" are cultural products that, like informal health-care delivery systems and traditions, are determined by social, cultural, political, and economic factors.[7] My approach is informed by recent work in medical anthropology and sociology, which extends scholarly perspectives beyond arguably biased categories and polarities—"learned" versus "folk" medicine; "professionals" versus "laypeople"; "scientific" versus "popular" viewpoints—and benefits from interdisciplinary methods and theories.[8] I presume that each pair of categories, rather than being necessarily polarized, inhabits a common space, where overlaps are the rule rather than the exception, and polarization may itself be a manifestation of power dynamics both observed and used by participants in the process.

In fact, many health-related concepts and tasks are shared among occupational experts and nonexperts, and the experience of these groups changes relentlessly in response to broader trends. Thus, as societies alter as a result of, say, industrialization or the Women's Movement, their conceptualization and management of birth, illness, injury, disability, and death also change. Furthermore, biomedicine itself is not unitary, but rather includes both elements common among national and regional Western health cultures (e.g., acceptance of the germ theory of disease causation) and differences that reveal demographic, political, economic, and cultural diversity (e.g., management of childbirth).[9] My intention is to add a regional case study to a growing and eclectic body of research on health culture, of which *Hearts of*

Wisdom, Emily Abel's work on family caregivers, and *The Gospel of Germs,* Nancy Tomes' "ethnoscience" research on social responses to germ theory, are but two outstanding examples.

Despite the trends favoring social history and history told from the "bottom up" that began in the 1960s, the history of health and illness has continued to be dominated by a focus on physicians—their ideas, professional development, and relationships with each other and the wider society. Even histories of nursing, hospitals, public health, disease, and the "patient's view" are often composed in terms of their association with doctors—regardless of the fact that most experience of ill-health and care occurs when doctors are not present, and involves the ideas and participation of a great many non-physicians.[10] This is not surprising, given the power of professional medicine in Western societies. However, because scholars are also products of these societies, to a large degree the physician has been exempted from cultural analysis except in somewhat splendid occupational segregation. Sociologist Deborah Lupton explains that scholars "have tended not to view medicine as a product or part of culture, but as an objective body of scientific knowledge external to culture (where 'science' is seen as the antithesis of 'culture') . . ."[11]

Nonscholars share this perspective. Oral history interviews I have conducted with laypeople in both the United States and Britain reveal a durable preoccupation with "the doctor." Although informants described a rich and multifaceted health culture, when asked "What did you and your family members do when someone got sick?" the answer invariably indicated whether or not a physician was consulted. Only after follow-up questions (e.g., "Would you, perhaps, try to deal with an illness at home before calling the doctor?") did informants discuss a broader scenario of decision making and care. I argue that the centrality of the physician in the historical scholarship reflects the gendered and class-stratified society in which he achieved hegemony.[12]

In the twentieth century, biomedicine became perhaps the most effective tool of state, professional, gender, and class power in the industrialized world. Less contested than capitalism, technology, or any religious doctrine, and linked to the dominant scientific worldview, for approximately 100 years biomedicine has been seen and employed as an unalloyed good. It's most visible agents, allopathic physicians (particularly those trained after about 1910), have represented both scientific progress and wise altruism. Thus, in an historical study of community experience and management of ill-health, it is a struggle not to repeat the formulaic account in which doctors occupy center stage, other care providers are invisible, and "patients" are passive beneficiaries of professional expertise.

Although this book provides a good deal of information about McLean County's medical practitioners, it views doctors, other health-care workers, and "laypeople" as sharing a shifting spectrum of expectations concerning life experiences and concepts (both "popular" and "learned") regarding health, ill-health, and therapeutics; and negotiating for power, resources, and status in a dynamic affected by science, politics, economics, gender, and social relationships. This reconceptualization strengthens the voices and perspectives of other county residents and health-care workers, at the same time enabling a more nuanced perception of physicians' own experiences—in part, because the doctor is only expected to speak for him- or (more rarely) herself, rather than on behalf of the entire health-care system or community. Due to resource limitations, in this book, the voices of laypeople, nurses, and doctors are loudest. Furthermore, this book focuses on childbearing and physical ills, leaving mental disorders for the attention of other researchers. This is not a history of professional or institutional medicine. Rather, it considers the impact of institutional and professional medical development, together with other factors, on community health experience and culture in the twentieth century.

Sources and Methods

This book represents the final stage in a journey that began in 1992, when I agreed to serve as guest curator for a temporary museum exhibit on the history of medicine in McLean County. Nine community volunteers and several members of the McLean County Museum of History's professional staff worked with me on archival research, oral history interviews, and collection of objects. As research progressed, it became clear that we had far more information than the exhibit required. Thus, I wrote a book, *A Matter of Life and Death: Health, Illness and Medicine in McLean County, 1830–1995*, to allow more in-depth exploration of our research topics and expansion of the amount of material—particularly from oral history interviews—that could be made available. That volume provided the foundation for the present work.

This book benefits from the perspective of a decade during which major national and international debates have influenced scholarship about health, medicine, and society, which offered an opportunity to get what my now-adult sons used to call a "do-over"—to address some of the limitations in the first book and take some new risks with familiar evidence. It also enabled me to focus, in this new study, on the period between 1880 and 1980.

This is, of course, a work of local medical and public health history. It joins an established historiography that includes research conducted by both professional and nonprofessional historians.[13] Exploring the experience of McLean County residents, this book considers rural, small-town, and small-city health cultures. Urban historians recognize that their field "tends to focus on the development of large cities, and relatively few historians have considered the history of small towns and cities, particularly those in the Midwest."[14] At the same time, they note that there were many more small than large cities in the United States in the late-nineteenth and twentieth centuries.[15] In terms of its urbanization, McLean County followed the national pattern of more than 50 percent of its residents living in rural (populations of fewer than 2,500) places before 1920 and more than 50 percent of its residents living in urban (larger than 2,500) places after 1920. However, these arbitrary statistics mask the fact that throughout the twentieth century, county population continued to be distributed in more than twenty hamlets as well as "out in the country." Also, although the majority of residents' health-care needs have been met within the county, proximity to Chicago (120 miles away) and other large Midwestern cities offered additional health-care resources. Thus, in contrast to works focusing on large cities, this book arguably illuminates the diverse community environments, as well as care and treatment options, that would have been familiar to a majority of Americans during the period under consideration. It also suggests an alternative to the conventional polarization of rural and urban, considering that during the study period McLean County residents, although never more than a mile away from farmed fields, also routinely used urban amenities—public transportation, downtown shopping, public libraries, educational institutions, and health-care facilities—and tended to consider themselves neither isolated rural- nor big city-dwellers.

In contrast to works regarding a single component of formal health-care provision—nursing, professional medicine, hospitals, or public health—this book takes an inclusive approach that, while exploring development of those elements of local health-care delivery, also views community residents not exclusively as passive "patients" automatically accepting services offered to them, but as individuals active in defining and addressing their own health-related needs. And, in contrast to community studies in which health and medicine are minor facets of a much larger picture, this research employs health culture as the lens through which to explore other aspects of the wider social world.[16]

Research for this book benefited from the loving preservation and maintenance of archival collections by the McLean County Historical Society and the Sisters of the Third Order of St. Francis. Particularly useful were McLean County Medical Society records for the years between 1891 and 1910; accounts, admission, and medical staff records for St. Joseph's Hospital from

1880 to 1906; and personal documents illuminating the experiences of both sufferers and healers.[17] Its real strength is, however, oral history evidence, which has the unique capacity both to fill gaps in the information supplied by written sources and offer alternatives to the perspectives of professional and institutional medicine.[18] Twenty-nine interviews were conducted specifically for the museum exhibit project by nine community volunteers and myself (see appendix). The volunteers included three nurses, a home economist, a lawyer, a physician, a student, and two others whose occupational backgrounds are not known. Three were male. Volunteers ranged in age from their mid-thirties to over eighty. Interviews were tape-recorded, transcribed, and subject indexed.[19] It is noteworthy that, although we expected interviews with doctors and nurses to elicit information about healing, and interviews with laypeople to elicit information about suffering and receiving medical care, in fact health-care practitioners often talked about their experiences as sufferers and patients, and laypeople described providing care and treatment to loved ones.

Interview informants were born between 1894 and 1938. They included eighteen women, eleven men, two African Americans, twenty-seven whites, thirteen laypeople, eight nurses, six physicians, one dentist, and one public health sanitarian. Eighteen informants had spent most of their lives in Bloomington or its twin city, Normal; ten had mainly lived in rural McLean County; one came from a small town in another central Illinois county. Informants were selected to provide specific perspectives (e.g., general practitioner, specialist, public health nurse, graduate of an early bachelor's degree nursing program, etc.) that the group believed should be represented in our study. Interviewees had a range of socioeconomic and educational backgrounds. They gave permission for their real names to be used in publications resulting from our research.

In addition to interviews conducted specifically for this project, this book also includes oral evidence collected for other research purposes. A graduate student gave permission for us to use her interviews about childbearing with three women from different generations of her family.[20] I also consulted interviews with nine African-American county residents conducted in the 1980s by members of the Bloomington-Normal Black History Project, which shed light on black experience of ill-health and care in McLean County during the long period before civil rights legislation and changing social norms ended formal racial discrimination in health-care provision.

Interview recordings and transcripts are the only historical evidence deliberately created by the historian. Although the scholar's charge is always to select and interpret evidence professionally, the oral historian bears additional responsibilities. S/he devises the questions, selects the informants, guides the interviews, assesses the meaning of what has been said, and selects the evidence to be incorporated into the historical work. The relationship between the interviewer and the informant is important. Within any interview situation there are both power dynamics and the desire of the informant to present him-or herself in the best possible light.[21] The resulting interview is invariably "the product of both the narrator and the researcher"—an issue that was complicated, in the research under consideration, by involvement of multiple interviewers.[22]

Every oral historian must decide how to refer to the people who contribute their memories to a research project. The usual choices are "interviewees," "respondents," "narrators," or "informants." The terms *interviewees* and *respondents* reflect one truth—that interviewers ask questions. However, these terms also ignore the more important truth that people who are interviewed control what they say. A "narrator" is a person who tells a story about a situation or event in which he or she may or may not have participated; oral history includes more than stories, but always involves personal experience and point of view. Thus, the term *informant*, which I mainly use in this book, implies the speaker's discretion about the content and attributes credit for the evidence provided.

Another, more important, challenge in using oral history is the issue of memory. How accurate are accounts of events and emotions of the some-times distant past? How much of what is remembered takes on the qualities of myth or mantra? In this study, lay informants hark back nostalgically to a time when people were healthy and medical attention was personal and cheap; nurses fondly recall an era when bedside care took up most of their time; and physicians remember old-fashioned patient-doctor relationships that had not yet been corroded by lay criticism and malpractice litigation. These accounts say as much about an experienced present as they do about a past reality. However, so often are they repeated that they reveal elements of community health culture that are as important as "facts." By contrast, informants reported common experiences—of home quarantine, for ex-ample, or of private duty nursing—that, though repeated, do not appear to mythologize the past, but instead offer a glimpses of a real health culture that has nearly been forgotten.[23] Thus, insights emerged from comparison of informants' accounts and identification of representative or contrasting stories, which are used in this book with other evidence as "textual verifica-tions of a historical interpretation."[24]

There are limitations in the oral evidence used for this book. In contrast to my work with the life histories of 239 working-class residents of three northern English cities, resource constraints limited this study to far fewer interviews.[25] Interviews with members of additional health-care occupations—pharmacists, hospital administrators, technicians, and mental health professionals, for example—would certainly have enriched this research. In addition, the ages of informants affected the quantity and quality of information about the experience of suffering, caring, and healing during different parts of the twentieth century; thus, interviews with nurses and laypeople are strongest about the interwar period, whereas interviews with the physicians, dentist, and public health administrator are most informative about the post–World War II era. Furthermore, the ethnicity of respondents affects perspectives offered in this book; African American and native-born white perspectives are comparatively well represented, but European and Latin American perspectives are lacking, despite the significant number of immigrants who lived in McLean County throughout the study period. In addition, black informants came from well-established local families, arguably representing a social elite within the county's African American community. By contrast, the perspectives of comparative newcomers who arrived in the county after World War I are not included.

Despite these limitations, oral history evidence enriches and strengthens this book. In contrast to works based on institutional or professional medical records, this evidence documents the experiences of nurses and sufferers. Furthermore, *how* informants talked about their pasts is informative. Nurses' repeated accounts of standing when doctors entered a room before the 1960s represented many other changes in this important relationship during the post–World War II years. Laypeople remembering being very healthy as children, despite having suffered from serious ailments including scarlet fever, whooping cough, and rheumatic fever, indicated changing conceptualization and expectations of health and illness. Older physicians—particularly general practitioners—criticizing younger doctors for being "in it just for the money"—suggested a downside to professional progress more often discussed in triumphal terms. Furthermore, what informants did *not* say is also important. For example, despite the large numbers of nurses trained and employed in McLean County, few laypeople or physicians mentioned nurses as part of the health-care environment; similarly, doctors' preoccupation with medical malpractice litigation rarely appeared in laypeople's and nurses' accounts.

For these and other reasons, oral history evidence is quoted at length in this book. I do not adhere to what might be called the Studs Terkel school of letting the informant speak for him- or herself. Rather, I use other source material to help contextualize and interpret informants' accounts—a technique I learned from Dr. Elizabeth Roberts at the Centre for North-West

Regional Studies at Lancaster University (United Kingdom) when I served as her research assistant in the late 1980s.[26]

Organization

This book is organized thematically rather than chronologically to enable the voices of nurses, physicians, public health professionals, and laypeople to be clearly heard and to enable the reader to focus on these distinct perspectives. Disadvantages of this choice include potential confusion about chronology and some overlapping of topics among chapters. Furthermore, it could be argued that segregating perspectives of doctors, nurses, and people who do not work in health-care occupations perpetuates the conventional polarity between "expert" and "lay." There can be no doubt that this distinction exists, both in legal and professional designations, and less formally in social relationships and cultural meanings. However, I hope that the structure I have chosen will not privilege one perspective over the other, but will facilitate a fuller, more textured view of community health culture.

The book begins by setting the scene. In 1880, McLean County's urban heart and its rural communities were well established. Yet, conditions and choices dating from earlier years helped to shape the environment for change in health care after that date. Chapter 1 introduces late nineteenth-century McLean County, providing information about population, economy, morbidity and mortality, health-care practices and resources, and collective responses to ill-health.[27]

Chapter 2 considers the development of hospitals in McLean County, using St. Joseph's Hospital as a case study to explore their late nineteenth-century formation as charitable substitutes for sufferers' homes and going on to document their mid-twentieth-century transformation into specialized technology-driven factories of health. In McLean County, as elsewhere, this transition exemplifies changes in the expectations and experiences of health-care providers and consumers. The county's hospitals also became both visible signs of its modern development and centrally located services attracting patients from a large rural region.

Closely related to the establishment and expansion of McLean County's hospitals was the development of nurse training programs and of nursing as a respectable and popular occupation for local women. Chapter 3 discusses the hospitals' early dependence on the labor of student nurses and the mid-twentieth-century shift toward hospital employment of graduate nurses. It considers the changing pattern of nurses' careers, from private duty in the first half of the century to work in hospitals and doctors' offices after World

War II. It argues that nurses were important translators and mediators of biomedicine for sufferers.

Chapter 4 focuses on the work lives of physicians in McLean County. It observes the shift from general practice to specialization and from home- and office-based practice to increasing dependence on hospital privileges, which was linked to the evolution of organized medicine in the county. It also explores increasing expectations of biomedicine, which, on the one hand, enhanced physicians' status and incomes but, on the other, exposed them to growing risk of malpractice litigation.

Chapter 5 discusses public health provision during the twentieth century. Selecting for particular attention Fairview Tuberculosis Sanitarium, the Co-operative Extension Service's Home Bureau, and development of government-supported public health infrastructure, services, and enforcement, it explores changes in collective efforts to prevent disease in the county.

Chapter 6 explores lay health culture between about 1880 and the late twentieth century. It observes changing patterns and expectations of ill health, from traditional reliance on home care and nursing in the early twentieth century to increasing dependence on professional institutional attention as time went on. It considers differences in county residents' attitudes toward, access to, and use of professional medicine according to gender, race, social class, and place of residence. It also discusses rising expectations that converted medical care from a luxury to a necessity.

The final chapter offers conclusions about changes in McLean County's health culture that are organized around three central themes: changes in the *place* of treatment, care, and prevention; in *agency and authority* regarding these matters; and in the *interpretations and expectations* of health experiences and management. It closes with a brief discussion of health-care needs and resources in McLean County at the end of the twentieth century.

1. Living and Dying in Nineteenth-Century McLean County

The County

First settled by migrants of European and African heritage during the 1820s, the area that became McLean County in 1830 is located in north central Illinois, 120 miles southwest of Chicago.[1] Early settlers encountered a flat grassland, interrupted by occasional groves of trees that sheltered and named many of the area's earliest communities—Keg Grove (later renamed Blooming Grove and, still later, Bloomington), Twin Grove, Cheney's Grove, Funk's Grove. There were no navigable bodies of water—only creeks that flooded during spring rains and almost disappeared in the heat of late summer. The county's natural wealth was its soil—black, deep, stoneless dirt deposited by the same glaciers that carved out the Great Lakes. Unlocked by the steel moldboard plow, the corn planter, and the reaper, introduced between 1842 and 1853, that heavy fertile soil produced grains and livestock that enriched the county's farmers and supported growth of its towns and cities.[2]

In addition to agriculture, McLean County nurtured industries, foremost among which was rail transportation. In 1851 the Illinois Central railroad broke ground for a line to connect the Great Lakes with New Orleans and the Gulf of Mexico. Midway between Chicago and St. Louis was McLean County's largest town and county seat, Bloomington (incorporated in 1843), where, as a result of local political and financial influence, both the Illinois Central and the Alton and Sangamon (later renamed the Chicago and Alton) railroad lines arrived in 1853. In the same year, the Chicago and Alton Company opened a Bloomington facility to manufacture and repair equipment. The presence of the railroad lines and works literally put McLean County on the map; between 1850 and 1860, the county's population increased from 10,163 to 28,772.[3] For the next century, the "Alton Shops" was the county's major employer, at its peak in the early twentieth century employing three thousand men and women.[4] Only after World War II, when the shops closed and State Farm Insurance mushroomed, would a larger number and proportion of county residents work for another employer.[5]

Attraction of the railroad lines and works suggests an important factor in the county's success—its political and business leaders, who had close ties with state and national powerbrokers. For example, Abraham Lincoln was personally and politically allied with the Fell family (local businessmen, lawyers, and politicians) and the lawyer David Davis (1815–86), whom he appointed to the U.S. Supreme Court in 1862.[6] On the other side of the political divide, Dr. Thomas Rogers (1812–99), a charter member of the McLean County Medical Society (founded in 1854), settled in Bloomington in 1849 because he learned from Stephen Douglas that the Illinois Central Railroad line was going to pass through the town. Retiring from medicine in 1867, Rogers continued to be active in Democratic politics, serving in the Illinois Legislature from 1872–80.[7] Jesse Fell (1808–87), a lawyer who arrived in the county in 1833, helped broker the deals that brought the Chicago and Alton Shops to Bloomington and established (in 1857) Illinois' first public university, Illinois State Normal University (ISNU), in Normal (incorporated in 1865).[8] Jesse's brother, Kersey H. Fell (1815–93), was one of the thirty local leaders who established the Methodist Illinois Wesleyan University in 1850.[9] Judge David Davis donated the land for both ISNU and the Soldiers' Orphans' Home (1865), Illinois' only residential facility for children of Union soldiers killed or disabled during the Civil War.[10]

Instead of being refugees from poverty or lack of opportunity elsewhere, many of McLean County's early residents should be viewed as entrepreneurs, gambling on the prospects of the new settlement. After all, before the mid-nineteenth century, it was by no means a foregone conclusion that Chicago and St. Louis (with 1840 populations of 4,470 and 16,469, respectively) would become the dominant regional cites.[11] The numerous Fells, who arrived in Blooming Grove in the 1830s, were descendents of the English family that helped found the Quaker faith and ancestors of Adlai Stevenson I and II.[12] James Allin (1788–1869) moved from North Carolina to Kentucky, Indiana, and southwestern Illinois before realizing "that a line drawn from the rapids of the Illinois River to Cairo would pass through Blooming Grove. It was also on a direct line from Chicago to Alton and St. Louis." In 1830, Allin built the first house in Bloomington, advocated passage of a bill in the state legislature to found McLean County, and donated twenty-two and a half acres for the new county seat.[13] These examples suggest that the county's development was crafted by people expecting to gain from its success.

Members of this elite conformed to what Timothy Mahoney calls a "booster ethos."[14] Attraction of railroad lines and works fostered other enterprises including a coal mine, manufacture of heavy agricultural equipment, tile and brick works, and nursery businesses.[15] Trains linked the county with regional and remote markets. Left comparatively unscathed by the Panic of 1857, and avoiding the dependence on a single product that undermined many local economies in the late nineteenth century, by 1880 McLean County was both self-sufficient and well connected to other population centers in the region.[16]

In that year, 60,115 people lived in the county; of these, just over one-third lived in the city of Bloomington (20,484) and its much smaller "twin" city, Normal (2,470). The remaining 36,161 residents lived either on scattered farmsteads or in the county's twenty small settlements.[17] Mirroring national trends, McLean County's population remained predominantly rural until after 1920.[18] (See Table 1.)

Although there were African American residents in the county from the earliest days of settlement, its population has been predominantly white, native-born, and of European heritage; between 1880 and 1900, 1.5 percent of the county's population was nonwhite and between 1910 and 1960, approximately two percent of the county's population was nonwhite.[19]

The development of McLean County and its communities exemplifies relationships discussed by urban scholars in terms of "central place" and "network

Table 1: Populations of Bloomington, Normal, and McLean County, Illinois, 1880–1960

Census Year	Bloomington	Normal	McLean County
1880	20,484	2,470	60,100
1890	23,286	3,459	63,036
1900	25,768	3,795	67,843
1910	28,725	4,024	68,008
1920	30,930	5,143	70,107
1930	32,868	6,768	73,117
1940	34,163	6,983	73,930
1950	36,271	9,772	76,577
1960	39,992	13,357	83,877

Sources: The Illinois Fact Book and Historical Almanac 1673–1968 (Carbondale: Southern Illinois University Press, 1970); *Blue Book of the State of Illinois,* 1910–1960 (Springfield, Ill.: Office of the Secretary of State); United States Censuses, 1880–1960.

systems" models.[20] McLean County's twin cities, Bloomington and Normal, served as central places for a region extending beyond county boundaries. An administrative, commercial, transportation, educational, and social hub, the cities generated wealth and provided services that expanded, after 1880, to include health care.

Health and Illness in Nineteenth-Century McLean County

In the early years of settlement, Illinois had "the reputation of being one of the most unhealthful portions of the United States."[21] As was generally true before the mortality transition, which occurred in the United States in the late nineteenth and early twentieth centuries, the major challenge to health consisted of communicable diseases in epidemic or endemic forms.[22] Visitors (including Charles Dickens) and settlers remarked particularly on the fevers infesting the region.[23]

It is impossible to obtain accurate morbidity and mortality statistics for most of the nineteenth century, because cause of death was not reported before the 1850 Census and there was no standard state mechanism for reporting or maintaining information about the incidence of contagious diseases until about 1885. Indeed, before 1918, one expert estimated that the state's mortality figures were between 60 and 80 percent incomplete.[24] Furthermore, mortality data—however complete—are only a crude guide to incidence of illness and resulting impact on quality of life. Nonetheless, imperfect statistics together with contemporary reports provide an evocative impression of the health conditions of early McLean County residents.

Most of the agues, chills, autumnal, bilious, remittent, and intermittent fevers settlers reported were probably malaria.[25] Several variants of the ailment flourished in Illinois' low, wet, undrained terrain, which bred clouds of insects.[26] Residents recognized an environmental cause for these fevers, but explained this in terms of the miasma rising from newly broken soil or lurking in the dangerous night air. Intermittent fever was an expected part of life in the region. Mrs. Tillson, recalling her 1821 experiences in Pike County (Western Illinois), wrote, "An illness native in the prairie country was fever and ague. There was burning fever following chills which left the patient so weak he could not work. It came with perfect regularity."[27] An early McLean County poet reflected on the prevalence of fever, writing, "I'd rather live on a camel's rump / And be a Yankee Doodle beggar, / Than where they never see a stump / And shake to death with fever *ager*."[28] Both professional and lay observers associated fevers and fluxes with "seasoning"—the process of adapting to new conditions, establishing a home, and cultivating the soil.[29]

Ague sufferers became depleted and depressed as the illness lingered.[30] And, although the quinine nineteenth-century Americans took for all fevers was actually effective in controlling the symptoms of malaria, the disease caused significant mortality in Illinois, which declined only with the draining and tiling of agricultural lands during the last half of the nineteenth century.[31] As towns grew, however, other communicable diseases, including smallpox, cholera, typhoid, diphtheria, tuberculosis, diarrheal diseases, and ailments now known to be caused by streptococci, including scarlet fever, erysipelas, and puerperal fever, increased in incidence and mortality.

Always endemic and sometimes epidemic in Europe and Africa, small-pox was an early import from the Old to the New World. Although Jenner's vaccination technique was well known by the early years of the nineteenth century, many people feared it, and vaccination tended to be used mainly in response to an outbreak rather than as a preventative measure.[32] Before 1878 Illinois required isolation of smallpox sufferers, but not vaccination. Thus, its communities displayed the familiar pattern of regular rare incidence of the disease, interspersed at intervals with epidemics that disfigured sufferers it did not kill. As late as 1925, a Bloomington outbreak sickened 109 people.[33] Although it produced lower local mortality than other disorders, includ-ing malaria, tuberculosis, and diarrhea, smallpox as one of the few diseases generally presumed to be contagious was feared out of all proportion to its danger. Thus, for example, in the 1830s or '40s, Dr. Henry sheltered in his Bloomington home an eight-year-old girl and her mother who were suffer-ing from smallpox to save them from being expelled from the settlement by the terrified residents.[34] Things had not changed much by 1882, when a honeymoon couple and several other migrants showing smallpox symptoms arrived in Bloomington and were blamed for an epidemic that killed 2,641 people in Illinois that year.[35]

Cholera came to McLean County in 1834, two years after its first appearance in North America. Thereafter, local incidence mirrored national outbreaks of the disease until 1873. The worst McLean County epidemic occurred in the summer of 1855, when at least seventy-two sufferers died.[36] Cholera was feared, in part, because it killed so quickly. Describing the 1849–52 outbreak in Henry County (also in central Illinois), one observer wrote, "Men would go to work in the morning in good health and be dead before sundown."[37] Thus, newspapers tracked its movements, and communities took measures to prevent local sickness. Based on the miasma theory of disease causation, they cleaned their streets; associating outbreaks with the arrival of strangers, they banned the entrance of travelers from afflicted areas.[38]

Tuberculosis was a leading killer in the United States for much of the nine-teenth century. Until its bacillus was discovered by Robert Koch in 1882, the disease was not generally regarded as contagious.[39] Although it was generally believed that hard physical labor and fresh air helped to prevent and cure tuberculosis, involuntary outdoor therapy did not keep the disease from affecting McLean County's early residents; at least eight of the seventy-eight deaths reported in 1850 were due to consumption, with the likelihood that five more attributed to ailments such as "inflammation of the lungs" and "lung disease" brought the real total to nearly 17 percent. In 1860, of three hundred McLean County deaths, twenty-eight were from consumption, eleven from "lung fever," and two from congested lungs, suggesting that at least 14 percent of local deaths may have been caused by tuberculosis.[40] Death rates per one hundred thousand population in Illinois from tuberculosis were 113.7 in 1860, 145.6 in 1870, and 150.9 in 1880.[41] Tuberculosis took a long time to consume its victims, stealing their energy and ability to function before taking their lives.[42] It thrived in the crowded conditions of pioneer and low-income households, reducing the productivity of workers and burdening caregivers. It also complicated many pregnancies, thus inflating the number of postpartum maternal deaths.[43]

Not identified as a specific disease until 1829, typhoid was often confused with other fevers, including typhus and malaria (sometimes called typho-malaria). Carried by water and milk supplies contaminated by human and animal wastes, typhoid was more common when people relied on private wells and backyard privies than it became after installation of public sewage systems and water supplies.[44] In 1860, eight McLean County residents died of typhoid. In 1880, 1,487 Illinois-dwellers outside the City of Chicago died of the disease.[45] Regarded as a disease of filth associated with decomposing organic matter, means of transmission were not understood until the early twentieth century.[46]

More common and deadly than typhoid were diphtheria (often also reported as croup), scarlet fever, measles, and whooping cough. Diseases mainly afflicting children, they were endemic in McLean County, but flared up in devastating epidemics every few years. For example, scarlet fever caused fifty-seven (19 percent) of three hundred McLean County deaths in 1850. Although the diphtheria bacillus was identified in 1883, and antitoxin introduced in 1895, diphtheria continued to cause fatalities until the mid-twentieth century.[47] The same was true of scarlet fever, measles, and whooping cough, which killed 233, 346, and 367 Illinois residents respectively in 1926.[48]

More dangerous than any other contagious disease, but less feared, was diarrhea. A symptom often associated with other disorders, such as malaria, typhoid, or cholera, "the flux" on its own was not generally taken very seriously. Indeed, subscribers to humoral or antiphlogistic theories (including both most physicians and laypeople in early Illinois) were more likely to worry about constipation than "looseness"; indeed, laxatives were among the most common remedies used in nineteenth-century America, and their operation was regarded as central to prevention and treatment of most disorders.[49] Nonetheless, diarrhea and dysentery were both common and deadly in Illinois throughout the nineteenth century. Epidemics tended to occur in the late summer. Describing an 1860 outbreak of dysentery in the McLean County community, LeRoy, Dr. J. W. Coleman wrote, "No class, age, or sex were exempt. About one patient died out of each fifteen sick, but five miles from LeRoy on the Bloomington road, twenty cases developed of whom six died."[50] Diarrhea particularly attacked young children, helping to account for the high infant mortality rate, which in 1880 still hovered at approximately 200 per 1,000 births reported in Illinois.[51] Thirty-eight of the seventy-eight deaths reported in McLean County in 1850 were of children under age five.

Diarrhea and dysentery mystified physicians of the time. Even Abraham Jacobi, founder of pediatrics as a medical specialty, believed that "cholera infantum" resulted from heat-induced paralysis of the nervous system.[52] Many medical writers thought diarrhea was associated with malaria and advocated dosing children with quinine to prevent it.[53] Some advocated the prophylactic use of emetics.[54] However, only after the introduction of public sanitation and changes in domestic hygiene related to popularization of the germ theory after about 1880 did Illinois' mortality rates from diarrheal diseases decline—from a high of 188.3 per 100,000 in 1870 to 28.1 per 100,000 by 1924.[55]

Beginning in the last quarter of the nineteenth century, mortality from contagious diseases declined and was gradually replaced by mortality from chronic disorders mainly affecting the elderly. Infant mortality also plummeted, from 218.8 per 1,000 reported births in 1881 to 69.3 per 1,000 reported births in 1926, whereas the average age of death rose from the forties in the late nineteenth century to the sixties by the mid-twentieth century.[56] These changes had a tremendous impact on McLean County residents' expectations, life experience, and health culture that, in turn, affected individual and collective approaches to prevention, care, and cure of ill-health.

Public Health

Community responses to illness depends, in part, on prevailing ideas about the causes and transmission of diseases. However, the relationship between health culture, action, and outcome is always complicated. Some activities that had a positive impact on general health in McLean County—tiling and draining fields, for example—were only coincidentally beneficial; although mid-nineteenth-century Westerners associated swampy areas and stagnant water with fever, they did not perceive a link between water, mosquitoes, and malaria and did not tile fields for health reasons. Nonetheless, this measure, undertaken to ease farming and improve agricultural yields, undoubtedly eliminated some of the fevers that had made the Illinois country dangerous. Other collective activities performed to prevent disease reduced morbidity and mortality even though the theory underlying the actions was later superseded by other theories; for instance, town clean-ups to reduce dangerous miasmas when cholera epidemics threatened may have also "worked" in terms of germ theory. Still other behaviors—for example, the practice, prevalent in McLean County in the late nineteenth and early twentieth centuries, of building houses with basements in order to trap dangerous sewer gases below stairs—probably had little impact on health.

As indicated above, to prevent spread of the few ailments generally believed to be transmitted directly from one person to another—smallpox, for example—early McLean County residents used the time-honored approach of isolating the sufferer or denying entrance to the community to strangers showing signs of disease or traveling from afflicted areas. New communication and transportation systems aided such prevention attempts. After about 1870, in years when an expanding range of contagious diseases were known to be epidemic elsewhere, it was not uncommon for public officials to forbid passengers to disembark from trains coming from the direction of infected areas.[57] A smallpox outbreak in Shirley (five miles from Bloomington) in the mid-1870s stimulated both the quarantine of the township and vaccination of all school children.[58] To isolate cases, in 1878 a house on the outskirts of Bloomington was adopted as a "pesthouse" for people (including migrants) who could not be quarantined in their own homes.[59]

Growing urban population and changes, after the mid-nineteenth century, in people's perception of the danger posed by animal and human waste resulted in a series of public health initiatives.[60] An ordinance was passed to rid Bloomington's streets of roaming farm animals.[61] To aid street cleaning, paving was initiated in Bloomington in 1869 with the laying of crushed gravel on a stretch of Grove Street, a thoroughfare that ran through the business district and a prosperous residential neighborhood. Several other streets were paved with wood blocks, which were abandoned in favor of bricks beginning in 1877.[62]

Until the 1870s, all McLean County households made individual arrangements for water supply and human waste disposal—wells, cisterns, and privies, located "out back." "Wells were always uphill (if possible) and a safe distance away from the privy, and were generally more convenient to the house."[63] Only Philadelphia, New York, and Boston had public waterworks before the 1860s. Many other cities depended on lakes and rivers. The lack of a large natural water source was an ongoing matter of concern to McLean County's city-dwellers. According to a late nineteenth-century historian, "The dry year of 1854 caused great distress for water in this part of the State, and Bloomington people were very much exercised with fears that the location and building of their rapidly growing city might, after all, have been a serious mistake."[64] During an 1863 attempt to find a local coal supply, the drill struck an underground water source, which in 1869 was tapped by the Chicago and Alton Railroad Company for its own uses.[65] This success stimulated the city to solve its water problems by digging a well—a project undertaken in 1874 "at the end of a series of four very dry seasons":

> On Christmas Day, 1874, the whole population that wished, examined the fountain—the well having been finished the day before. As a sample of what had been discovered, the engines were kept at work, throwing the water in a stream, which, as it flowed off, was equal to a good-sized brook. There was but one opinion, and that was that the fountain was large enough to justify the erection of a system of water works; and in the summer of 1875, the stand-pipe was erected, 200 feet high, an engine and pump placed in position at the well, two miles and half of pipe laid in the streets, and a full system of water works inaugurated, which has since been enlarged by additional pipes and more machinery. The total cost of the whole, up to April 30 1878, has been $86,944.83. This includes about eight miles of water-mains, the engines and machinery, the stand-pipe, four drinking fountains, seventy hydrants and everything connected with the Water Department.[66]

Although this development was publicly lauded, many homeowners were unwilling to install the expensive new plumbing necessary to connect their houses with the public water supply. Indeed, in August 1878, only fifty families drew water from the city well and three thousand continued to use private wells and cisterns.[67] Acceptance of public services was gradual and tended to be associated with new construction.

In the third quarter of the nineteenth century, most Bloomington households kept horses for transportation and livestock for food; virtually all depended on backyard privies to dispose of human waste. As towns became more crowded, available space for outhouses, stables, and animal pens was increasingly limited and pollution of water sources inevitable. An 1875 article in Bloomington's daily newspaper, *The Pantagraph*, indicates concern about this threat:

> The local order is to usually locate your house in front, the well in the rear of the house, and the stables, pig pens, privies, etc. in the rear of the well. Often the privies and wells are higher than the house for access to the street. Such

results in a chronically damp cellar from the stable and privy fluids. The distance between well and privy is generally 30 feet. The instances are very numerous in which the poison of typhoid fever has been traced to water that had traversed the soil many feet.... In view of the way porous soil extends in this city ... are we not compelled to the inference that our wells are impure and unsafe.[68]

The first American patent for a flush toilet was awarded in 1833, and by the 1850s many upper- and middle-class households in eastern cities had installed them.[69] However, McLean County was slow to follow this trend. "Clover Lawn," the mansion built by Judge David Davis and his wife Sarah (1814–79) in Bloomington in 1872, was apparently the first home in the county to have a flush toilet.[70] At about the same time, city leaders were considering the question of public management of waste water and sewage.

Before the 1870s, all kinds of garbage and human and animal waste had been thrown into the "North and South Sloughs," which "became a ... sodden pool of stench that was the breeding place for disease ... because it drained sewage into the community's primary water source, Sugar Creek."[71] The nuisance and perceived health risk motivated Bloomington in 1874 to begin constructing a sewerage system. "The unsightly holes of the North and South Sloughs were covered by large tile pipes that carried the sewage underground away from the City.... Hotel builders and private landowners paid the cost of their own installation. Other buildings were drained through plank or box sewers which were installed from year to year. The box sewers were square wooden ducts running underground from a business or residence to a larger box collecting drain."[72]

Bloomington's public works built on long-term interest in public health; the community established a City Health Board in 1842, when fewer than two thousand people lived there. However, paralleling developments elsewhere, the city became more active in public health administration during the last quarter of the nineteenth century. In 1877 the Illinois State Board of Health was established to administer the Medical Practice Act, which regulated the professional practice of medicine, and the State Board of Health Act, which took charge of sanitation, quarantines, and collection of health statistics. A leader in this effort was Dr. Elias W. Gray (1821–96) of Bloomington, who presented a paper on the sanitary control of disease at the 1876 meeting of the Illinois State Medical Society, and became the state board's first secretary.[73] In 1880 Bloomington's City Council formed a Health Committee that employed a health officer, Hiram Greenwood, for $40 per month. Exemplifying the link identified by David Armstrong between public health services and control of people's behavior, his responsibilities included "abatement of nuisances and the enforcement of garbage removal regulations. He had police powers and . . . was responsible for removing to the 'pesthouse' persons found in the community with smallpox."[74] Greenwood held his position until 1898.

As was the case elsewhere, tension developed between local physicians and public health authorities. For example, McLean County Medical Society's records indicate that in 1891 members were offended by a city regulation requiring them to report cases of diphtheria to the health officer, and allowing that official to visit sufferers in the absence of their doctors.[75] Organized medicine resisted public infringement on private practice and public provision of health-care services, viewing public health officials as competitors, and prevention activities as threats to doctors' practices and incomes.[76] However, Bloomington's physicians opted to control local health administration, rather than fight with it. In 1897 the Medical Society organized a committee to advocate appointment of a physician as medical officer. Dr. Dwight O. Moore (1838–1901) was hired in 1898. Serving under him was a sanitary policeman who undertook the nuisance abatement and enforcement activities previously performed by Greenwood.[77] This new structure eased relations between the Medical Society and the Bloomington Health Committee, although as we shall see, tensions between physicians and public health officials resurfaced from time to time.

Home Care

What did nineteenth-century McLean County residents do when they became ill? The answer to this question varies depending on the time period, socioeconomic class, and geographic location of the person concerned. Nonetheless, it is fair to say that for them as well as many other Americans before about 1920, health care took place at home and was administered by women. Along with basic cooking, sewing, and other housework, young girls traditionally learned how to prepare remedies, help after childbirth, and nurse the ailing. Adult women became medical authorities within their families and settlements and managed health maintenance; infant and childcare; pregnancy and birth; injury, illness, and death.[78] They determined when sickness was present, diagnosed, decided when consultation of other authorities was necessary, and took charge of the sickroom. Their expertise depended on several overlapping traditions—oral, maintained through ethnic and family memory, which included magical and religious beliefs as well as other traditional theories and practices; semiofficial, transmitted through published home medical manuals and cookbooks, as well as through advice from doctors; and empirical, based on successful experience. Their tools included herb lore; prayers and charms; recipes for home remedies; "patent" (prepared over-the-counter or mail order) medicines; instruments used for minor surgery and childbirth; plasters, poultices, bandages, and binders; and special food and clothing used to prevent or treat illness.[79] Early Bloomington residents including Aunt Jane Hendrix, Aunt Ann Dawson, and Mrs. Gardner Randolph treated their neighbors' ills.[80] According to one source,

> Mrs. Randolph . . . brought . . . an assortment of dried herbs, a bottle of Number Six—a villainous compound of pepper, camphor and other hot substances, administered in alcohol, and quite taking the skin off an ordinary throat, as I know to my sorrow—and the seeds of numerous other herbal remedies, such as thyme, madder, comfrey, elecampane, catnip, horehound, and various other nauseous plants which spread over the neighborhood, and all of which she administered without stint or hesitation to such unfortunate victims as fell in her power.[81]

Women were thought to have a natural capacity and obligation to deal with the health problems of family members and neighbors. Furthermore, women and men shared, to a large extent, the health culture—if not the demeanor and social authority—of the almost exclusively male trained physicians, and applied do-it-yourself medical attention to themselves and household members.[82] John Berry Orendorff, born in 1827 in Blooming Grove, offered a dramatic example:

> Major [Seth] Baker was a remarkable man. A true type of the early pioneers of Blooming Grove. He had a steady nerve with a wonderful will power, always ready and willing to face all obstacles. As proof of this . . . [I] will state one case—He had a very sore toe that was very painful to him. He couldn't get it to heal, so he decided the toe had to be cut off, but there was not a surgeon or surgeon's tools in McLean County. He asked several men to take a chisel and cut his toe off. They were all afraid to do it as he might bleed to death. He got his chisel, made a keen edge to it, placed his foot on a solid block of wood, then placed the edge of the chisel to the diseased toe, then one stroke with the mallet severed the toe from the foot. He dressed the wound and gave it close attention till it healed up, and that was sooner than anyone expected. I think that was the first surgical operation by white people at Blooming Grove.[83]

This account, of course, is exceptional. Nonetheless, early county residents expected to deal independently with health problems, often supported by "the old-time family medicine book that along with the Bible used to be on the table of sitting rooms in many a home in the United States."[84]

Nineteenth-century McLean County families had a variety of reference books from which to choose. Cookbooks routinely contained a few recipes for remedies. For example, *The Home Cook Book of Chicago* (1874), based on recipes provided by Illinois housewives, suggested the following treatments:

For Sore Throat.—Cut slices of salt pork or fat bacon; simmer a few moments in hot vinegar, and apply to throat as hot as possible. When this is taken off, as the throat is relieved, put around a bandage of soft flannel. A gargle of equal parts of borax and alum, dissolved in water, is also excellent to be used frequently.

Healing Lotion.—one ounce glycerine, one ounce rosewater, ten drops carbolic acid. This preparation prevents and cures chapping of the skin, and at the same time bleaches it. It is also excellent for sore lips and gums . . .

To Stop Bleeding.—A handful of flour bound on the cut . . .

To Restore From Stroke Of Lightning.—Shower with cold water for two hours; if the patient does not show signs of life, put salt in the water and continue to shower an hour longer.[85]

In addition to cures, the expanding genre focusing on home medical treatment tended to offer information on anatomy and physiology, diagnostic approaches, and therapeutic advice, thus providing "official" medical education to home caregivers and linking formal and informal health cultures.[86] Continuing to be published in the twentieth century, these works reflected the expectation that mothers made health-care decisions and nursed the sick.[87]

Some mid-nineteenth-century publications offered sectarian alternatives to the heroic medicine practiced by "allopaths," even attacking the "regular" medical profession for trying to confuse laypeople with complicated theories and long words.[88] Others, following a tradition dating back at least to seventeenth-century England, argued that formally trained physicians were largely unnecessary.[89] This argument appealed both to the ethos of hardy self-reliance and to the slender pocketbooks of many Midwestern families. However, most home medical books encouraged sufferers to consult physicians if possible, but when professional help was unavailable, to dose themselves with the same violent purges, opiates, and metallic remedies that regular physicians generally proscribed. Thus, families kept medicines normatively including calomel, jalap, ipecac, castor oil, laudanum, and quinine. Adults (particularly women) developed a good working knowledge of what were thought to be appropriate doses of these powerful substances, and even as late as the 1920s were expected by physicians to mix their own compound prescriptions.

Use of strong medicines sometimes had unintended consequences. According to an early settler, two Blooming Grove children, Omen and Catherine Olney, got "the itch" when very young. "Friends recommended Red Percipity. They used it, had to go out in the rain, got wet, both got deaf, and Catherine lost her speech."[90] She lived into her late thirties, remaining deaf and mute. Like residents of Sugar Creek in nearby Sangamon County, nineteenth-century McLean County residents also experienced the "toothless gums and uncontrolled drool, symptoms of the mercury poisoning that occurred as a result of regular doses of calomel or mercurous chloride."[91]

McLean County medicine chests were fed by the expanding patent medicine business, stimulated in the mid-nineteenth century by development of industrial production methods; improved transportation and postal systems; and proliferating advertising vehicles.[92] Nostrum factories sprang up all over the country, profiting by both the heroic dosing common among regular physicians and laypeople, and by the opposition to heroic remedies among medical sectarians.[93] Patent medicines were sold during performances of traveling medicine shows, where consumers received both entertainment and hope of relief for the price of a bottle. Bloomington annually hosted many of these troops, which in the 1880s included Bigelow's Kickapoo Indian Shows and Healey's Kickapoo Indian Shows.[94] Nostrum makers also advertised in newspapers, popular magazines, and their own publications, such as the almanacs published annually after 1860 by Bloomington's leader in the patent medicine trade, "Dr." Cyrenius Wakefield (1815–85).[95]

Wakefield's factory, opened in 1850, produced remedies including Blackberry Balsam, Cathartic Liver Pills, Cherry Pectoral, Egyptian Salve, Golden Ointment, Rheumatic Resolvent, Worm Destroyer, Worm Lozenges, and Wine Bitters.[96] By 1874, Wakefield employed

> forty persons in his medicine business (one-half of whom are females) and his annual sales amount to $100,000. He converts twenty-five tons of paper into almanacs every year for free distribution, for the purpose of advertising his remedies. His largest sales are made where fevers are most dangerous and most common, particularly in new[ly settled] countries where he is glad to know that his remedies are the means of doing great good. . . . the Doctor has made himself quite independent by the judicious advertising of good and reliable remedies.[97]

His advertisements, featuring testimonials from satisfied patients, followed a conventional pattern that highlighted the failure of attention from regular physicians and the cheapness and efficiency of Wakefield's remedies, even in cases of incurable diseases including tuberculosis.[98]

In addition to using prepared medicines, McLean County residents made their own. Many knew the healing properties of plants that were either cultivated for that purpose or grew wild in the fields and forests of the area; like familiarity with drugs, herb lore was shared by doctors and nonphysicians. For example, Dr. Silas Hubbard (1821–1917) who practiced in the McLean County village, Hudson, paid local residents to gather the medicinal plants he used in his therapies.[99]

McLean County residents also made remedies from household ingredients. Every family had its favorite recipe for cough syrup. Goose grease and flannel cloth were applied to congested chests. Warm oil was poured into sore ears. Like Jack in the nursery rhyme, people plastered bruises with vinegar and brown paper. They used soap and sugar poultices to "draw" boils; mustard plasters to provide counter irritation for pneumonia and other lung ailments; and fabric to bandage wounds. Obvious fractures were splinted; burns were buttered; bleeding was staunched by a variety of mechanical and medicinal means.

Despite this arsenal of practical knowledge, little could be done to cure the legion of diseases threatening early McLean County dwellers; thus, attention focused on care. Nineteenth-century ailments, when they did not kill immediately, lasted a long time. Home nursing involved intensive hands-on service from relatives and (among the prosperous) servants; no formally trained nurses were available in the county until the 1890s. Women spent long days and nights watching fever sufferers. Determined caregivers forced foul-tasting draughts down unwilling throats. The struggle to keep the ailing clean was Herculean because all clothing, bedding, and dressings had to be washed by hand in water drawn and carried from wells or streams, heated on stoves or open fires, and carried again to be poured away. Special meals demanded by tradition had to be prepared. In settlers' small cabins and the cramped quarters inhabited by the poor, the nineteenth-century sick shared rooms and beds with the healthy. Thus, people were familiar with the sights, sounds, and smells of illness and death. Often without recourse to a physician's presumed expertise, caregivers depended on their own knowledge and skill, taking responsibility for all decisions and outcomes.

This was especially true regarding childbearing, which was traditionally an exclusively female matter. Nineteenth-century American women were often pregnant. Indeed, in 1800, white American women bore an average of more than seven live children, presumably undergoing several additional pregnancies ending in abortion, miscarriage, or stillbirth. At the end of the century, this number had been reduced to an average of 3.56 babies; however, African American women still bore an average of more than five children in 1900.[100] John Mack Faragher comments on the extraordinary fertility of women living in early nineteenth-century Sugar Creek.[101] There is no reason to presume that McLean County women were less fertile.

Although McLean County doctors delivered many babies, neighbor women and informally trained midwives served as authorities on pregnancy and managed many births throughout the nineteenth century.[102] Like illness and death, virtually all county births took place in the mother's home; indeed, before about 1920 there was no local alternative. Women sent for a midwife or doctor when labor began—in this era of social childbearing often also summoning women friends or relatives.[103] They stayed in bed, when possible, for the customary ten days or two weeks following delivery, believing it to be dangerous for a woman to get up too soon. During the lying-in period, the housework and care of older children was done by female relations, friends, or hired practical nurses. Thus, regardless of who delivered the baby, the environment within which birth took place differed dramatically from that of the hospital deliveries that became customary during the next century.

Whether managed by professional or domestic caregivers, the outcome of birth or illness often was not good. Indeed, death was considered to be the "natural" consequence of many ailments and even certain times of life. Stillbirth and maternal death in childbirth or old age were so common that census records routinely recorded these conditions as causes of death. Some illnesses (such as tuberculosis) were regarded by both physicians and non-physicians as incurable.[104] In early McLean County homes, the sickbed often became the deathbed. The final service rendered by the caregiver was often preparation of the sufferer's body for burial.

Calling the Doctor

When physicians were available and there were serious health problems, McLean County residents consulted doctors, and were prepared to travel many miles under difficult conditions to get their assistance. For example, "In 1830 the doctors were not so numerous as at present. Young Esek [Greenman] remembers some horseback exercise when he rode to Pekin, a distance of 33 miles, without saddle or stirrups, for the doctor. On his return with the doctor he forded the Mackinaw on the upper side, so that, if swept from his horse by the current, the doctor could catch him."[105] Surgical skills were especially needed. The early county resident, John B. Orendorff, remembered the experience of a neighbor boy, Simon Olney, one Thanksgiving Day. Having been left alone with his younger siblings, Simon "decided to have some jollification":

> He got the powder flask and . . . commenced to sprinkle powder on coals that was scattered on the hearth and was having a gay time till he happened to extend his hand over the burning coals so the burning powder flashed in the flask. It went off and up through the ceiling with a crash and a report that was heard a long ways. It tore the thumb of his right hand so it was turned clear back on his wrist just like it had been cut with some sharp instrument. The thumb hung perfectly loose. They sent to Bloomington for Dr. Henry. He replaced the joint

and sewed up the wound so it healed up in course of time, but his thumb was as stiff as a bone, couldn't bend it a particle.[106]

Nineteenth-century county residents fondly remembered doctors whose effectiveness was arguably based on long relationships with whole families. Orendorff wrote of a physician who began practice in Bloomington in the 1840s:

> Doctor Espy had a very extensive practice for a great many years, I think between 35 and 40 years. He was considered the leading doctor of Bloomington—was very successful in chills and fevers. . . . The night was never too dark or stormy for him to go, then he was very moderate in his charges. . . . He was our family doctor for a good many years. I remember well going after him one terrible stormy night for my mother that was suddenly taken ill with something like the bilious colic. All the home remedies were of no avail. Her suffering was terrible. We all felt very much alarmed about her—the nearest neighbor was a mile away. I was the oldest of the children, then 14 years of age. Father says to me, "Can you go after Doc Espy." I says yes . . . In less than five minutes I was on my way. As I mounted my horse, Father says, "Berry, let your horse go, your Mother's life may probably be saved if you make good time."

In this case, which took on the formulaic structure and drama of myth, the doctor was roused from his own sickbed and treated Mrs. Orendorff, who recovered.[107] It is noteworthy, both that the family also apparently relied on neighbors in times of illness, and that the sufferer in this case was also the mother—the household's medical authority and main caregiver, whose illness thus required external expertise.

Generally speaking, people did not *expect* doctors to cure them or their loved ones. However, physicians were called when other means had failed or when sudden illness appeared to be potentially fatal. Laypeople expected doctors to have special knowledge of medical theories and therapies. Physicians also were expected to assume responsibility for the patient, thus easing the burden of relatives. Doctors were expected to look the part and radiate confidence; it helped if they were middle-aged. Consequently, new young doctors encountered some suspicion. An account of the career of Dr. John M. Major, who practiced medicine in Bloomington between about 1849 and 1867, said,

> In January 1850, Dr. Parsons [Major's much older medical partner] was called to go twenty miles in the country, and, as he did not wish to face the intense cold, sent young Dr. Major. He gave the latter a letter of introduction to an old widow lady, whose children were very sick with pneumonia. Dr. Parsons had been the old lady's family physician, in whom she had great confidence, and she

was much disappointed with the juvenile appearance of Dr. Major. . . . But when this juvenile, adding a year or so to his age, told her he was 25, she allowed him, with some misgivings, to prescribe for her children. He was successful in curing them, and she was quite as well satisfied as if the old doctor had been present, for she had thought it was age that made the doctor, and not the man.[108]

As the century progressed, McLean County residents—particularly town-dwellers and the prosperous—depended increasingly on doctors' advice. Even the smallest communities supported physicians—a situation that continued into the mid-twentieth century, but changed as medical services were concentrated in urban areas.[109]

Doctors and Doctoring before 1880

Early McLean County settlers included several trained physicians. The 1850 census lists sixteen men identifying themselves as doctors. Although some of these may not have been full-time practitioners and others not formally qualified by later standards, this was a large number for a population then totaling 10,163.[110] As was typical of American physicians of the time, their preparation for practice varied. For example, Dr. William Cromwell (1812–74) had "graduated in medicine and surgery at University of Maryland," Dr. Harrison Noble (1812–70) had "read medicine one summer at home and attended Ohio Medical College the fall of 1846 and received his diploma the following spring in 1847. In 1851 Rush Medical College of Chicago conferred on him an honorary diploma and degree of Doctor of Medicine."[111]

Medical work was performed almost exclusively in sufferers' homes and involved significant travel and frequent visits during the often lengthy course of nineteenth-century illnesses. Dr. Charles Ross Parke (1823–1908), who practiced in Bloomington between 1857 and 1902, remembered of his early years:

> One great difficulty the pioneer doctor had to contend with in traveling over the prairies was the absence of landmarks—so much sameness. Then, again, at certain times great districts in the neighborhood of sloughs were enshrouded in dense fog, making it impossible to locate one's self, especially at night. Every pioneer medical man had more or less of this experience. During a practice of fifty years in McLean County I was lost three different times and wandered around until daylight, frequently was obliged to alight and feel for the roads, especially when riding a livery horse—they will invariably take to the grass when given the reins. The doctor's usual mode of travel in those days was on horseback with saddle-bags strapped on behind the saddle.[112]

Pioneer physicians, like the families they served, also dealt with and made imaginative use of very basic care environments. John Orendorff provided a rare early account of mental illness, where both Dr. Espy and Mrs. Omen Olney's family members had to care for Mrs. Olney, a "large muscular woman . . . [who] weighed over two hundred pounds and was possessed of wonderful strength":

> She had a hard spell of bilious fever for some time. She was not expected to live, but after lingering some four or six weeks between life and death, she took a turn to get well and gained very rapid so she was able to be about her household work again. But all of a sudden she became very weak and violently insane, and for six weeks she was a raving maniac. The doctor said the insanity was caused by her fever. They had to place a lock and chain to her ankle and with a staple fastened at the other end of the chain that was spiked to the floor. Also had her bedstead nailed to the floor. . . . One day while Dr. Espy was treating her, at an unguarded moment she gathered him and jammed him and his head under a forestick of a big burning fire into a red hot bed of coals and would have burnt him to death if some parties that was just coming in had not hastened to his relief and dragged him out of his perilous situation. . . . After she became sane again, she then kept rational as long as she lived.[113]

The daybooks kept by Dr. Thomas P. Rogers (1812–99) between 1839 and 1854 offer a window through which to observe some aspects of the working lives of early McLean County physicians.[114] Rogers was born in Ohio. His medical training combined apprenticeship with a practicing physician and an academic course in Philadelphia. He began his practice in Decatur in 1838 and moved to Bloomington in 1849 because he expected the city to prosper after the railroad came through. Although medical fees in his day were not large, Rogers did well, retiring in 1867 at the age of 55 to "engage in agricultural pursuits" and politics.

Although he kept an office, Rogers spent much of his time making house calls. His pattern was to visit patients at least once a day during the course of their illnesses. Rogers dispensed, and probably mixed, the remedies he prescribed. Most of the clients who visited his office apparently came to purchase medicine. Rogers's daybooks do not provide information about symptoms or diagnoses. Rather, they record the names, sex, and sometimes ages of patients; remedies and services provided; and fees charged.

Most of Rogers's business was what would now be called internal medicine. Prescriptions indicate that he treated many fevers, chest infections, and gastrointestinal upsets. His therapeutic approach was typical of allopaths of his day, using laxatives, emetics, and bloodletting to produce evacuation and reduce inflammation.[115] Frequently prescribed medical ingredients included senna, castor oil, antimony, cream of tartar, camphor, and calomel, in addition to unspecified tonics, bitters, cathartics, and pills. Rogers sold patent remedies including Doverspowder and Rockwell Salts. He also prescribed opiates for many conditions and quinine for fevers. He let blood, sometimes therapeutically, sometimes prophylactically. In addition to practicing internal medicine, Rogers treated skin diseases, pulled teeth, and delivered babies.

Rogers's charges for individual services were modest. House calls in town cost $1.00; rural and night visits added to the fee. For example, for a night journey of nine miles in January 1840, he charged the patient's husband $7.00, which included medications (an emetic and "oil"). Canny clients often asked him to attend more than one patient in the household during a visit, thereby incurring only a single charge for the call. Rogers charged 50 cents for a simple dental extraction and $5.00 to deliver a baby. Despite Rogers's moderate fees, lingering ailments and regular house calls meant that his patients ran up substantial tabs. For example, Mrs. Charles Baker incurred charges of $22.50 for nearly daily attendance during September 1851—a considerable sum at a time when the annual expenditures of a working family of five was estimated at $538.44.[116]

Rogers's success owed more to his political and business talents than to the profitability of nineteenth-century medical practice. In cost-benefit terms, doctoring in the period was an inefficient and uncomfortable route to prosperity. Without surprise, a local historian remarked of two of McLean County's early medical settlers, "Dr. Haines died in 1838 and Dr. Anderson in 1842, both believed to have succumbed to overwork in the hard conditions and much sickness of the time."[117] It is no wonder that many physicians, like Rogers, left medical practice to use their superior educations and social status in more comfortable and lucrative ways. Before retiring from medicine, however, Rogers participated in a significant professional development activity, in 1854 becoming one of fourteen charter members of the McLean County Medical Society.

As was true elsewhere, physicians in McLean County were highly individualistic and competitive. According to a recent study, "A Bloomington, Illinois, practitioner reminded his fellows in 1889, 'The hustler gets to the front. However well-qualified a man may be for any avocation in life, he can not sit down and wait, Micawber-like, for business to turn up. If he does, the chances are, some one less qualified will soon be so far ahead in the race, that to overtake him will be impossible.'"[118] However, as self-interested as they were, mid-nineteenth-century allopaths organized national, state, and local medical societies to increase their competitive advantage over burgeoning numbers of "irregulars," including homeopaths, Thomsonians, eclectics, and others, and raise standards for regular practice. Only rudimentary information survives about the McLean County Medical Society's first thirty-seven years in existence.[119] However, records kept by the society for the years between 1891 and 1910 provide a detailed account of its activities during that period.[120] This source will support discussion, below, of the Progressive Era changes in McLean County health care—including the increasing professional importance and influence of "organized medicine."

Conclusion

In 1880 McLean County was prosperous, growing, and increasingly healthy. Infant mortality and deaths from contagious diseases were declining. Public sanitation infrastructure and administration were expanding—in Bloomington, at least. More than sixty allopathic physicians practiced in the county, of whom approximately one-half worked in Bloomington, while the others served in outlying hamlets.[121] Health-care decisions were made, services offered, and nursing care provided in sufferers' homes. However, this situation was about to change. During the next forty years, development of hospitals and trained nursing; location of medical services in doctors' offices; specialization of medical services and identities; and uncritical acceptance of biomedicine on the part of the general public transformed health culture in McLean County.

2. No Place Like Home

Hospitals and the Development
of Institutional Care

Hospital as Home Away from Home

When Mrs. Rosie Flanagan became St. Joseph's Hospital's first patient on March 22, 1880, she encountered a care environment that was entirely consistent with Bloomington's health culture at the time. The facility was in an old house, grander than the dwellings of most of its patients, but less than suitable for hospital uses. It offered nursing care in an unspecialized environment typical of what Joan Lynaugh refers to as the "domestic" era of hospital development—an era that continued, in Bloomington, until the 1920s.[1] The forty-five-year-old Flanagan, a married Irishwoman suffering from breast cancer, was the hospital's only patient for the first four days of her stay and shared the facility with just five other patients before she was released on April 5, "recovered."[2] During its initial year of operation, at any one time St. Joseph's generally accommodated fewer than four patients, who were nursed by four nuns, including their Superior, Sister Augustina. The new hospital conformed to a model described by Lynaugh, where "Nuns and nurses cared for patients, did laundry, cleaned, prepared food and medicines, and assisted at surgery. They also admitted and discharged the patients, raised funds, and managed the institution."[3]

The addition of a purpose-built hospital building in 1883 expanded St. Joseph's capacity to forty-two beds and made it possible for the old building to be used as a residence and chapel for the nuns. The nursing staff also grew, by 1886 including twelve sisters.[4] However, the domestic care environment continued—even in the hospital's appearance. According to an 1887 medical staff account, "Since our last report of a month ago, the sisters, especially

Sister Ludovica, aided by Mr. Rothmann, teacher in the German school, have painted and frescoed all the wards and nearly all the departments of the hospital in a style that would do credit to our best painters."[5] The homelike atmosphere extended out of doors. According to a founding medical staff member, Dr. Parke, in 1890:

> Large trees in great abundance afford shade and shelter. In the summer time the beautiful lawns, decorated with flowers and laid out by walks; the sisters dressed in their black and white garments walking hither and thither, followed by a faithful dog; here and there sitting at the foot of some tree patients sufficiently recovered to be out in the open air; the singing of the birds and the quiet that reigns about the neighborhood all remind one of those ideal refuges pictured in story books.[6]

Parke's description projects both the ideal of home care and desire to allay the fears of county residents for whom hospitals were both unfamiliar and threatening.

Most patients came from farms or households where vegetables and livestock were raised for family consumption. In this matter, too, St. Joseph's conformed to a familiar domestic model. The building was located on the edge of town, in the midst of "several acres of rich, high land upon which is raised nearly all the vegetables used in the institution."[7] The nuns and hired men, paid between $18 and $25 per month, farmed this land and took care of the hospital's livestock, which generally included a cow, several horses, and chickens.[8]

Like both traditional housewives and new women consumers, St. Joseph's nuns produced goods for this household and managed its budget.[9] Very little money changed hands in early days. For example, during April 1880, the hospital received $168.35 and spent $174.52. Income came from patients' fees, charitable donations, and contributions from the sisters' order. Expenditures were for medicine, shoes, dry goods, animal feed, groceries that could not be grown on the property (including regular payments for oysters!), workmen's labor, utilities, sisters' travel to collect donations and visit the mother house in Peoria, and building projects. A major factor in keeping costs down was that the nuns were not paid.[10] In this respect also, the sister nurses exemplified a normative model of unpaid female labor in the home—mother as housekeeper and budget manager, sister as obedient handmaiden. When student nurses entered the picture in 1921, they took on the equally familiar roles of low-paid apprentice housemaids whose time, labor, and choices belonged almost entirely to their employers.[11]

The nuns augmented St. Joseph's income through the traditional professed religious activity of fundraising, collecting money from individuals and businesses, including Bloomington's coal mine (opened in 1868). Five dollars was a usual donation. However, hospital account entries also indicate regular collection of larger amounts: for example, Sisters Agatha, Theresa, and Joseph brought in $159 in October 1884; Sisters Vinzent and Walburga collected $100 in October 1886.[12] The nuns also ran raffles.[13] The only very large sums mentioned in hospital accounts were borrowed or donated for building projects. During its second expansion, in January 1888, St. Joseph's owed $4,000 to the Mercantile National Bank, $2,000 to Mr. Fred Ruppenkamp, $1,160 to Rev. B. Baak, and $615 to Mrs. Sarah Adams. Aside from this debt, the hospital's cash balance was $443.57.[14] However, at the same time significant contributions were coming in. In May 1889, Reverend Mother Theda collected $900 "for new addition"; in August of the same year, Father James Orth and the Patient's Board provided $1,448.[15]

St. Joseph's was not long the only home away from home for McLean County sufferers. Two additional Bloomington hospitals soon opened—the Kelso Home Sanitarium (1894), a proprietary facility founded by homeopathic physicians George (1860–1935) and Annie (1858–1927) Kelso, and the Deaconess Hospital (renamed Brokaw after its principal donor in 1902), established in 1896 as a charitable Protestant alternative to the Catholic institution.[16] Like St. Joseph's, these late nineteenth-century facilities were initially located in former private residences and provided care in consciously homelike environments. This was also true of hospitals established in the early twentieth century: Mennonite Hospital, first located in the Harber family residence in 1919 before moving into the Kelso Home Sanitarium; the small cottage hospital operated in rural Arrowsmith between 1921 and 1948 by local physician, Dr. L. M. Johnson, to serve his own patients; and the nine-bed Bloomington "Clinic" run by the osteopath Dr. Fuller between 1930 and the early 1940s in a house where his family also lived.[17]

There were social class and ethnic dimensions to early McLean County hospital missions, services, and clienteles. St. Joseph's and Brokaw hospitals were originally founded as charities to serve poor people who lacked the family, accommodation, or resources for home care.[18] St. Joseph's especially focused on the needs of a growing Roman Catholic immigrant workforce, which was generally low income and socially marginalized.[19] Although physicians were essential to hospital establishment and operation, most contemporary medical care was delivered in patients' homes, and successful medical careers were achieved without hospital staff appointments; thus, charitable hospitals were established to meet social and moral goals. Because the stigma of indigence remained strong in late nineteenth-century Illinois, identification of the hospital with a welcoming home that opened its arms to the community's needy—yet virtuous—residents helped to distinguish charitable general hospitals from McLean County's Poor Farm, established in 1860.[20] By contrast, the Kelso Sanitarium, which also marketed its services with reference to ideal domestic characteristics—"A place for health-building with the distinguishing characteristics of simplicity, cheerfulness, and a home-like atmosphere"—targeted as its clientele the middle- or upper-class "nerve-wracked business man . . . [and] woman grown weary of social demands."[21] All of Bloomington's hospitals collected fees, although St. Joseph's and Brokaw charged on a means-related sliding scale, and the Kelso Sanitarium's charges were approximately double those of the charitable hospitals. The pay system helped both to undermine potential association of hospitalization with pauperization and to increase the sense of agency and choice on the part of patients and their families in this unfamiliar care environment.

The home care model projected important aspects of health culture related to conceptualization of the ailing body; dynamics and power relationships among formal health-care providers, family caregivers, and sufferers; and popular anxiety about using hospitals. The individual sufferer's body, cared for at home, retained its social identity and wholeness in a way that the hospitalized patient's body did not.[22] At home, the sufferer was a named individual, rather than a case, a bed occupant, or a disorder—often of a single body part (e.g., fractured leg, ruptured appendix, heart attack). S/he wore her/his own clothes, occupied her/his own room and bed, saw visitors (unless quarantined) according to personal and household interests, and consumed familiar food and drink. Because it was usual for "sick" people to stay in bed, lay female caregivers governed access to the sickroom; compliance with doctors' orders; administration of treatment; personal and domestic hygiene; and supply of meals, linens, and any special consideration the ailing person received.[23] In early hospitals, nurses and matrons assumed responsibility for these matters. It is, perhaps, not coincidental that Bloomington's first trained nurses were nuns and (at Brokaw before 1907) Protestant "deaconesses"—women whose religious profession separated them from the traditional association of nursing with domestic service and low social status, and also attributed to them the authority and virtue of mother or a higher power.[24] Hospital patients became residents of the nurses' "homes."

Strict hospital rules and divisions between patients and their families, on the one hand, and hospital personnel, on the other, did not develop fully in Bloomington until the interwar period, undergoing a long transition marked by families' increasing dependence on hospitals and the growing size, specialization, and power of hospital staffs. Thus, for example, at St. Joseph's

Hospital in 1894, there was a party during which, "Father Donavan, a well known former clergyman of this city, who is now a patient at the hospital, and Dr. Godfrey gave a violin duet, assisted by Miss Mayme Schell, who is also a patient. The gentlemen are talented players, and the trio gave a charming concert. Mrs. Dr. G. R. Smith, who has an excellent voice, sang several selections sweetly. Dr. Corley also sang a solo."[25] Furthermore, as Emily Abel has also noted, during the early twentieth-century transition to professional institutional care, family members continued to participate in hospital-based decision making and care.[26] During the winter of 1922–23, Fanny Weaver's infant daughter, Florence, suffered from both colds and digestive problems:

> We found a Dr. Edmund Behrendt who advised barley water. He called in Dr. Gerald Cline, the first child specialist who was a new arrival in the community. She was in [Mennonite Hospital] at the advice of Dr. Behrendt and Dr. Cline studied her all night. He came up with the conclusion she was suffering from ruptured appendix and advised immediate surgery. I was permitted to stand by Behrendt and through the efficiency of those responsible for her care [she] recovered.[27]

As Lynaugh reminds us, "Domestic-era hospitals for paying patients developed in the private sector as a way of creating an accessible, safe place in which to be sick."[28] They also helped to bridge the gap between local perception of hospitals as unnecessary and disreputable, and developing belief that hospitals offered superior care environments to homes—particularly for surgery and childbirth. McLean County's hospitals, therefore, can be viewed as part of an educational and marketing effort to sell professional medical treatment to County residents in the late nineteenth and early twentieth centuries.

Suffering away from Home

What do we know about the first McLean County residents who received hospital care? Admissions records kept by St. Joseph's Hospital between 1880 and 1906 provide some information about the patients who were accommodated during that time. Comparable information is not available for other early hospitals in the county; however, with the likely exception of religious affiliation, there is no reason to believe that Brokaw's patients were different from St. Joseph's patients in terms of socioeconomic status, reason for hospital admission, or fees paid. As indicated above, the Kelso Sanitarium targeted prosperous clients and aggressively marketed surgical and obstetrical services; thus, its patient profile was probably different from that of the other two hospitals.

Between 1880 and 1906, sex was not indicated for 5 percent of the 4,695 patients admitted to St. Joseph's Hospital; of the remainder, 41 percent were female and 54 percent were male. Patients' ages ranged from two weeks to ninety-five years. However, very few children were admitted; indeed, only 3 percent of patients were under age 10. The mean age of patients in this period was forty-one, with the largest concentrations being of people in their twenties and those over age sixty-one.

Many early St. Joseph's patients were Catholic and foreign-born. However, as the only area hospital for more than a decade, St. Joseph's also admitted patients from a wide range of ethnic and religious backgrounds. Of those indicating religious affiliation, 44 percent were Catholic and 21 percent were Protestant. In 1880, 14 percent (8,557) of McLean County's 60,100 residents were foreign-born; however, only 40 percent of patients appearing in the admissions records during the period under consideration were born in the United States.[29] Approximately one-third was Irish and one-sixth was German. The hospital also admitted English, Swedish, French, Polish, Chinese, Belgian, Scottish, Danish, Canadian, Italian, Bohemian, Syrian, and Welsh patients. In addition to these foreign-born sufferers, St. Joseph's admitted at least thirty-five African Americans during the period under consideration.

St. Joseph's mission was to provide care regardless of recipients' ability to pay.[30] In fact, however, from the beginning most patients paid something toward the cost of their care. The county paid for hospitalization of paupers.[31] Only a few patients, identified by an early staff physician as "those who had neither home, money, or friends," were admitted free of charge.[32] The proportion of patients in this category ranged from less than 1 percent in some years to 8 percent of those treated in 1900.

Charges ranged from $1 to more than $600. Larger sums were paid for "a home for life" rather than for medical services. The median fee was $5, regardless of treatment or duration of stay. However, between 1880 and 1906, the average charge for hospital care rose. (See Table 2.)

Most of this money covered patients' "board"; very little went toward other expenses, such as medicine.

Diagnoses were not recorded for 65 percent of the people admitted to St. Joseph's. For the remaining 1,438 cases, reasons for hospitalization fell within twenty-two broad categories, of which six occurred most frequently: miscellaneous surgeries, fever, injuries, alcoholism, contagious diseases, and miscellaneous ailments (see Table 3).[33]

The large number of alcoholics admitted suggests that St. Joseph's served as the drunk tank for Bloomington-Normal. The inebriated occupied basement rooms which, "although not as handsomely furnished as those on

Table 2: Average Charges for Care at St. Joseph's
Hospital in Selected Years, 1880–1905

Year	Amount Most Patients Paid
1880	$3.00
1881–1895	$5.00
1899	$7.00
1903–1905	$10.00

Source: St. Joseph's Hospital Admissions Records, 1880–1906
(Archives of The Sisters of the Third Order of St. Francis,
Peoria, Illinois)

Table 3: Reasons Patients Were Admitted to St. Joseph's Hospital,
1880–1906

Diagnosis	Percent of Patients
Miscellaneous ailments	7.4
Alcoholism	3.5
Injuries (excluding fractures)	3.1
Miscellaneous surgeries	2.7
Miscellaneous contagious diseases	2.7
Miscellaneous fevers	2.2
Joint, back, and nerve problems	1.6
Mental illness	1.5
Local infections (e.g., abscesses)	1.5
Respiratory illness (excluding tuberculosis)	1.3
Tuberculosis	1.3
Gastrointestinal problems	1.2
Dropsy	0.8
Fractures	0.7
Heart problems	0.7
Cancers	0.6
Amputations	0.5
Boarding (i.e., living in the hospital)	0.4
Poisoning	0.4
Epilepsy	0.1

Source: St. Joseph's Hospital Admissions Records, 1880–1906 (Archives of The
Sisters of the Third Order of St. Francis, Peoria, Illinois)

the other three floors . . . are very comfortable and may be used in a case
of necessity."[34]

Noteworthy are conditions that do *not* appear among reasons for hospital
admission. Fewer than five babies were delivered at St. Joseph's during the
period under consideration. No tonsillectomies were done; this surgery did
not become a routine curative or prophylactic therapy until the interwar
period, when it became the most common type of operation performed on

young children.[35] The only cancers treated were of the breast and uterus. However, the hospital also dealt with some conditions that were rarely or never seen in McLean County after the mid-twentieth century, including malaria, smallpox, and erysipelas.

Most of the patients admitted between 1880 and 1906 were discharged as "recovered" (46 percent) or "improved" (12 percent). Many (7.1 percent) "left" the hospital, either without being officially discharged, or without change in their condition. Some were discharged as "incurable" (2.3 percent). Of the 3,683 patients for whom outcomes are known, 479 of them (13 percent) died in the hospital.[36]

Not all "patients" were ill. For instance, on January 9, 1900, nine-year-old Jim Dolan and his two-year-old brother, Archie, were admitted because they were "orphans" and stayed at the hospital for 181 days.[37] In addition, several elderly people purchased a home for life at St. Joseph's. For example, in August 1884, Mrs. Kath Weismuller paid $410 and in March 1889, Mrs. Anne McHugh paid $620 for this accommodation.[38]

Between 1880 and 1906, length of hospital stay ranged from one to 1,821 days. Chronic physical and mental disorders, general debility, and old age called for longer hospital stays, whereas patients suffering from alcoholism, injuries, conditions requiring surgery, fevers, and gastrointestinal ailments tended to be discharged in fewer than fourteen days. Generally speaking, hospital stays were much longer than they became in the course of the twentieth century, in 1891, averaging fifty-two days.[39]

The care environment resembled that offered by contemporary middle-class homes. St. Joseph's had few private rooms and no private baths. Bedrooms lacked specialized equipment. Patients came to the hospital for nursing care.

Doctors and Hospitals

The relationship between McLean County's early hospitals and its physicians was very different than it would become after about 1920—and, further, differed between proprietary and charitable hospitals. The Doctors Kelso ran their Home Sanitarium as a business, admitting only fee-paying patients. As homeopaths, the Kelsos were marginalized by local allopaths and lacked staff privileges at St. Joseph's and Brokaw hospitals; consequently, their sanitarium, open until 1919, when it had eighty-five rooms and sixty patient beds, offered their only local access to hospital facilities.[40] Their hospital made it possible for George to perform surgery in up-to-date convenient surroundings, while Annie led the local trend toward hospitalization of childbirth. As was also true of the charitable hospitals, day-to-day management, patient care, and housekeeping were done by a matron, a few graduate nurses, and the student nurses enrolled in Kelso's nurse training school, which opened in 1894.

By contrast, the physicians associated with Brokaw and St. Joseph's hospitals in the early years of their operation joined these staffs, not to augment their incomes, but to demonstrate their civic mindedness and expand their resources for surgery and nursing of private patients. Unlike the pattern that began during the interwar years when young doctors undertook emergency call to build their practices and strengthen their relationships with older practitioners, before the 1920s hospital staff physicians tended to be well established in the community. St. Joseph's Hospital's medical staff records kept between 1885 and 1902 offer physicians' perspectives on relationships between McLean County doctors and hospitals during the domestic era of hospital development.

When Reverend Mother Frances and Sister Augustina visited Bloomington in 1879, they discussed their hospital proposal with two physicians, Dr. Charles R. Parke (1823–1908) and Dr. John Sweeney (1840–83). Dr. Parke was then in his late fifties and had been practicing in Bloomington for over thirty years. Having trained at the University of Pennsylvania during the 1840s, Parke moved west to Whiteside County, Illinois, in 1848. In 1849 Parke joined a company of gold seekers bound for California. In the early 1850s, he returned to Illinois via Central America, only to leave again in 1855, becoming a surgeon in the Russian army during the Crimean War. Parke journeyed back to the United States by way of Berlin, Paris, and London, where he followed a pattern common among American physicians by augmenting his medical education.[41] In 1857 he settled in Bloomington and started a practice specializing in diseases of the eye and ear and in general surgery.[42] Nearly a generation younger than Parke, Dr. John Sweeney attended the "session of 1859 and 1860" at Albany Medical College in New York—training that was amplified by service as an assistant surgeon with the Union Army during the Civil War. He arrived in Normal in 1865 and was appointed the first medical attendant of the Soldiers' Orphans' Home. He later became Dr. Parke's partner.[43] These doctors gathered a medical staff for St. Joseph's Hospital.

This staff included Doctors Parke and Sweeney, A. H. Luce (1816–93), T. F. Worrell (1821–87), William Elder (1826–95), R. Wunderlich (1833–93), and Lee Smith (1832–1911). Each agreed "to serve without pay, except, of course, private patients whom they may recommend to the hospital for the superior nursing."[44] The new hospital was run by nuns; staff physicians made no administrative decisions, although they did make recommendations. St. Joseph's annual report for 1887 noted, "One or more members of the medical staff visits the hospital daily."[45] However, these visits were generally made only to the physician's own patients (both private and assigned upon admission), since the staff had agreed the "necessity and propriety of patients keeping one physician for an attendant"—a decision that supported private practice and reduced potential competition among practitioners.[46]

The medical staff's primary contribution to hospital management during the 1880s and 1890s was to provide a sanitary inspector, who made regular reports. For instance, in November and December, 1885, Dr. A. T. Barnes (1832–1901), "reported the drug room, operating room, halls, wards, and private rooms, water closet, outhouses, etc., as in excellent condition. The patients are doing well and well pleased. He thought the washroom ought to be supplied with a steam washing machine and a mangle, and the kitchen with a steam table for vegetables that the sisters might be able to work to better advantage." At the following month's meeting, Dr. Barnes recommended that the hospital purchase an elevator, a suggestion that was reiterated by Dr. William Elder (1826–95) when he served as sanitary inspector in 1886.[47] The sanitary inspector reported when the hospital was connected with the city sewer system in May 1886, and recommended the use of disinfectants in water closets.[48]

Reports illustrated the association between professional medicine and theories of disease causation.[49] Although McLean County Medical Society records indicate that conversion to the germ theory was slow among local physicians, there were many places in the hospital that either miasmata or germs could lurk. Due to their responsibility for the hospital's sanitary condition, St. Joseph's staff physicians were somewhat defensive about deaths occurring there, ascribing unusually high mortality figures in 1890 (twenty-two deaths of 216 admissions), 1891 (twenty-two deaths of 192 admissions), and 1893 (twenty-eight deaths of 244 admissions) "to the septic condition of the atmosphere due to presence of 'grippe' [i.e., flu]."[50] The physicians also explained fatalities by noting that patients were often admitted to the hospital "in a dying condition, living only a few hours."[51] In addition, doctors distinguished between preventable and inevitable deaths (revealing assumptions about the limitations of medical intervention), in 1888 reporting, "We have had only sixteen deaths during the last year out of 234 patients admitted, and of these, eight were necessarily fatal. Two with cancer, two old age, three phthisis pulmonalis [tuberculosis], and one a shoulder crushed under the railroad cars, leaving only eight cases legitimate subjects for medical and surgical treatment, a little over 3 percent, which compares favorably with any hospital record."[52]

Low mortality was attributed to good hospital sanitation. For example, the sanitary inspector found the hospital "in excellent sanitary condition" in

October 1888, "notwithstanding the fact that most of the time every bed has been occupied by patients, a large proportion of whom have been surgical cases, [but] there has not been a single case of hospital gangrene or erysipelas occurring among them."[53]

In addition to the reports of the sanitary inspector, medical staff meetings also provided a forum for discussion of physicians' needs regarding hospital facilities, chief among which was surgery. In 1893, the medical staff planned a new operating room:

> It is the intention to supply the new room with a complete set of new and im-
> proved instruments supplemented by a fine operating table which, being con-
> structed entirely of glass and iron, will leave no infection after being cleansed.
> The interior of the apartment will be conveniently arranged and the floor will
> probably be cemented. After being used, the instruments will be boiled and
> placed on a rack and kept so that contamination will be impossible. Everything
> that is possible according to the most approved methods will be done to con-
> tribute to the efficiency and safety of the room, and it is probable that when
> completed it will be equal in appointments to the best in the state.[54]

The room was built in 1895 to specifications informed by antiseptic theory: "To prevent septic poisoning the walls were constructed of glass and steel, the floor of cement. Thorough drainage was secured, and the rooms can be flooded with super-heated steam, thus reducing the danger of sepsis to the minimum." St. Joseph's paid $88.25 for the operating table and $325 to the carpenter.[55]

Medical staff members also occasionally made suggestions regarding the sister nurses' activities that indicated relative powers in administrative decision making. For example, in 1891 one physician proposed that a blank form for keeping consistent patient records "be placed before the sisters for their adoption."[56] In 1897 the staff used a scientific argument to request additional nurses and recommend that the nuns devote their time solely to nursing, rather than to other household tasks, "thus enabling them to keep their hands and clothing in as perfectly an aseptic condition as possible."[57] This suggests that turn-of-the-century physicians were becoming less tolerant of the domestic model, moving toward new standards of efficiency and specialization.[58]

Paradoxically, among physicians the home care model retained its association with morality and familiar comfort. For example, responding to the negative image clinging to hospitals, Dr. Parke observed in 1888, "The character of the hospital itself has gradually changed from that of a general public hospital to that of a sanitary home for the sick and invalids."[59] Staff physicians took pride in St. Joseph's appearance, donating trees for its grounds, and praising its interior, claiming in 1887, "There is not a room in the building which any citizen of Bloomington could not occupy with comfort and satisfaction."[60]

Regardless of the lingering domestic model, McLean County doctors were reconceptualizing the local practice of medicine to include hospitalization, and reconceptualizing hospital services according to principles of appropriateness, efficiency, and specialization.[61] Although several staff physicians had experience in military and mental hospitals, none of them had previously been associated with a charitable general hospital. Thus, they arguably helped pilot the transformation of community hospitals that was under way throughout the United States.

Physicians discussed the kinds of health problems that should appropriately be dealt with in the hospital—something about which there was no local consensus. For example, although there was general agreement that surgical cases should be admitted, there was disagreement about whether St. Joseph's should treat emotional illnesses. Despite the fact that admissions records indicate that the emotionally ill were routinely accommodated by St. Joseph's, in 1895 the medical staff decided that it was "not for the best interest of other patients that insane persons should be admitted."[62] In 1898 Dr. Parke called for construction of a separate facility for the mad. However, McLean County never built one and, despite its doctors' objections, St. Joseph's regularly admitted patients with diagnoses including "monomania," "acute mania," "nervousness," "neurosis," and "insanity."[63]

As indicated previously, St. Joseph's provided "a home for life" to some paying residents—thus offering a respectable middle-class alternative to the McLean County Poor Farm.[64] By the end of the nineteenth century, staff physicians began to question whether this was an appropriate hospital service.[65] However, local hospitals continued to offer this accommodation into the 1930s. For example, in 1936, Mr. John L. Lampe made arrangement with the board of directors for a permanent home and care in Brokaw Hospital, after which he occupied "Room 109 in exchange for some real estate and securities." During his stay, Lampe improved the hospital's amenities, paying for installation of new wall sockets and light fixtures in all of the old building's rooms, improving the patients' call system, having a new bathtub installed in the men's room, and purchasing a gasoline-powered lawn mower.[66] This example illustrates the extent to which the domestic model endured in McLean County hospital, coexisting with the medicalized configuration that was beginning to emerge in the early twentieth century.

The wide range of needs addressed at St. Joseph's and other McLean County hospitals in the late nineteenth and early twentieth centuries reflected both their traditional unspecialized care environments and the fact that their staff physicians were all general practitioners—regardless of the adoption by several of informal specialties. Both hospital physicians and hospitals exemplified a community health culture that was on the brink of change.

Hospitals and Nurse Training

All of McLean County's major hospitals had nurse training schools.[67] Although this topic will be discussed at greater length in the next chapter, nurse training was so central to hospital services, operations, and finances that it is appropriate to say something about it here. The proprietary Kelso Sanitarium and charitable Mennonite Hospital (which took over both the Kelso building and its nursing school) began training nurses when they opened in 1894 and 1920 respectively. After a brief unsuccessful attempt to support hospital needs with first Mennonite, then Methodist deaconesses after its establishment in 1896, Brokaw Hospital also opened a nurse training school.[68] Supplied with trained sister nurses by the mother house of the Third Order of the Sisters of St. Francis, St. Joseph's Hospital operated without student nurses until 1921, when expansion and growing utilization made it impossible for the order to meet the hospital's labor needs.

From the beginning, McLean County's hospitals followed the nationally typical model of employing graduate nurses as superintendents and supervisors, and using student labor for most patient care and housekeeping duties.[69] This enabled hospitals to keep their own costs and charges low and helped the charitable hospitals fulfill their service missions. Hospitals continued to depend on student labor until the 1940s.

Student nurses were important links in the transition from home to hospital care. As Barbara Melosh points out, late nineteenth- and early twentieth-century nursing students came from respectable middle- or working-class homes and, due to ongoing racial discrimination, were disproportionately white.[70] Thus, they were from the same farming, small business, craft manufacturing, and professional backgrounds as the patients McLean County's hospitals hoped to attract. Students' scrubbed faces, demure hairstyles, white caps, starched aprons, and sensible shoes evoked the normative respectful and capable daughters and housemaids in the ideal middle-class home. Consequently, the presence of student nurses in domestic-era hospitals reassured first-time patients and their families, helping them to feel at home. Indeed, because both students and staff nurses lived in hospital accommodation, the institution was in fact home to them. Nurses' presence encouraged the sense that hospitals were safe and respectable places for sufferers to be—and for families to place them. Furthermore, this hospital atmosphere encouraged physicians, dependent on client families' good opinion for their professional success and incomes, to send increasing numbers of middle-class patients to the hospital. Trained to defer to medical authority, but fresh from traditional home health culture, student nurses became transmitters of biomedicine, translating, advocating, and carrying out doctors' orders in a controlled environment where question or disagreement—from either student nurse or patient—became unthinkable.[71]

Bloomington's hospitals hugely increased the number of trained nurses in McLean County.[72] Each hospital nurse training school graduated between fifteen and thirty nurses per year. Since hospitals employed few staff nurses before the late 1940s, virtually all of these graduates went into private duty—working either in patients' homes or as "special" nurses serving private patients in hospitals.[73] Thus, they helped to bridge hospital and home care environments, carrying hospital routines, biomedical theories and therapies, and presumptions regarding professional medical authority into local households. Many student nurses came from rural backgrounds, trained in urban hospitals, but did private duty throughout the county, thereby linking country and city and aiding a transition in rural health culture to routine hospital care after the 1930s. Finally, unlike the general practitioner making house calls, the trained nurse was something new—arguably a representative of modern medicine in a way that the family doctor could not be.

Hospital Management

Before World War II, McLean County's hospitals were run by people without formal hospital administration qualifications, although management structures differed.[74] St. Joseph's Hospital was administered by a Mother Superior, who managed communication with her order's headquarters in Peoria, dealt with the medical staff, and supervised the work of nursing sisters, student nurses, and other hospital employees. Supported by the Order's rules and its financial backing, St. Joseph's administration was patterned on a long tradition of Roman Catholic charitable institutions.

By contrast, until the late 1950s, Mennonite Hospital—a new venture into the health-care arena by local Mennonite congregations—was run by married couples referred to as the "superintendent" and "matron." These managers lacked medical backgrounds; the hospital's second superintendent, Noble Hoover, had been a farmer and electrician before he was hired in 1927 because of his "business experience."[75] Despite Mennonite's transition to a modern care environment during their nearly 30 years of service, the Hoovers continued to exemplify an unspecialized domestic approach to hospital management. In addition to dealing with the financial challenges of the Depression, Nobel Hoover "took a working interest in all operations of the hospital work, for example, soon learning to take X-rays so he could relieve the only X-ray technician during the nights, every other Sunday, and holidays."[76] Esther Hoover became the business office manager, receptionist, and supervisor of the hospital's housekeeping, laundry, and kitchen staff—a challenge that increased as the staff grew from fewer than 15 in 1927 to 130 by the end of her career.[77]

Before 1924 Brokaw Hospital and its School for Nurses shared a superintendent, who was responsible to the board of directors. Early superintendents were graduate nurses with some experience in hospital and nursing administration. In a revealing 1939 comment, Maude Essig, Brokaw's first separate director of its School of Nursing said of Lula Justis, superintendent between 1907 and 1924, "She was a most economical manager and was a valuable assistant to the board of directors in helping to pay off the bonded indebtedness on the new building. This she did perhaps at the expense, sometimes of patients' comfort, since it is a generally recognized fact that one cannot take in from patients more than enough to meet the actual running expenses of the hospital and in most hospitals the latter is impossible."[78] Brokaw's administration was arguably more like that employed in other domestic-era hospitals than was Mennonite's.[79] Until its first male business manager was hired in 1938, Brokaw was run by nurses, who, according to David Rosner, "with their claim on the household and emotional lives of the community, made excellent candidates for administrative positions."[80]

Transition to Scientific Efficiency

During the interwar years, McLean County's hospitals evolved from approximations of home to increasingly specialized factories for clinical intervention.[81] Linked to changes in medical theories and therapies; professional development of medicine and nursing; Progressive-Era emphasis on science and efficiency; and sufferers' expectations of health, ill-health, and medical intervention, this transformation was a central component in the new community health culture. *Transformation* is, perhaps, the wrong word, because change occurred gradually and affected different aspects of hospital development and utilization at different times in different places. There was a large and long overlap between domestic-era and what might be called institutional-era hospital cultures. For example, the same 1916 promotional pamphlet that advertised the Kelso Sanitarium as "A place for health building with the distinguishing characteristics of simplicity, cheerfulness, and a home-like atmosphere" also proclaimed, "Kelso Sanitarium is strictly scientific and its methods, its apparatus, and its medical staff are recognized as particularly efficient by the medical profession."[82]

There was also a gap between popular and biomedical perspectives on the need for hospital care. So, at the same time as Brokaw Hospital asserted that "It receives patients from any locality, and its records show an increasing patronage each year by people who live in the country and small Illinois towns," oral history respondent Richard Finfgeld (born in 1906) said that when he broke his leg playing baseball in 1924: "They took me home and the doctor came to the house and set my leg there at the house . . . so I think I graduated from high school on crutches . . . I never knew anybody from Lexington that was in a hospital. . . . Nobody ever went to the hospital. When people died, they died in their homes."[83] In the 1920s Brokaw's pamphlets continued to emphasize the hospital's "wholesome, homelike atmosphere," while also arguing that, "Caring for the sick in the average home is a burden to the family, and with the most loving care of the home folks a patient cannot have the scientific treatment and sanitary surroundings, and plainly speaking does not have the chance for a quick and complete recovery that he would have in a modern equipped hospital."[84] Despite rising admissions, hospitalization remained an unusual experience for most McLean County residents.

Surgery enjoyed an early victory of hospital over home treatment—a development that can be partially explained by the inconvenience of home operations. For example, Dr. Rhoda Galloway Yolton, who practiced in Bloomington from 1887–1932, remembered "spending the day before a surgical operation tearing off the paper from the walls of a room in the patient's home, washing the walls and baking necessary linens and bandages in the oven, preparatory for the operation."[85] However, it is also arguable that new hospital surgical facilities contributed to the skyrocketing demand for and status of surgery.[86]

Early McLean County hospital staffs disproportionately included surgeons. In 1921 Brokaw had five operating rooms; ten of its twenty-four medical staff members were surgeons.[87] Proliferating surgical specialties focused on specific body parts, sometimes creating a kind of assembly-line hospital practice that filled beds. For example, in the 1920s and '30s, local hospitals profited from "the continued efforts of E. P. Sloan. Many goiter patients came to Mennonite [Hospital] . . . from all over Illinois and Kentucky to receive his care. Dr. Sloan often had as many as five goiter surgeries in one day at the hospital."[88] Dr. Watson Gailey did eye surgery; Dr. Herman Wellmerling held fracture clinics. Surgeons sent their patients to hospitals, increasing both the demand for hospital accommodation and the number of operations performed there. In 1931 Mennonite Hospital admitted 891 patients and performed over six hundred surgeries.[89] As Rosemary Stevens has pointed out for the United States generally, by the late 1930s, there was no local alternative to hospital-based surgery.[90]

Surgery brought members of all social classes to the hospital, undermining the longstanding association between hospitalization and poverty. It increased the age range of hospital patients, developing, for example, new routine demand for tonsillectomies that, in turn, helped to create a need for children's wards. It also created for the general public a visual and experiential connection between scientific medicine and what Joel D. Howell calls "the use of shiny new machines."[91] This connection rapidly spread beyond surgery to create other opportunities for local hospital services.

Science and technology fueled arguments for hospital birth. In an influential article published in 1920, Chicago's Dr. Joseph DeLee described the hazards of unaided birth.[92] He advocated the use of forceps and episiotomy in normal birth to protect mother and baby from injury—advice that encouraged the trend toward hospital delivery by specialist obstetricians. Before 1920 most McLean County babies were born at home. However, with medicalization of birth, the trend, led by middle-class urban mothers, favored hospital deliveries. The Kelso Sanitarium addressed this market, appealing to biomedical authority and class identity and prejudices:

> In order to meet this trying and critical period with more success, we have fitted rooms especially for this purpose. They are large, sunny, and furnished in pleasing taste. There is an aseptic delivery room in connection which is completely equipped. . . . The fact that every detail can be carried out under the supervision of the physician makes it in every way more desirable and much more satisfactory to the patient [than home confinement]. We believe that our success in the handling of this class of patients is due to the fact that our physicians deeply appreciate this delicate condition and every attention is given and alert vigilance observed in order that the mothers may have a minimum of stress and a better chance for an excellent recovery. This plan relieves the mother of all domestic and social cares during her seclusion and convalescence, and results in a more satisfactory return to health and a more correct beginning for the child.[93]

Other local hospitals appealed to a broader population, projecting some physicians' opinion that the hospital was the best place for *all* babies to be born. Although home deliveries continued, particularly in rural areas, through the interwar period, the tide had turned.[94]

The rhetoric of birth as dangerous and pathological, requiring attendance of a medical specialist, influenced first area doctors, then members of the general public. Thus, James Welch (born in 1915), a rural general practitioner who attended home births in the 1940s, said, "We [doctors] preferred to get them into the hospital because of the complications."[95] Russell Oyer (born in 1920), another general practitioner who did obstetrical work when he started his rural practice soon gave it up because, "Women in this general area . . . wanted to go to the obstetrician. . . . Here nobody was making home deliveries when I came in '54; they went to the hospital."[96] Rebecca Rittenhouse (born in 1941) indicated the degree to which mid-twentieth century central Illinois women internalized concerns about the dangers of childbearing, on the one hand, and belief in hospital delivery as a type of insurance, on the other: "People now [1990s] are even having children at home, which I don't think is a good idea. Things can happen so quickly, and it is really scary to think people would take that kind of a chance with a life they had planned on for nine months. To knowingly not be where that technology can be helpful."[97] When she had her first baby in 1962, "They told you what hospital you would go to and you would call the doctor and he would meet you there."[98]

Scholars including Charles Rosenberg and Rosemary Stevens have pointed out that the hospital itself was medicalized in the early twentieth century.[99] This change included both use of hospitals for medical and surgical interventions and scientific theories and technologies that motivated and supported those interventions. At the same time, doctors were becoming increasingly hospitalized.[100] Home care had been as much a part of physicians' expectations and experience as of sufferers'. However, after about 1920, it became professionally important for McLean County doctors to have staff privileges at one or more community hospitals. Hospitals helped physicians develop relationships that both strengthened professional esprit de corps and enhanced medical practices and incomes through emergency call, consultations, referrals, and (until the 1950s) fee splitting.[101] Like the contemporaneous transition from home- to office-based practice, the hospital pay system enabled physicians to charge private patients for care provided in the hospital; the opportunity to visit multiple patients during rounds made admissions cost-efficient. Hospitals supported specialty practice; in turn, specialists determined numbers of patients and types of conditions treated in hospitals, ultimately influencing hospital design and allocation of space. The hospital was the medical specialist's home as patients' households had been the primary professional arena for general practitioners.

Leading local specialists, such as the goiter surgeon E. P. Sloane, became stars in interwar-era hospitals, both attracting patients and catalyzing profes-

sional rivalries. Thus, in the 1920s, when Mennonite Hospital was establishing itself,

> there was a real medical rivalry in the Bloomington-Normal community. The
> Sloane Clinic was significant in Bloomington, and in Normal there was a group
> of physicians of about equal age and ambition, which caused some tension.
> This situation was pronounced enough that outlying doctors, when referring
> patients to a hospital, sent them to a hospital connected with the physicians
> or specialists that they were associated with. This helped cause an occupancy
> problem at Mennonite Sanitarium.[102]

Similarly, as we will see in Chapter 4, staff privileges and increasing external regulation of hospitals affected status relationships among physicians.[103]
Having dominated McLean County medical practice, in the interwar period
general practitioners began to lose ground to specialists—a transition that
was completed during the 1950s and '60s in part because of a growing sense
that G.P.s were unfit to perform surgery and deliver babies.[104]

At the same time, physicians assumed major decision-making powers
within hospitals. Before the 1920s, as we have seen, hospital management was
done by matrons and supervisors; in the 1960s, professional administrators
gained the upper hand. But during the middle years of the century, according
to Paul Theobald, who began medical practice in the 1940s, "The doctors
more or less ran the hospital. They didn't own it or anything, but they had
enough power to do most anything they wanted to."[105] Medical practices and
local hospitals were joined at the hip; their successes were interdependent.

Advent of the institutional era of hospital development also affected student and graduate nurses. With increasing emphasis on scientific medicine
and the use of technology, the academic component of nurse training increased as did hospitals' demands of nurses' skills. As the Depression eased
and demand for hospital care increased during World War II, local hospitals
followed national trends by hiring graduate nurses.[106]

It is noteworthy that the mid-twentieth-century institutionalization of ill-
health and growth of professional medical power were fostered by a survival
from the home care tradition—the practice of keeping patients in bed for a
long time in situations where authority and tradition limited contact between
the sick and the well and enhanced the ailing person's dependence on caregivers. Long stays were partly due to limited efficacy of contemporary therapies.
Dr. Albert Van Ness, born in 1926, remembered of his clinical training at
Indianapolis General Hospital in the 1940s, "The pneumonia ward had . . .
60 beds in it. You can imagine what it used to be like back in the '40s in the

winter. . . . Fifty percent of the men recovered and they were out for . . . six months with empyemas and all that stuff."[107] Jane Tinsley, born in 1924, who finished nurse training at Brokaw in 1945, remembered,

> If a man had hernia surgery when I was in training . . . they were there about two weeks and they were not allowed to turn themselves. You turned them. They weren't allowed to get up on . . . one elbow or be rolled up in bed to feed themselves; they were fed . . . An appendectomy stayed a week. They didn't even dangle on the edge of the bed until about the fifth day. Then they went home on the seventh . . . If you had a baby, you stayed ten days before the war. They were flat on their back for six or seven days, they dangled one day, then they sat in a chair, and then they went home about the tenth day.[108]

This care environment depersonalized and disempowered hospital patients. It correspondingly empowered doctors, nurses, and hospitals.

As hands-on care providers, nurses were the agents of hospital and medical authority. Their training emphasized development of a somewhat distant professional demeanor; their authority was enhanced by their white uniforms and quasi-military ranks.[109] Perhaps more than doctors, they represented the new hospital as an authoritarian, hierarchical institution that discouraged the social care people experienced at home. Margaret Esposito, born in 1923, remembered her obstetrician presuming that the nurses at St. Joseph's Hospital would object to her husband's presence in the delivery room when their daughter was born in 1947.[110] Ralph Spencer, born in 1914, had a similar experience with Lena Maxwell, superintendent of nurses at Mennonite Hospital from 1944 to 1966, when his wife gave birth in the 1940s:

> I and the head nurse there at Mennonite . . . her name was Maxwell. She was the head of the thing. I had been in there with an appendectomy and when my wife went in for delivery, she said, "I want my husband with me." The nurse said, "Yeah, sure, sure, sure, sure." I stood out in the hallway and waited, and when nobody showed up, I just opened the door and went in. Maxwell was there and she said, "You can't come in here!" I said, "Well, I'm in there." "You can't come in here without a cap and gown on!" I told her she better get one, because I wasn't going anywhere. And I did. I stayed right there when the baby was born.[111]

Not until the 1970s, when broad-based social movements challenged authority and criticized biomedicine, would hospital rules be revised.

Local expectations of medical intervention and hospital utilization rose after World War I, even before antibiotics offered the first effective treatment for infection. In 1925 there were 250 hospital beds in Bloomington; by 1943, there were 464 beds.[112] Mennonite Hospital records indicate a 70 percent increase in admissions between 1933 and 1936—despite hard economic times. During this period,

> patient beds were often placed in the halls. A bed was once placed in the emergency operating room to accommodate a patient. At times, dresser drawers were used as bassinets. The office of the superintendent of nurses was used so often that she moved out to permit its regular use as a patient room. Beds were set up in the board room on occasion with three patients once cared for there simultaneously. By the end of 1937, the emergency room was being used as a patient room and patients had to be turned away because of lack of space.[113]

From facilities marketed to the public as imitations of their own homes, in the 1940s McLean County hospitals were viewed as facilities necessary for county residents' safety and quality of life.

In the years after World War II local hospitals grew enormously, supported in part by the 1946 Hill Burton legislation that funded development of community hospitals.[114] (Here we see national policy both driven by and driving changes in community health culture.) The postwar years also witnessed further expansion and specialization of hospital services, spaces, technologies, and staffing—changes with important implications for community employment opportunities, appearance, and identity. As the visible symbols of modern medicine in a progressive city, Bloomington's hospitals both provided and represented service and safety to a population extending beyond county borders.

Finally, in the second half of the twentieth century, McLean County hospitals made the transition from charitable operations run on a financial shoestring to multimillion-dollar businesses. This transition also affected community health culture. Childbirth offers a useful illustration of changes in cost of care. When Martha Ferguson, born in 1916, had her first two children at home in the 1930s, "The doctor and the nurse came for $25 and stayed the entire time."[115] By contrast, Linda Rohm's (born in 1966) two children were delivered in the late 1980s:

> For Robert—it was $1,200 for a vaginal delivery and $1,400 for a C-section. For Kelly—it was $1,475 for a vaginal and $1,600 for a C-section. So it increased some $200 within those two years. For the hospital—both times I was in the hospital in those two years it was $250 a day per mother and per child: $1,000 for two days in the hospital. . . . But we got lucky because . . . the Sisters of St. Francis had a fund for people with insurance, but have a big amount left over to pay. We only paid $500 for Kelly.[116]

Rohm exemplified both general awareness and significance of health-care costs and lay internalization of biomedical concepts and terms in the late twentieth century. She questioned neither the place nor the expense of child-bearing, rather viewing these matters as necessary and natural components of adult life, thus highlighting the centrality of hospital care in community health culture.

Hospitals were also central to the County's economy after World War II, becoming major employers and wielding important influence in county decision making regarding matters such as land use, traffic patterns, and discretionary welfare provision. Hospitals also became significant amenities invoked to attract new residents and businesses to McLean County. However, the county's hospitals, always competitors, were playing for ever-increasing stakes. When, in the early 1960s, the three institutions asked the State Bureau of Hospitals for just under $1 million each from Hill-Burton funds, local concerns were expressed about duplication of services and pressure grew for collaborative planning and possible merger. Although the grant applications were reluctantly approved in 1964, concern about cost-efficiency remained.[117] In 1984 Brokaw and Mennonite Hospitals merged, becoming BroMenn Healthcare, which also absorbed Eureka Hospital (in adjacent rural Woodford County), reducing the number of local hospitals to two.

3. Nursing, Gender, and Modern Medicine

Nurse Training and Careers in McLean County

Nursing has always been central to a good woman's role. In most times, places, and cultures, wives, mothers, and neighbors have cared for the sick, attended births, and laid out the dead.[1] However, before the late nineteenth century, nursing was only respectable when it was unpaid. With the exception of professed religious nurses, occupational nurses had low social status and bad reputations. Employed by almshouse-era hospitals or hired temporarily to work in private homes, nurses were untrained and paid little to deal with the messes and miseries that servants refused to handle. Although Charles Dickens's Sairey Gamp was a caricature, mid-nineteenth-century readers would have recognized her as representative.[2]

With development of formal training after the Civil War, the image of the nurse changed.[3] In contrast to its traditional association with ignorance, poverty, dirt, and vice, nursing was increasingly linked with cleanliness, competence, and personal refinement. McLean County's nursing schools contributed to the trend for nursing to become a respectable career choice for women living in rural and small-town America. Like teaching, nursing offered a white-collar alternative to domestic service, factory work, or dependence on a father or husband. And, because of the residential supervised character of nurse training programs, parents were willing to allow daughters to attend them.

The training programs that opened at Brokaw (ca. 1897), Kelso (1896), Mennonite (1920), and St. Joseph's (1921) hospitals emphasized character, discipline, and physical strength, rather than academic preparation. In 1921

Brokaw Hospital School for Nurses required only one year of high school; however, the school demanded a reference from the applicant's pastor, together with a physician's certificate of health.[4] Most Mennonite students "came from the rural areas and small towns around Bloomington-Normal. . . . Most of the girls came from strongly religious, Protestant backgrounds."[5] This description would also have characterized students at other McLean County nursing schools, with the exception that some St. Joseph's students were Catholic.

The training offered by Brokaw and Mennonite hospitals illustrates contrasting developments in twentieth-century American nursing education. Both schools extended their diploma programs from two to three years during the 1920s. However, perhaps in response to the 1923 Goldmark Report, which called for more academic rigor in nursing education, in that year Brokaw affiliated with Illinois Wesleyan University to offer students the option of obtaining a bachelor of science degree.[6] In 1956 Brokaw's program changed its name to Brokaw Hospital School for Nursing of Illinois Wesleyan University. In 1962 this school graduated its last class, and Illinois Wesleyan University opened its own nursing program.[7]

In contrast to Brokaw's untypically early development of a bachelor's degree, Mennonite Hospital's School of Nursing retained its three-year diploma program long after the bachelor of science in nursing (BSN) had become the standard qualification. Although in 1945 the academic component of its curriculum was enhanced by course work at Illinois State Normal University, until the late 1960s Mennonite's nursing school provided "an apprenticeship style of training based on a strong learning-by-doing philosophy."[8]

Until the mid-twentieth century, although they attended lectures given by medical staff and graduate nurses, student nurses devoted most of their time to hospital work. Nursing and housekeeping tasks were learned by repetition.[9] Students were paid stipends that rose as their skills grew. As Susan Reverby points out, this attracted women to nurse training; it also distinguished nursing education from more academic postsecondary education.[10] As the academic component of nurse education grew, stipends dwindled. By the late 1930s, McLean County's nursing students were paying tuition.[11]

McLean County's graduate nurses joined the Illinois Graduate Nurse's Association (founded in 1901) and the 6th District of the Illinois State Association of Graduate Nurses (founded in 1914), thus becoming registered nurses.[12] Registration controlled employment—either on hospital staffs or as private duty nurses. Bloomington's hospitals maintained "registers" that assigned private duty jobs to nurses (giving preference to graduates of their own schools) on a rotating basis. In addition, physicians called on favorite nurses to care for their own patients.[13] Private duty, though demanding, was well paid. However, this work conferred lower status than hospital staff positions. Furthermore, in the mid-twentieth century, the market for private duty nursing declined and the swelling population of registered nurses was chronically underemployed. Only the emergence in the 1940s of demand for graduate staff nurses by community hospitals and doctors' offices eased this situation. With the introduction after World War II of hospital intensive care units, the "special" (privately-employed hospital) nurse virtually disappeared, and hospitalization for a growing range of conditions almost eliminated the market for home-based private nurses.[14] At the same time, along with clinical medicine, graduate nursing was institutionalized in hospitals and doctors' offices.

This is not to say that all graduate nurses made the transition from full-time private duty to full-time institutional employment. Nurses' work-lives, like those of other women, were diverse, accommodating shifting individual needs, social norms, and occupational standards. Before about 1950, hospital staff nurses could not be married. Many graduate nurses gave up work or worked part-time after marriage, cobbling together careers that combined hospital, private duty, and contract work.[15] Never-married, divorced, or widowed nurses were more likely to undertake long-term, full-time employment. Oral and other personal evidence helps to flesh out the lived experience of nurses during the mid-twentieth century.

Personal Accounts

As Margarete Sandelowski points out, "Anyone embarking on a history of nursing is soon confronted with the problem invisibles pose, that is, with how to study the relatively unseen. . . . Because there are fewer traces of what everyday nurses thought and did, a history of nursing requires special acts of reading and writing."[16] Furthermore, traditional histories of nursing, like traditional histories of medicine, offer formulaic accounts of professional heroines and steady progress toward a late-twentieth-century golden age. Because of these challenges, oral history offers a particularly useful tool for exploring the past experiences of nurses—especially at the local level.

This study depends on life history interviews conducted with eight nurses born between 1909 and 1938, which elicited information about their family and educational backgrounds, nursing educations, and experiences as graduate nurses. The oldest informant, Ruth Carpenter, was admitted to Brokaw Hospital Nurse Training School in 1928. The youngest, Sally Wagner, joined the diploma program at Grant Hospital, Chicago, in the late 1950s. Sister Theonilla, born in 1912, was the only informant to attend a two-year diploma program. Five informants had completed three-year programs. Evelyn Lantz received a scholarship in 1935 to attend the five-year bachelor's degree course jointly offered by Brokaw Hospital and Illinois Wesleyan University. Three informants earned bachelor's degrees; one went on to get a master's degree in nursing. All spent most of their working lives in McLean County except Sister Theonilla, who arrived from Pontiac in 1961, and Alice Swift, who came to Bloomington in 1972. Several had short or interrupted careers, either giving up work or working part-time in order to focus on family responsibilities. Their job experiences ranged widely within nursing, from hospital staff to public health, private duty, nursing home, factory, doctor's office, and blood-mobile nursing. (See Table 4.)

Career Choice

Young women became nurses for cultural, social, and pragmatic reasons. For several informants, nursing was a dramatic heroic career. Some chose nursing for religious or altruistic reasons. Other informants followed admired role models into the occupation. For still others, nursing was a practical alternative to marriage. Some interviewees' families supported their choice; others objected for reasons including a lingering association between nursing and vice, and worries about the physical demands of the job.

Table 4: Oral History Informants: Nurses

Informants	Birthdates	Nursing Schools	Qualifications
Ruth Carpenter	1909	Brokaw	Diploma, 1931
Sister Theonilla	1912	St. Joseph Hospital, Keokuk, Iowa	Diploma, 1940
Evelyn Lantz	1918	Brokaw/ Illinois Wesleyan	B.S., 1940
Roberta Holman	1921	Brokaw	Diploma, 1944
Sister Judith	1922	School in Dusseldorf, Germany	Diploma, 1946
Jane Tinsley	1924	Brokaw	Diploma, 1945
Alice Swift	1927	Eastern Mennonite College, Virginia Washington University	Diploma, 1948 B.S., 1957 M.S., c. 1965
Sally Wagner	1938	Grant Hospital Nursing School, Chicago	Diploma, 1959

Roberta Holman was attracted to nursing because of its romantic image. She remembered, "It was a dream thing. . . . I wanted to be a nurse when I was ten years old. I thought being a nurse just sounded wonderful. And then when I had occasion to visit people in the hospital . . . I'd see these nurses walking down the hall in these beautiful, white, starched uniforms and, ah—that must be wonderful! You know! I wanted to wear one of those white uniforms."[17] Similarly, Jane Tinsley said, "I think I thought I was going to be by somebody's bedside in a little white uniform just taking care of them, making them well. It was the only thing I ever wanted to do. I never even thought about anything else."[18]

From World War I onwards, idealized images of nursing were generated by fictional nurse heroines, such as Sue Barton, Cherry Ames, and many characters in romance novels and magazine stories targeting girls and women.[19] They were also fostered by popular films featuring nurses and doctors.[20] The fictional nurse, always beautiful and self-sacrificing, but also knowledgeable and powerful, became a strong marketing tool for nursing and biomedicine.

Real role models were also important. Ruth Carpenter followed a friend she admired into nursing. Carpenter grew up on a farm in Vermilion County, Illinois. Her mother died in childbirth when Carpenter was four. Thereafter, she spent several years in the Cunningham Children's Home in Champaign, Illinois. At the children's home, her closest friend was a girl who became a nurse and sparked Carpenter's interest, which her father discouraged, "because in those days nurses were pretty low on the totem pole as far as respectability is concerned. . . . In the early '20s . . . a lot of nurses were just not respectable."[21] Nonetheless, she stuck with her childhood ambition and, after a year of teacher training at Illinois State Normal University, enrolled in nursing school.

For Sister Theonilla, of the Sisters of the Third Order of St. Francis, the decision to become a nurse was linked to her religious vocation. She was born in Dortmund, Germany; her father was a skilled factory worker, and her mother was a seamstress. She finished the standard eight years of education, then looked after her father's household for two years after her mother's death. Conversations with her aunt, who was a member of the nursing order she eventually joined, influenced Sister Theonilla's decision to enter the convent at age nineteen. Previously, she had no career ambitions and "never thought about getting married." She was sent to the order's hospital training school in Keokuk, Iowa, where she completed a two-year diploma course that also trained lay nurses.[22]

In contrast to Sister Theonilla's experience, Sister Judith's interest in nursing pre-dated her religious vocation, although she had had a childhood interest in being a missionary. Born in Düsseldorf, Germany, she began her nurse training in 1942 during World War II because, "I saw the work. One time I was in the emergency room and I saw the work they were doing to help people, so I decided I would like to work as a nurse to help people. These were compassionate and helping people. I think this was the reason for doing this."[23] After the war ended, Sister Judith entered the convent and applied to serve in the United States.

Like Sister Judith, Evelyn Lantz became interested in nursing because of childhood exposure to the work:

> My grandfather Garner developed diabetes and he was in the hospital in Quincy. ... My mother would take me with her to visit her father, my grandfather, in the hospital. I was about three years old. There were no rules or regulations about children being in the hospital. I was sort of a pet of the nurses and they would let me follow them around. I would sort of just tag along and I became very interested in what was going on in the examining rooms when they were cleaning them. Not when patients were in there, but when they would clean them, and just up and down the hall and that kind of thing. As I grew older, then I played nurse, you know, with a red cross on your head, or a dishrag to sort of wrap around your head or something or other to look like a nurse's cap.[24]

She was also attracted by the status and demeanor of nurses. "Their families were respected families. They always seemed to be very much in control and, how shall I say it, dignified. . . . It wasn't that they were reserved or anything of that kind, but very much in command of the situation."[25] Nursing and teaching were the only occupations that were available to women and offered them this kind of authority.

Alice Swift's decision to become a nurse was based on a practical assessment of the opportunities available to her. Swift grew up in an Iowa Amish Mennonite community that viewed marriage and housework as the appropriate destiny for girls and "really opposed higher education, anything beyond elementary education." However, Swift liked to study and thought it was unlikely that she would marry young, since "somehow I never had dates." She said, "I did not look forward with anticipation and pleasure to the thought of doing housework the rest of my life if I wasn't going to get married." Swift persuaded her parents to send her first to a Mennonite high school in Virginia and then to a nursing school in Lancaster, Pennsylvania. Swift went on to take both a bachelor's degree and a master's in nursing.

Training

In 1921 the Brokaw Hospital School for Nurses advertised that it, "Offers to women desirous of becoming professional nurses, a course of practical and theoretical instruction. The practical knowledge is gained by actual care of patients, under the supervision of the superintendent and her assistants. The theoretical course is of the best. . . . Each student is given many opportunities for the special nursing of private patients, a work especially fitting her for duty as a graduate nurse."[26] Students could be admitted at any time of year. They were instructed to bring with them to the school, "Three wash dresses simply made, six large white aprons, several plain white collars, two bags for soiled linen, and a good supply of plain underclothing. Each article must be distinctly marked with the owner's name in full. Each nurse will be required to have her own watch, also to wear rubber-heeled shoes. If teeth are out of order, they should receive the necessary attention before entering."[27] Students were given material for uniforms, textbooks, and stipends of $8 per month in their first year for the months following the three-month probationary period, $12 per month in their second year, and $15 per month during their final year.[28]

The curriculum was organized into junior (first-year), intermediate, and senior courses. In theory, course work was evenly divided between "practical" and "class and lecture" work. In practice and when it was possible, classroom education and study time were sandwiched in between ward duties. (See Table 5.)

Nurses' uniforms and caps indicated occupational status and training-school affiliation. Like military dress, their ritualized changes, well understood by nurses but incomprehensible to laypeople, also marked the transitions from individual to group identity and between ranks within the group. Oral history informants provided detailed descriptions of their student nurse uniforms. When Ruth Carpenter began her training at Brokaw in 1928, "We had to make our own uniforms, . . . blue and white chambray with a belt and a full skirt. . . . Of course, they gave you the apron and you wore that for six months and then you got your bib and cap and that sort of thing. And then they had white cuffs. We got the cuffs that were detachable. . . . And sometimes we got to wear white shoes."[29] By the time Evelyn Lantz began training at Brokaw in 1936, student uniforms were provided. She described the changes in her uniform from her acceptance at the school to "capping,": "I think it was three months that we were considered probation nurses. We didn't have the bib and the cap. Our uniform [was] chambray blue and white stripe, princess style, with the white starched collar that you had to pin on

Table 5: "Class and Lecture Work," Brokaw Hospital School for Nurses, 1921

Junior Course	Intermediate Course	Senior Course
Practical: 4 months medical, 4 months surgical, and 6 weeks house work.	*Practical:* 4 months senior floor work, diets, massage.	*Practical:* 2 months assisting surgical nurse, 2 months in charge of operating rooms, 6 months senior medical work, 2 months obstetrics, 3–4 months head nurse work.
Primary Anatomy	Preparation and after care of major surgical and obstetrical patients	Surgical and Medical Emergencies
Physiology and Hygiene	Bacteriology	Care of Children
Materia Medica	Surgical and Operating Room Technique	Contagious and Nervous Patients
Practical Nursing, including the entire care of ordinary medical, surgical, and gynecological patients	General Medicine, Eye, Ear, Nose, and Throat	Massage and Electricity
Urinalysis	Dietetics, theoretical and practical	Instruction by the superintendent of Private Nursing Supplies
Cost and care of hospital supplies		Hygiene and isolation in private homes

Source: Brokaw Hospital pamphlet, 1921, 18–19.

Note: Subjects offered by local nursing schools varied. In 1925–28, Mennonite's school covered these subjects, but also offered courses in history of nursing; hygiene and sanitation; urinalysis, chemistry; eye, ear, nose and throat; infant feeding; and gynecology. See *Mennonite School Commemorative History,* 19–20. The lack of standardization of local programs nationally is typical.

and cuffs that had to be pinned on. After you passed your probationary period, you were given a cap, the cap of the school, and a bib to go over your shoulders and cover the front of your uniform."[30]

Nurses' caps and uniforms remained important after World War II. Sally Wagner, who finished training in 1959, remembered a uniform similar to the ones her older colleagues wore twenty years before, "When we went in . . . our uniforms just consisted of a striped dress and a little pinafore. And then, when we had been there . . . six months, they had a capping ceremony where you received your cap. And then, when you were a junior, you got a stripe on your cap, and then . . . when you were a senior I think the stripe came off, but you got a pin or something different. Then when you graduated, you had your nursing pin and they had the graduation ceremony."[31] Graduate nurses continued wearing their school caps. Alice Swift, who graduated in 1951, associated the competence of nursing instructors at her Pennsylvania training school with their caps, "I particularly admired the math and physiology teacher. She was so clear. I enjoyed her instructions very well. . . . She was short and petite and she wore all those fluted nursing caps. They wore their uniforms to teach in. Then the nursing arts professor, she was an older person. I didn't get quite as excited about her. . . . She was a likeness to a general hospital cap. A very orderly pointy cap."[32]

Their pristine uniforms contrasted starkly with the tasks student nurses performed—beginning with cleaning hospital buildings and equipment.[33] When Ruth Carpenter began her training in 1928, "The first place I went to for any kind of service was in surgery. And we were taught to scrub anything that didn't move and some things that did move. We scrubbed everything— surgical instruments and the floors and the woodwork . . . [with] soap and water."[34] Eleven years later, Roberta Holman's introduction to training at Brokaw was similar. "Back then the first thing you learned was cleanliness. If you didn't know it, you learned it then. They had all the pictures of all the former nurses there. Every day we scrubbed their faces—shined the pictures. We cleaned cupboards, we cleaned beds; that was when we were 'probies' our first six months of training. You learned to clean."[35] In the 1940s, Alice Swift remembered, "We had to always empty the wastebaskets. And we had a little hot water sterilizer where we had to boil our syringes and needles and sharpen them and store them in alcohol containers. We had to wash all the enema cans and rectal tubes and rubber gloves, and boil them, and we boiled all the bedpans. We had a song about bedpans. At night we'd always collect everybody's bedpans and we had to sterilize them."[36]

Although Evelyn Lantz began her nursing education in the 1930s, her introduction to training was different from that of her contemporaries because she was admitted to the five-year degree program jointly offered by Brokaw Nursing School and Illinois Wesleyan University. Lantz remembered that nursing degree students were accepted more easily by Illinois Wesleyan students than by diploma students at Brokaw, "It was a matter of sort of like teasing—you know, 'Those college girls, they think they're so smart'—and they would play tricks on us which were hurtful. I remember one of the little incidents. We always had dirty linen, you know, when you're working with patients. I was told that I had to wash that out by hand and carry it down to the laundry room and give it to the head laundry man. Of course, that wasn't true, but I didn't know it. It was that kind of thing."[37] In this account, the diploma student's obligation to scrub represented difference from—and punishment of—the degree student, illustrating local and national tensions within nurse training.[38]

Despite her participation in a diploma rather than a bachelor's degree program, Sally Wagner's introduction to nursing in the late 1950s was very different from that of her older colleagues. She recalled,

> We would have class all day long, and then we were expected to work in the evening . . . another six to eight hours. . . . We had anatomy, microbiology, chemistry, history of nursing, and just all the courses that I think they have now, except now I think when you get your bachelor's degree you are also taking English courses and math courses. . . . This was five days a week, and you never had a day off during the week that you weren't going to class or working. A lot of us worked even on Saturday or Sunday for extra pay.[39]

The classroom component of nursing education had grown by this time and, although student nurses were still expected to do a lot of hands-on patient care, they were doing less scrubbing.

In addition to cleaning, before the introduction of disposable medical supplies, student nurses made many materials used in patient care. Ruth Carpenter remembered, "We made our own cotton balls and squares, two-by-two squares and four-by-four squares and abdominal pads and then we made toothpick applicators [i.e., Q-tips]. I know I made enough toothpick applicators to reach from here [Shirley] to Bloomington [five miles away] twice."[40] Sister Theonilla said, "We made all those things. . . . You took cotton and rolled it up into balls. . . . You made all your bandages. You just bought a ball of cotton and a ball of gauze. . . . We washed our instruments, too, that weren't used. . . . There was nothing disposable. . . . Like IV tubings, and all that. . . . That was a job to clean."[41]

More important than cleaning and making supplies, however, was bedside care. Ruth Carpenter recalled, "If a patient came in with pneumonia, you didn't figure he'd get out except from three weeks to four. It would take three weeks to pass the crisis. Everything took a lot longer then. They didn't have any antibiotics."[42] Home care traditions, medical theories, and hospital customs combined to keep hospital patients in bed doing very little for themselves. Because few hospital rooms had private bathrooms, nurses passed bedpans and bathed patients in bed. They gave back rubs and watched patients through the night. Jane Tinsley, who attended Brokaw's nursing school during the 1940s, described a typical day for a nursing student:

> Well, there were lots of times we did what they called split shifts. . . . In other words, you worked an eight-hour day, and they usually planned your work so your class time wouldn't come out of your work. . . . We used to get up and eat, then we had chapel where you sang a couple of songs and had a poem read or

whatever—people took turns leading chapel. Then, when we went out, we had to have a check of the cloth on your collar—you couldn't have your hair on your collar. And you went to your respective floors whatever they happened to be. Of course you rotated, you spent so many times on each floor—so much on medical, so much on surgical, so much in O.B. Usually you listened to reports, and if you were just on a general floor, you were assigned so many patients to do their baths. And you did their baths, even if they went home that afternoon, you gave them a bath. . . . If the individual needed an enema, they got the enema somehow worked in between all the other baths and what have you. . . . When I first went into training, if somebody had surgery, you made up the bed for them. They brought them down from surgery and transferred them into the bed, and then you sat with that patient in his room and took pulse and respiration until he woke up and [was] really responding and knowing what he was doing and where he was before you could leave him.[43]

Students learned to tolerate the sights and smells of ill-health while preserving a professional demeanor.[44] Indeed, as Barbara Melosh points out,

Graduates from the 1920s and the 1950s retell their experiences of training in strikingly similar ways: common perceptions and values blur the actual historical differences in their educations. These are narratives of initiation, of a journey from innocence to knowledge. As they begin the narrator is an outsider describing the initial strangeness and threat of the hospital world. The trials and rituals of ward duty challenge her, and gradually she learns the skills and discipline of a nurse.[45]

All nurse informants for this study supplied versions of this narrative. For example, Roberta Holman said, "I'll never forget we had this bachelor up from Lexington who had a ruptured appendix. Our rooms then were just like little bitty cubicles. . . . The man died, of course. We did not have penicillin . . . But with dressings—the odor was so bad, we didn't have all these things to kill odor then like you do now. But I had to do it out by the door. I could not stay in the room. The odor was just horrible."[46] Ruth Carpenter remembered that "One of the first things I had to do when I was a student was up in surgery, and they were amputating a leg, and I got to hold the leg. . . . They didn't have anything else to do with it. Somebody had to hold it. They didn't want to let it just fall on the floor in a floor pan."[47]

Students also had to put aside normative maidenly modesty and shame to do their jobs. Roberta Holman said, "This was embarrassing for 18, 19, 20–year-olds. We had to prep everybody. Surgery didn't do that, and we didn't have orderlies. Now, you get in a 19, 20, 30, 35–year-old man and you have to go in and do a prep for an appendectomy—it wasn't easy."[48] Sometimes embarrassment undermined professional demeanor. Roberta Holman remembered the first time she tried to administer a milk molasses enema:

> Our supervisor said to one of my classmates and I, "Go up and give an enema to that [patient]. . . ." We said, "We've never been checked on enemas." She said, "It's all right, 'cause you're gonna give one now. . . ." And to top it all off, it was on a fracture bed, and the man was laying here, and his bottom came through. . . . So Charlotte and I went in to give this milk molasses enema, and we did not know what to do, seeing this fat bottom down there. So, here we were, underneath the bed. We were looking at each other under there, and we'd get tickled. We were just two "probies," you know, and so we go back in this old room where we got the bedpans, and Charlotte doubles over laughing. So we go back in with a straight face and we get that tube. I made her take it, and so finally I tried, and she tried. I finally made it. I got it in, but I didn't get it in far enough. We let that old milk molasses run in the tube and out. . . . Molasses went everywhere![49]

This account illustrates a challenge associated with staffing hospitals with students; the crisp uniform, some classroom education, and practice sessions with each other did not transform schoolgirls into mature nurses overnight. In addition, the account replicates a theme, also common in accounts of medical school training, where the macabre or disgusting became a vehicle for humor—as well as an initiation rite and badge of honor for those who persevered to graduation and licensure.

The example also shows that students trained before World War II were taught already outdated remedies. Both Ruth Carpenter and Evelyn Lantz learned to make mustard plasters. Evelyn said that in the 1930s, "We were taught how to make a mustard plaster to the degree of redness to draw the blood to the surface as a counter-irritant. You could put it on the back if you had a headache, or on the chest. This was in our Nursing Procedures and we were taught how to do it. I never did it for a patient."[50] Ruth, trained a decade earlier, had more experience with this therapy, remembering that, "Of course you had to be real careful with those. Some people, blond people, if you put too much mustard, oh, you'd get a big fat blister. Oh. You could be sicker with that than you would with what you were using the poultice for."[51] Roberta Holman, trained during the 1940s, remembered using hot packs on the chest for pneumonia.[52] Sally Wagner, an obstetrical nurse trained in the late 1950s, recalled, "A lot of nurseries would have a bottle of whiskey so if a baby's heart rate were a little slow, or if they felt the baby needed to be stimulated a little bit, you would have an eye dropper and you would give them a couple of drops of whiskey."[53] These examples illustrate the enduring overlap between "modern" and "old-fashioned" theories and therapies and the porous boundary between "popular" and "learned" medicine.

Student nurses worked very long hours.[54] They went to school year round, and rarely had more than a half-day off at a time. Sister nurses experienced even greater demands on their time than lay students. Regarding her training in the 1930s, Sister Theonilla remembered, "I got up early in the morning, sisters do. We had early morning prayers together, mass together, breakfast together, and then we went on duty and nursed all day. There was no time off. . . . The [lay] nurses had their days off, you know. I never really did. I was always there, day and night. That was just the way it was . . . that was the Sister's job. As a Sister, you look at that a little different."[55] Unlike lay students, nuns did not expect their roles to change once they had finished their training. Sisters did not do private or special duty. Having not been paid as students, they were not paid as graduate nurses. They continued to work in hospitals affiliated with their order. Change for them came in the forms of new demands (e.g., use of emerging technologies, mounting types and quantities of paperwork), increasing expertise, and rising levels of assigned responsibility.

The stipends paid to lay student nurses helped to compensate for the long hours and unremitting work. However, beginning in the late 1920s, stipends decreased, according to Maude Essig, Director of Brokaw's training school, "to offset the cost of instruction. During this year [1928] the case study method of learning was instituted. Graduate staff nurses were added to relieve the students of many responsibilities previously accorded to them and to provide a more stable nursing service."[56] During the Depression, both student stipends and the salaries of staff nurses dropped. By the time the economy improved, nurse training had begun the transition from apprenticeship to academic preparation. Evelyn Lantz says of her own class of 1938, "We were the last ones to receive a stipend. The next class that entered didn't have a stipend. I can't remember what it was, but it was just enough to pay for our books. . . . Probably around $5–$6 per month."[57] In the early 1940s, Roberta Holman's parents paid $100 a year for her training, which "paid for our tuition at Wesleyan, it paid for all of our books . . . our uniforms. . . . Of course, remember you work [in the hospital] and that pays for your room and board."[58]

Indeed, schools continued to provide free housing, and even some support to students who lived at home. For example, Jane Tinsley remembered that in the 1940s, "I lived there [the nurses' quarters at Brokaw] at first, but when they got crowded and I was in my junior year, I lived at home. . . . I remember now, they gave my mother so much a day to feed me, but I think she had about 28 cents left by the time I paid for my bus ride."[59] This lingering financial commitment suggests the slow reduction of student labor as a central component of hospital workforces. It also illustrates the long association of nurse training with what Barbara Melosh, quoting Erving Goffman, calls a "total institution" where "the usual social boundaries between public and private life collapse. 'Inmates' of total institutions sleep, work, and play under a single pervasive authority" that governs, exploits, and supports them.[60] Not until after the war, when hospital work was done by graduate nurses, schools moved out of hospitals, and students paid for both tuition and housing, would the financial interdependence of McLean County's nursing students and hospitals dissolve.

How did student nurses learn to do their jobs? Practical nursing was taught by graduate staff nurses or supervisors, with invariably exacting standards. Ruth Carpenter said of Maude Essig,

> She was very straight-laced. And she was only trying to make good nurses of us.... And I..., well, you treated her with respect.... She was very particular about how we kept the patients' rooms.... And she had certain ways that she liked the linens put in the drawers.... You wanted them so that the closed end was toward the drawer beginning when you opened the door. So it would be the closed end of a sheet, or a pillowcase or a towel.... And if you didn't do it right, you got to go do it over so you learned after awhile.... She was strict.... Everybody liked her in a sense of the word, but she, when she said, "No," and "Do this," you did it that way. You didn't ask why, you just did it.[61]

Sally Wagner recalled of her instructors in the 1950s, "They were very professional. They were there to teach you and they expected you to learn. Some of the instructors were very strict, so they were not like a buddy-buddy-type instructor. They were all business."[62] Jane Tinsley commented on etiquette among nurses in the 1940s, "Anybody that was senior to you, you were supposed to stand up. You gave them your seat, or whatever."[63]

A few nurse instructors had bachelor's degrees. However, according to Sally Wagner, in the 1950s,

> I think most of them [her instructors] had on-the-job training and became instructors by being offered the job. It was probably about four to five years after I graduated that they started making a lot of rules and regulations about instructors needing to have a degree. Then they even wanted them to have a master's degree. I can't remember for sure, but probably 10 years after I graduated they closed the [Grant Hospital] School of Nursing because they did not have enough instructors that were qualified with degrees ... because they had made the program different.[64]

This change, driven by nurse leaders, was paralleled in the job market for nurses.[65] Although most were diploma-qualified when Sally Wagner began her career in 1959, by the mid-1990s, "In this [Bloomington] hospital, they claim . . . that they do not discriminate, you know, if people graduate from three-year, two-year, or bachelor's, that they get the same starting salary. That may be true, but when job positions become open they are probably going to pick the person that has the degree or the master's degree over somebody that might be from the three-year or two-year school."[66] However, despite qualification inflation, nurse training retained much of its original learning-by-doing format well into the second half of the twentieth century, supporting a long overlap between apprenticeship and academic preparation.

Student nurses practiced new skills on dummies (the ubiquitous "Mrs. Chase," who appeared in Bloomington as well as elsewhere in the country), each other, and, finally, patients.[67] Sally Wagner remembered,

> We had clinical instructors that would sort of follow us around. . . . Each new procedure—we would be expected to demonstrate that we could do it, and they would check us off to make sure that we knew what we were doing. We also had classroom instructions when we'd have to give each other baths, shots, wrap bandages, practice on each other, but they would also check us out on patients too. We were not expected to do it until we were okayed by the instructor. We really never had the supervision that these students have now. You know, once they checked you off on a procedure, then you were free to do it as many times as was expected.[68]

Until the 1960s, staff physicians provided much of the clinical instruction for student nurses, at the same time inculcating an inter-professional etiquette based on the complete authority of doctors and the unquestioning deference of nurses. Jane Tinsley remembered of the 1940s, "And, of course, any time a doctor walked into the room you immediately stood up; they were 'God,' practically."[69] Sally Wagner's account of the late 1950s indicates both the comparative status of medical and nursing students, and the authoritative position of physicians vis-à-vis students and patients:

> They were very good teachers and they expected you to listen. When the doctor talked everybody just was quiet and he would make rounds. The interns and residents would go and the [nursing] students would go and he would teach at the bedside. He would come to the patient and he would tell us what the problems were in front of the patient and he would say what he was going to do, and . . . then he would ask questions to the interns and residents, but the nurses were never asked questions. We were just there to learn.[70]

As time went on, students took more classes from university professors, although Alice Swift recalled that in the late 1940s, "Our books were tiny compared to what the students have now. They weren't hard at all. . . . The books were so simple and easy compared to college."[71]

In addition to local training, McLean County students traveled to affiliated hospitals for specialized clinical rotations. For example, in the late 1920s, Ruth Carpenter studied pediatrics at a hospital in Indianapolis. In the late 1930s, Evelyn Lantz recalled, "We affiliated with Milwaukee Children's Hospital and the nurses taught us pediatrics. We did not have doctors teaching us. The courses were all taught by nurses. Then we affiliated with Peoria State Hospital, which is in Bartonville, for our psychiatric work. We had physicians teach us there and the Nursing Arts Instructor taught us how to care for what we had to do."[72] Generally speaking, nurses remembered rotations as highlights of their training. For many it was the first time they had been far from home; thus, the experience was liberating. It could also be frightening. Roberta Holman remembered of her rotation at the mental hospital in Bartonville during the 1940s:

> I was scared to death when I first went over there. I almost got kicked out of training, too, over there. . . . I was pretty much a homebody. To be gone and not be able to see my folks and stay all night with them for six months was unheard-of, you know. So Abby and I decided we were going to go home. . . . We were dressed and in bed, and after this mean old woman checked us at night, we went out a window. . . . We thumbed a ride, got into the car with some drunks, we were scared to death, and there was a tavern down the way, so we told them we wanted a drink . . . would they buy us a drink. So they stopped at this tavern, and we had to go to the restroom. We walked right out of that building, went out, thumbed a ride and got a ride home. . . . The next day at class, the teacher said, "I understand there were two girls who hitchhiked to Bloomington, and I have no idea who it was." Of course they didn't! There was only two there from Bloomington. "And unless they report to us immediately, they will be expelled from school." We about knocked those people over getting up there. We were—what is it you call it?—we couldn't leave, we couldn't go anywhere the rest of the time we were there. Anyway, it's a part of growing up.[73]

Nursing school rules were strict, designed to protect the reputations of the students, the school, and the profession. Ruth Carpenter recalled Brokaw's regulations in the 1920s:

> Well, you didn't get married. That was the head of the list. You didn't get married because if you did, you went out on your toot. And you had to be in at 10:00. And, if you were on call, you couldn't leave the campus. Your boyfriend

could come to see you if he wanted to, but you couldn't leave the campus. And you had to go to Chapel and . . . our uniforms had to be halfway respectable looking. . . . We didn't wear jewelry. No earrings. None of that sort of thing. No jewelry in uniform. And we didn't smoke in uniform. . . . And you didn't wear your cap off campus.[74]

Brokaw's rules relaxed somewhat by the 1940s; however, students' behavior was still closely monitored. Jane Tinsley remembered,

In one of the areas, you had to be in by 10 p.m. And then, you had so many 11 p.m. times per month that you could sign out for. Then, about two overnights and a couple of midnights. But you had to get permission before you signed out, you didn't just sign out. [This] entailed if you were going home or where were you going and when. If you didn't get permission . . . you ended up staying in. . . . I know when the war was on, some of the gals who were in love and wanted to get married before they were shipped overseas had to get special permission to marry.[75]

Students lived in the hospital, in purposed-designed residence halls, or in private homes supervised by housemothers. In early years, student accommodations were a low priority. Jennie Miller, who graduated from Brokaw Hospital's School of Nursing in 1906, remembered, "When the nurses lived on the top floor of the old Brokaw building, there was such a dire need for patient beds that the nurses moved into tents on the hospital lawn. We undressed in the hospital and scooted out to the tents in our night clothes."[76] Not until May Mecherle Hall was constructed in 1941 did Brokaw's student nurses have purposed-built accommodation.[77]

In the late 1930s the accreditation of Mennonite Hospital School of Nursing—and, indeed, the hospital itself—was threatened by inspectors' finding that nurses' housing was inadequate.[78] However, in 1943, the school's more than fifty students were still living in five houses, "The accommodations were extremely crowded. Much of the time there was no money for badly needed repairs. The roof would leak, the rooms were drafty, and there were never enough bathroom facilities. In the house known as Hawk House, between the years of 1943 and 1946, seventeen girls and a housemother shared one bathroom. The Chestnut home with fourteen students in 1941 was a paradise by comparison—it had two bathrooms."[79] The four-story Troyer Memorial Nurses Home, opened in 1946, accommodated seventy-five students and also included a library, recreation room, lounge, chapel, and classrooms. A tunnel connecting the home to the hospital "meant that the nursing students were never really separated from their duty on the hospital floors."[80]

Students worked, lived, and played together; strict supervision and rules supported both development of *esprit de corps* and separation from the world outside the hospital. Throughout the study period—long after graduate nurses moved out of hospital accommodations—students in diploma programs were required to live in training school housing. Nonetheless, despite hard work, Spartan living conditions, and strict discipline, nurse informants remembered their training with nostalgia. Ruth Carpenter said of her days at Brokaw's training school,

> We had a lot of fun. My roommate, she was as crazy as I was so we got along real well together. She had an old ukulele and of a night we'd come off duty, maybe in the summertime, and we lived on the Southwest corner . . ., and we'd have a concert. So she got her ukulele out and I and all the rest of us had combs with tissue or toilet paper or them, and we had a concert out on the little patio there, the fire escape. . . . And there was a nurse, and she was a World War I nurse, and she was very sedate; straight-laced as all get out. . . . And, oh, she raised Cain, but the patients just loved it.[81]

Like the rituals associated with interaction with doctors and changes in uniform at various milestones of training, student high jinks built group identity that nurses carried with them into strong relationships with alumnae organizations.

Nursing Careers

Nurse training ended with graduation and, for most McLean County nurses, formal registration with the State of Illinois, although nurses trained before the 1920s sometimes failed to take that step, which was not mandatory in any state until 1938.[82] Evelyn Lantz remembered an older private duty nurse worrying in the late 1930s about the fact that she was not registered: "Dr. McCormick told her she didn't need to worry about registration because he would always have patients for her to nurse . . . So she was never a registered nurse, and she did private duty for Dr. McCormick. She was always busy. He kept his word."[83]

As time went on, registration involved taking a state board examination. Alice Swift first took her state boards in Pennsylvania in 1951: "I don't think they [the exams] were anywhere as detailed as they are today. Of course, we didn't cover near as many subjects then."[84] Nurses moving to Illinois from other states had to become licensed in Illinois before obtaining employment. Sister Theonilla was first licensed in Iowa during the 1930s:

INFORMANT: I got licensed in three states: Iowa, Illinois and Michigan . . .
INTERVIEWER: So when you moved, you had to take a licensing exam?
INFORMANT: Yeah. From Springfield. . . . You had to fill out some papers and
    then sign your name, and with a doctor's signature. Then I got my license.[85]

Licenses were renewed annually. Local nursing organizations, such as the
Sixth District Illinois Nurses' Association, with which McLean County nurses
affiliated, offered the opportunity for graduate nurses to stay in contact with
each other, upgrade their skills, and influence legislation and regulation.[86]
They also governed access to the job market.

Before the late 1940s, most graduate nurses went into private duty nursing.
This situation reflected sufferers' lingering preference for home care; general
practitioners' continued practice of visiting patients at home; and lack of
hospital jobs for graduate nurses. Hospitals did, however, serve as brokers
for both home-based and "special" (hospital-based) private duty. Brokaw
Hospital's "Registry Rules" indicated that "The Registry is to be conducted
at the Hospital under the supervision of the Superintendent of Nurses with
the approval of the Alumnae. No nurse is eligible to the use of the Registry
unless she is a member of the School Alumnae and the Sixth District." Nurses
were allocated jobs "in the order in which they register unless the Doctor in
charge or the patient expresses a preference."[87]

Before the Depression, private duty was comparatively well-paid. In 1920,
Brokaw's Registry published the following fees for services:

$42.00 per week [=$2,184 per year, full time] for general nursing
$7.00 per day for quarantine cases, mental, nervous, genito-urinary and last
    stages of carcinoma and tuberculosis
$7.00 per day for pneumonia and typhoid through critical period, and $6.00
    per day through convalescence
$7.00 per day for obstetrics
$10.00 per call for assisting with delivery
$42.00 per week from date of engagement to confinement
$5.00 to $10.00 for assisting with operations in the home
This fee in addition to charge if nurse remains on case.
$10.00 per week or $2.00 per day for each additional patient
When two nurses are employed, each shall charge the regular fee.
Nurses are entitled to six hours' rest at night and three or four hours off for
    recreation each day.
Traveling expenses including taxicab when needed at night to be paid by
    employer.[88]

At a time when the average annual earnings of employees was $1,342, and
railroad workers (many of whom lived and worked in McLean County) made

an average of $1,807, these figures suggest that nurses could earn more than many men—and, as women, earned particularly good wages—if they could get steady work.[89] However, by the early 1930s, private duty opportunities and fees declined. Ruth Carpenter explained, "Nurses were a dime a dozen. You couldn't hardly find a job." When she graduated in 1931, Carpenter took a room in a house where she could work for her board and room when she was not nursing. She put her name on the private duty register at Brokaw Hospital, "and maybe you'd get a case for three days, and then when you got off that case you'd go right down to the bottom of the register."[90] When she did get work, Carpenter was unhappy about the working conditions, calling private duty "a slave driver's trade. You'd work 20 hours for six dollars. Now, that's not much money. . . . And in 1931 and '32, people did not have private duty nurses unless they were just desperately ill. And you'd watch them, and we worked 20–hour shifts."[91]

Shortly after finishing her training, Carpenter was asked to take an erysipelas case by Dr. Minnick of Danvers, who picked her up with his horse and buggy to drive her to the patient's home:

> Well, this man was shaving one Sunday morning and there was a little pimple . . . right close to his nose. And by the end of the day, it began to get . . . worse. So the family was, they were not rich, but they were affluent enough they could afford to . . . have somebody to come to the house. And he [Dr. Minnick] came in to get me, and he said, "What were you trained to use for erysipelas?" And I said, "Well, the only thing I ever knew was hot Epsom salt packs." So . . . it took us three weeks to get this man well, but we got him well. . . . And of course it's an awful disease. It used to many times be fatal.[92]

This account indicates that even patients thought to be in danger of death were cared for at home during the 1930s. It also illustrates that, despite the physician's formal authority, doctors could accept—and even, in some circumstances, solicit—advice from nurses.

Carpenter assisted with home deliveries, learning to bake linens in the oven to sterilize them and to use a portable delivery table. On one occasion, "This young man came to me in the middle of the night and he said, 'Mrs. Carpenter, my momma is in confinement. Will you come and help her?' The aunt was going to do it, and they got pretty far along and discovered the cord was around the neck about two times, so I went out and helped."[93] These accounts illustrate both the private duty nurse's independence and the extension of traditional home care and neighborhood mutual aid patterns into the interwar period.[94] However, they also indicate the instability of Depression-era private duty work. In 1932 Carpenter took a pay cut to accept a general duty staff position at Brokaw Hospital.

Increasingly, home-based private duty became the province of the wealthy. Roberta Holman did private duty nursing after she graduated (and married) in the 1940s:

> I took special Mrs. W. H. Roland [whose family owned a local department store] in her home out at Country Club Place. That was in 1946–47. . . . Dr. Ed Stevenson called me and asked me if I would go take care of her. . . . And I took care of her for several months. I was pregnant . . . at that time, and it was really nice working in a home like that. . . . [But] finally I think I was getting on her nerves and she was definitely getting on my nerves. She had cancer, you know, and was very ill. And so I called Dr. Ed Stevenson and I said, "You know, I think she's getting tired of me and I'm getting tired period." And I said I would really like to be relieved.[95]

Despite its reflection of the nurse's independence, this example also suggests the parallel between private duty nursing and domestic service that undermined the nurse's status and authority.[96] The fact that the approved rates for private nursing charged in Bloomington-Normal in the early 1940s were not much higher than in 1920—$8 per day for round-the-clock patient care as opposed to $7 per day twenty years earlier—indicates the arguably declining status of this job.[97]

Special duty hospital nursing tended to be provided to very ill patients who required intensive individual care, or to the wealthy who retained traditional distrust of hospitals.[98] "Special" nurses worked in the hospital, but not with student and staff nurses or under the authority of nursing supervisors. According to Evelyn Lantz, in the late 1930s,

> At night, they would put a cot down in the room and they would sleep on the cot so they would be right in the room with the patient in case the patient needed anything . . . They all had to go down when they got the patient ready for bed, take off their uniform and put on a night dress and a robe. They didn't wear their uniform at night. They didn't lay down in their uniform. You know, you just didn't do that. You took the uniform off and you dressed, but in a night dress and a robe.[99]

They worked different hours from student and staff nurses, with whom they sometimes contested the care of "their" patients. Lantz remembered, "Private duty was a 20–hour position . . . Some of those private duty nurses didn't like probation nurses answering the signal if the patient had the signal or while they were gone. Sometimes we got in trouble. They wanted the older nurses on the floor to answer the signal because they felt you didn't know what to do and many times we didn't."[100] Lantz's comments reveal a widening cultural gap between a generation of nurses affiliated with the earlier domestic care model, and a younger more medicalized and institutionalized generation that would soon move into hospital nursing. For example, she remembered one nurse who "Did a lot of maternity nursing. She would go home with patients to take care of the baby and that kind of thing." Lantz said, "Some of those dear old souls I remember with great affection. So many of them were characters . . . Well, characters in the sense of being 'in charge' and very opinionated. They had high ideals, high standards, and were critical of young students."[101] By the late 1940s, as graduate nurses took hospital staff positions and sufferers grew accustomed to hospital care, private duty nurses faded from the local scene, disappearing entirely when postwar technology made it unnecessary for nurses to watch patients.

Graduate nurses had to be enterprising to cobble together a career and earn a living during the mid-twentieth century, when private duty opportunities were declining and hospital careers were not yet available. The career of Stella Reiner Bennett, who graduated from Brokaw's training school in the mid-1930s, illustrates this situation. Bennett worked as a private and special duty nurse, both in patients' homes and in Brokaw Hospital, where she dealt with a full range of age groups and diagnoses. In addition, from the late 1930s to the late 1950s, she worked for the Union Auto Industrial Association (an insurance company), paying home visits to employees who called in sick or left work due to illness, both recommending treatment and reporting the sufferer's condition to his or her supervisor.[102] This employment gave Bennett freedom from supervision and control over her time, tasks, and earnings. However, she was paid by the hour, and both worked long hours and traveled widely for small compensation—for example, making eleven calls to a senile patient in Downs (a rural community five miles from Bloomington) for $26 in 1944, and providing three hours of relief for another nurse caring for a patient with a fractured pelvis for $3 in the same year.[103] She finished her career as a part-time nurse at Brokaw Hospital, retiring in 1977.[104]

In the early twentieth century, hospital staff positions were available only to nursing's elite—unmarried women who had been trained in high-status nursing schools. A letter sent to an applicant for the position of surgical nurse at Brokaw Hospital in 1907 indicates then-current working conditions and personnel structure:

> My dear Miss Hartley,
>   I send you under separate cover a circular of our Hospital. We can accommodate nearly fifty [patients], at present we have twenty-four. Some days we have two and three operations, then again for several days we may have none.

My surgical nurse assists me with the housekeeping. We have two floor maids, cook, waitress and laundress. We send our flat work to the steam laundry.

The Surgical Nurse has a pupil assistant who assists her for a term of two months in the operating room. At the present time we have a very capable pupil nurse assisting, and I will keep her on for two weeks in October to assist the newcomer. At present, my surgical nurse is one of our own graduates and has completed a year's services. She is quite anxious to take up private nursing, hence her resignation.

Our work is general, and our nursing corps consists of myself; my first assistant who has charge of the nursing and is a graduate of the Henrietta Hospital of East St. Louis, Miss Justis, also took post-graduate work at the Presbyterian Hospital of Chicago, and is a very agreeable capable woman. I have a graduate night head nurse who has a pupil with her on each floor. I hardly think you could be more agreeably located in any small place. . . .

The salary is $40.00 per month with expenses. . . . It might interest you to know that two graduate nurses from your school are located here.[105]

Before World War II, staff nurses lived in the hospital. When they left their positions, they went either to the relative freedom of private duty or stopped nursing to marry.

Like private duty nurses, staff nurses suffered during the Depression. When Ruth Carpenter found private duty an unreliable source of income in the early 1930s, she worked for a time on Brokaw's staff. She remembered, "Times were rough. We had about five general duty nurses then. And she [Miss Essig] brought us all in for a meeting and she said, 'Now, I'm either going to have to lay some of you off or everybody take a cut.' So we decided we had board, room and laundry. Now, you can't hardly beat that. . . . [We] took the cut. I made fifty-five dollars a month."[106] At the time, it would have been hard to foresee growth in hospital demand for graduate staff nurses. However, after the beginning of World War II, the market for all types of medical personnel mushroomed.

The federal government responded to the need for military nurses by sponsoring the Nurses' Cadet Program. In 1944 a Nurses' Cadet Corps was set up at Mennonite Hospital. Members had their expenses paid and received stipends in return for a commitment to remain active nurses for the duration of the war.[107] Evelyn Lantz, whose bachelor's degree was conferred just before the war began, became an instructor for the corps. She commented, "To be an instructor, you had to have your degree, so I was hot stuff."[108] Lantz's career illustrates both the academic direction of nurse education and trends in nursing employment in the second half of the twentieth century. She took summer classes at the University of Chicago to enhance her knowledge and confidence as a teacher.

When the war ended, she worked as a hospital staff nurse and continued nursing for a time after her husband returned from military service.

Formation of the Cadet Corps stimulated growth in the number of nursing students during the war. However, a combination of military demand for nurses, increased hospital employment of graduate nurses, the marriage bar, and the trend toward women leaving paid work when men returned from active duty contributed to a postwar nursing shortage in McLean County. In 1946 a local newspaper reported, "1) Each of the three hospitals needs to double its present nursing staff; 2) The nurse per patient ratio is approximately 1 to 7 in Bloomington-Normal, whereas the normal ratio is 1 to 3; and 3) fewer students are entering nurses training now."[109] The Nurses Recruitment Committee set the goal of attracting 125 nursing students to local training programs in the autumn of 1946. In addition, hospitals began hiring graduate nurses under more favorable conditions than those prevailing earlier in the century. Wages increased and the requirement that staff nurses be unmarried and live-in was quietly dropped. Like teaching, nursing became a realistic lifelong career opportunity for area women.

After the War

After World War II, in McLean County as elsewhere in the United States, most professional nursing has been done in institutional settings including hospitals, doctor's offices, businesses, schools, and public health organizations. Like medicine, nursing became increasingly specialized and dependent on an expanding range of technologies and equipment, which were both nurtured by and, in turn, nurtured the growth of medical institutions. As Susan Reverby points out, "Nurses are now responsible for an array of new technologies and procedures from cardiac-monitoring devices to respiratory therapies. . . . Nursing, after all, is what is intensive about intensive-care units."[110] Margarete Sandelowski goes further, viewing nursing as, alternatively, a technology used, abused, and invisible in health care, and an antidote to the technology that depersonalizes sufferers, nurses, and care.[111]

These changes occurring on a national level also affected nursing in McLean County. As Sister Theonilla commented:

INFORMANT: Nursing has changed in a lot of ways. It's more complicated.
INTERVIEWER: In what respect is it more complicated?
INFORMANT: Well, all the equipment that you have nowadays, and the medications are much more involved. . . . And the IVs—all that. It's not what it used to be. And the treatment of the patients too is different.[112]

Jane Tinsley, who went into public health nursing, commented, "We got more specialized, not only in the hospital setting, but also in public health and some of the other agencies, in school nursing and what have you. All of a sudden, they have blood pressure monitoring and . . . heart monitoring where you are reading all these machines. Well, that was just unheard of. . . . If you had heard about this when I was in training here, it would have been like 'Buck Rogers in the Twentieth Century.' Unbelievable."[113]

Nurses see both positive and negative aspects in these changes. According to Roberta Holman, "Well, I think they [nurses] know so much more, or there's so much more for them to do. I mean, it's just progress. All of the machines and all of the fantastic things they can do now for people. But I think the nurses will tell you that we don't get the good bedside nursing. . . . And patients miss the bedside—they need that."[114] Informants agreed that although more nurses have degrees and advanced skills, they spend less time giving hands-on patient care. Illustrating the ongoing tension in nursing between professionalization and conceptualization of nursing as a woman's natural vocation, Sister Theonilla observed, "I don't think it takes a master's and doctorate degree to take care of a patient. What they need is a lot of good care and tender loving care. They don't need initials. As long as you know what you are doing and are responsible for what you're doing: that's the main thing, I think."[115] Furthermore, some nurses were alienated by the proliferating technology. Alice Swift said, "Well, the intensive care nursing was never the kind of thing I liked or went in for, so actually the more technology increased, the less I liked it. . . . As time went on, I got more away from that—into wellness, into gerontology, into teaching some of the basic techniques."[116] These examples represent a common theme in nurse informants' accounts, in which bedside care is "real" nursing, which depends on a combination of sympathy and skill—not academic knowledge or inanimate equipment.

Nurses' work changed in other ways in the postwar era. As the status and salaries of nurses increased, hospitals added to their housekeeping staffs and stopped expecting nurses to scrub buildings and equipment, clean instruments, do laundry, and make beds. Increasingly, nurses' aides and practical nurses did routine patient care, and registered nurses undertook management duties. Sister Theonilla said, "I think there is too much paperwork. Paperwork, well some of it is necessary; you have to keep accurate records. Sometimes you need to look back at that if a patient is having problems. But then, it's overdone I think."[117] This statement is formulaic and, indeed, extends beyond nursing: physicians also complained about paperwork and harked back to a remembered golden age when relationships between practitioners and patients were more direct and personal, and provision of care and treatment was more satisfying. In this narrative, the hospital inserts impersonal and unwelcome processes into an otherwise unproblematical nurse-patient or doctor-patient relationship.

Although hospital careers in many ways enhanced nurses' opportunities, increasing specialization, development of professional hospital administration, and growing stratification of hospital staffs limited nurses' scope of work and authority. Sister Theonilla remembered that, fresh from her training in the 1930s, she took over the surgery department in her Pontiac, Illinois, hospital: "We had very different training. We did more. We got more responsibility than the nurses now, I think. . . . We were just given a job, and you looked after that. The surgery, we took care of everything. We saw that everything was ready and everything was in order and the patients were well taken care of. . . . [Nowadays] it's too complicated. There are too many specialties. I mean, everything is kind of specialized now."[118] As a surgical nurse, of course, Sr. Theonilla participated in the trend toward specialization that many nurses—as well as general practitioners—felt damaged the satisfaction of dealing with a whole patient from the beginning to the end of his or her care.

With enhancement of the academic component of nursing education, upgrading of nursing qualifications, and development of the women's movement, relationships between nurses and doctors also changed. Evelyn Lantz remembered fondly the physicians who taught students at Brokaw's training school in the 1930s: "Many of those men felt they had a father-daughter relationship, and they felt that they sort of needed to take care of us. . . . It was a very, I don't want to use the word 'patronizing', but it was a family kind of thing."[119] However, there were less positive aspects of this relationship, where power was never equal. Nine years younger than Lantz and with a longer nursing career, Alice Swift said the following of the relationships between doctors and nurses in the 1950s and later:

INFORMANT: It was not as comfortable to be in nursing in large hospitals unless nurses knew how to assert themselves well. . . . Doctors were very abusive. They continued to be for a long time, as far as I was concerned. They liked to blame things on nurses. . . .

INTERVIEWER: How have nurse/physician relationships changed over the years?

INFORMANT: It depends on where you're located as far as I can see. And on your position. When you go over to [hospital in neighboring community], the interaction there is much more collegial than it was here in this community. . . . Here, nurses were not treated as well as they were over there.

Primary nursing put the nurse in a very different posture. It took an awful lot of strength in a nurse to know how to deal with some of the treatment doctors handed out.[120]

Jane Tinsley said about her early nursing experience in the 1940s and '50s, "Fewer doctors thanked you and made you feel like you were appreciated. Lots of times you felt like you were the invisible person there doing the job. He wanted it, and it was expected, and it should be ready. You anticipated. Some of them did appreciate what the nurse did. Many of them gave the feeling that the service was their due—they had studied and put in all the time and 'I'm saving this individual's life.'"[121] Roberta Holman, who began nursing in the 1940s, reflected on the change in the relationship between nurses and doctors during her career, "It was different then because, you know, they [nurses] were kind of the underdog as far as doctors were concerned. I mean, when a doctor walked in a room you jumped up because if you didn't you would be reprimanded. We looked up to the doctors like they were gods. Not anymore. Nurses got smart. You know they [doctors] are human beings just like everybody else."[122] Sally Wagner, nearly a generation younger, made a similar comment. Speaking of her early career she said,

> Even if you were busy doing something like charting. . . . you always stood up, and you never entered the room before them. You always let the doctors go into the room before you did. . . . I think now . . . most doctors stand back and let the nurses go into the room before they enter, so I think . . . it's a little more of an equal respect now than just one way. . . . I think it's different today. I think the doctors treat the nurses much better. I think they are on a social level too. They include us in some of their social activities. We know their families, they know our families. . . . [123]

The expectation that nurses stand when a physician entered the room, along with the decline in this ritual, recounted by almost all the nurse informants, contributed to a common narrative representing larger changes in professional status and the nurse-doctor relationships. The woman's movement and the professionalization of nursing brought changes in public demeanor projecting the argument that nursing was different from medicine, but equally necessary to care and healing.

Another alteration in nursing after about 1960 was the increasing diversity of nursing student bodies and the nursing workforce. Before this time, McLean County nursing schools were attended exclusively by young white women, most of whom came from rural or small town backgrounds. Neither nonwhites nor men were accepted. When Betty Ebo, an African American Bloomington resident, applied to St. Joseph's Nursing School in 1944, despite the national shortage of nurses she was refused admission because, "We've never taken a colored student."[124] She trained at the all-black nursing school run by St. Mary's Infirmary in St. Louis, later becoming a Dominican nun. St. Joseph's began accepting black students in the 1950s; Mennonite awarded its diploma to the first African American in 1978. The first male nursing student, Kenneth Unzicker, graduated from the Mennonite Hospital School of Nursing in 1963. Nonetheless, nursing remained a dominantly white female occupation in McLean County throughout the twentieth century.

Nurses and the Community

Considering the pervasive presence of nurses in McLean County, it is noteworthy that laypeople remembering their own health histories rarely mention nurses. Yet, the evidence reveals nurses' almost constant involvement in care situations. Evelyn Lantz remembered, "No doctor visited [hospital] patients without a nurse accompanying him. No doctor went into a patient's room without a nurse there."[125] Nurses were recognized as health-care authorities by their neighbors, bridging home and institutional care. Jane Tinsley remembered her friends and neighbors asking her for advice: "And penicillin, the great cure-all. That was in the age where, if you were a nurse, you kept some in your refrigerator—in fact, the doctor told you to. I used to give shots to two or three families in the neighborhood that had the same doctor I did. . . . Most of the nurses did that."[126] Similarly, Roberta Holman remembered administering penicillin shots, taking blood pressures, and advising friends and relatives outside of formal health-care situations, commenting, "Back then we had real personal contact. We got to know our people, you know . . . We got to know the families . . . it was different then."[127]

Occasionally, informants referred explicitly to the authority and competence of nurses. Caribel Washington, born in 1914, remembered one occasion when a local nurse was more capable than the doctor. Washington's son had scarlet fever, which the doctor did not recognize (perhaps because the child was black), but "Nurse Miller, who used to be the school nurse for so many years" diagnosed.[128] Evelyn Lantz described the nurse's continuing role in communicating with and caring for patients: "Nurses have a way of providing care that I think doctors are missing. There's so many things that [nurses] can do that really don't require a doctor . . . I always remember one of our pediatricians had a sister who was his office person and she was very good. She was just very good and very helpful to young mothers."[129] However, lay informants were more likely to mention the nurse as the rigid face of hospital authority or not not mention her at all.[130] Indeed, when asked about the role of nurses in home care during the 1920s, Richard Finfgeld, born in 1906, said he did not remember any nurses: "They weren't recognized as a profession."[131]

One explanation for this phenomenon is provided by Margarete Sand-elowski, who discusses the representation of the nurse as "physical or bodily extensions of physicians . . . as the physician's eyes, hand, and 'operational right arm'"; as "part of the homey room décor in print advertisements for hospitals"; or as "thermometers, barometers, monitors, information proces-sors, and human-machine interfaces."[132] This objectification dehumanizes the nurse and renders her invisible. In addition, however, it is also possible to see the trained nurse as an updated version of the mother, grandmother, or neighborhood authority who traditionally provided informal health advice and care outside of the physician's narrower sphere of operations. Like those other women, the nurse worked sometimes in opposition to, sometimes in support of, and sometimes as translator and mediator for "official" medicine. And, like the child told to "Wait 'til your father gets home" for punishment or reward, community residents perceive and remember the doctor's authority— not the nurse's activities. It is, therefore, ironic that the institutionalization and medicalization of health care characterizing the transformation of McLean County's health culture would not have been possible without nurses.

4. Doctors and Organized Medicine

The word *physician* has sometimes been used indiscriminately by both medical practitioners and historians, imputing to Western doctors of the past the same skills, knowledge, social relations, and status of their present-day counterparts. Although a flood of scholarship indicates that this conflation is inaccurate and misleading, the fact that the same words have been used to designate official healers for centuries, and thus appear in countless historical sources, perpetuates confusion. Furthermore, as John Burnham argues, occupational medicine has built its identity, legitimacy, and status on an idealized history of medicine, in which doctors of the past look remarkably like their descendants.[1]

In reality, the roles, reputations, and expectations of physicians have varied greatly from place to place and time to time—even within the same national (U.S.) and practice (allopathic medicine) contexts. Thus, for example, the Philadelphia and Chicago doctors who embraced scientific medicine and constructed professional elites in the late nineteenth centuries arguably had different concerns and led different work lives than the mid-nineteenth-century rural southern physicians whose identities and roles were crafted at the social bedsides of their patients.[2] Furthermore, some doctors not included in the conventional reference to "medical men"—women and nonwhites—had other preoccupations and experiences than their white male colleagues.[3] This chapter concerns the past century of official medical practice in McLean County, offering a specific local lens through which to observe related transformations in professional medicine and community health culture.

During those years, medicine in McLean County underwent the metamorphosis described by Paul Starr and George Rosen, from a highly individualized and not particularly well-paid occupation, competing with both traditional self-care and a horde of alternative practices and practitioners, to a corporate entity able to demand a monopoly over certain services and decisions, command a captive market, and control a significant portion of the economy.[4] Work lives of physicians in the county also changed environment and character, shifting from home-based general practice to institutionalized specialization, and from direct compensation by patients to dependence on third-party payers. At the same time, for laypeople, consultation of doctors shifted from one possible alternative during times of ill-health to an absolute necessity rivaling food, lodging, and heat. The power of professional medicine was expressed not only in political and economic terms, but in cultural and psychological influences on both everyday and life-changing decisions. Consumers' investment in and expectations of medicine generated increasing malpractice litigation, which, in turn, affected traditional relationships between individuals and "their" doctors. Thus, a new element of community health culture is nostalgia for an arguably mythical golden age of fee-for-service medicine, when patient-practitioner relationships were long, direct, and quasi-familial; doctors were altruistic, and their services inexpensive; and third-party payers were nonexistent. This chapter documents and explores these changes from the doctor's perspective. It will open with a snapshot of organized medicine in McLean County at the turn of the twentieth century, then use oral history accounts to flesh out physicians' experience of medical practice beginning in the interwar period.

The McLean County Medical Society

In 1880 the McLean County Medical Society (founded in 1854) had approximately sixty-one members, half of whom practiced in Bloomington while the other half lived and served in twenty smaller county communities.[5] The society's president, William Hill (1829–1906), had read medicine with an Indianapolis doctor, attended lectures in LaPorte, Indiana, and Ann Arbor, Michigan, received his M.D. from Jefferson Medical College in Philadelphia, and served as surgeon to the 48th Illinois Regiment Infantry during the Civil War. Thus, his qualifications were similar to those of a majority of American physicians of the mid-nineteenth century.[6] In 1880 Hill was at the height of his career, with a downtown Bloomington office and a large home two blocks away—"one of the majestic houses of the city." He was politically connected, a Democrat who served a term in the Illinois Legislature.[7] He was also an appropriate local leader for the allopaths' main occupational organization.

The times were good for professional medicine. In 1877 Illinois began to license physicians, at the same time cracking down on medical diploma mills and the many practitioners with inadequate or fraudulent credentials.[8] As a forum and advocacy group for allopaths, the McLean County Medical Society became part of the Progressive Era effort to both raise standards of practice and link county and state organizations with the American Medical Association (AMA) to form what, after 1901, became known as "organized medicine."[9] Records kept by the society for the years between 1891 and 1910 provide a detailed account of its activities during that period.[10]

Society members cultivated links with other county medical organizations and with the Illinois State Medical Society (founded in 1850). Although the McLean County Medical Society's constitution contains no mission statement, it is apparent that its primary purposes were to regulate the local practice of medicine by excluding irregular practitioners; inform members about scientific innovations, therapeutic controversies, and local cases of interest; support local sanitary improvements (as long as these were controlled by allopaths); and foster a network for professional consultations, social activities, and support of members and their families in times of hardship.

The society was open to allopaths conforming to a rarely articulated, but well-understood, code of professional behavior that reflected both late nineteenth-century efforts to upgrade medical practice, on the one hand, and tension between competition and solidarity, on the other.[11] Doctors were not to advertise their services, either in newspapers or by other means.[12] They must not refer to or consult with irregular practitioners. They must not sell or endorse proprietary medicines. They must not steal each other's patients. The society regularly updated a standard list of fees for the services most commonly offered, which individual practitioners ignored at their peril. Violations of these rules resulted in exclusion from the society.

How did a practitioner become a member? It apparently went without saying that applicants with degrees from reputable medical schools would be admitted once their credentials had been checked. However, recognizing that many practitioners did not have formal qualifications, the society's constitution required elected censors "to examine such applicants for membership as are not graduates in medicine and report to the Society upon their qualifications for membership." An applicant had to convince "the Censors that he has faithfully persevered in the study of medicine at least three years, and that he intends honestly and honorably to pursue the calling of his profession."[13]

Because members were determined to exclude alternative practitioners and quacks—to allopaths, one and the same—discussion of whether to admit an applicant sometimes became heated. For instance, in September 1891, Homer Wakefield was proposed for membership by James Branch Taylor, an informal

specialist in eye, ear, nose, and throat whose qualifications included graduation from the College of Physicians and Surgeons in New York City and attendance at medical lectures in Leipzig, Germany.[14] Wakefield had advertised his
services in the local newspaper. He also probably suffered from relationship
to his father, "Doctor" Cyrenius Wakefield, whose profitable Bloomington
patent medicine business had earned him both the contempt and the envy
of the regular medical establishment. The society's censors checked Homer
Wakefield's credentials, with the following results: At the November Medical
Society meeting, " . . . Dr. Little read a letter from Dr. Austin Flint, secretary of Bellevue Hospital Medical College, of which school H. Wakefield is
a graduate. He stated that Dr. Wakefield's name would be dropped from the
Alumni Catalogue and that he had no suspicion Dr. Wakefield would become
a quack."[15] The society denied admission to Homer Wakefield.

Dr. Taylor was enraged. In May 1892 he refused to serve on a committee
with S. T. Anderson, who had opposed Wakefield's membership, saying, "Dr.
Wakefield, a student of his [Taylor's], was refused admittance into this the
McLean County Medical Society on account of his newspaper advertisement
and claiming that Dr. Anderson was equally as guilty in advertising his Keely
Cure for drunkenness." At this point, William Hill raised the ethical ante
by accusing Taylor of advertising and consulting with a homeopath—thus
both threatening Taylor's position in the society and illustrating the extent to
which its members lived in glass houses. Apparently, the matter was amicably
resolved, because Taylor remained a member of the society. However, it is
unclear whether Wakefield was ever accepted for membership, because his
name does not appear among regular members in the society's *Biographical
History*, where it is noted only that in 1934 he was living in New York.[16]

Society members worked with external bodies to limit competition from
alternative practitioners. In 1898, for example, A. L. Fox solicited his colleagues' cooperation with the State Board of Health "concerning the intended
prosecution of irregular practicing doctors in the City [of Bloomington]."[17]
In 1902 the Society formed a Committee on Law to consider "the matter of
flagrant abuses of their privileges among itinerant and irresponsible practitioners" considered to be "violators of law and decency."[18]

In some cases, the society justified its actions by concern about the mis-
information and harm that might be inflicted by irregulars on members of
an unwary public. Thus, in 1908, the society called a special meeting "to take
some action concerning certain erroneous remarks which have been made
by one Flynn and his associate, Miss McIntire, who have been holding meetings in the churches of the city." Flynn was billed as a lecturer on hygiene

and a teacher of gymnastics. The society decided to "draw up resolutions denouncing Flynn and present same to the Ministerial Association."[19]

In other instances, the society was clearly protecting members' financial interests. For example, in April 1898 the Society

> resolved that it is the sense of the members of the McLean County Medical Society in annual meeting assembled that it is clearly a violation of the code of Medical Ethics of the American Medical Association by which we profess to be guided and governed for any member of this Society to associate himself with an irregular advertising quack doctor for the purpose of carrying on and managing a Free Clinic such as the one which is located at No. 106 W. Monroe Street.[20]

Like their colleagues elsewhere, society members perceived charitable clinics and dispensaries as unfair competition that threatened their clienteles and livelihoods.[21]

The society actually had more reason to worry about competition from qualified sectarians such as homeopaths, of whom there were nine practicing in Bloomington in 1908.[22] As indicated in Chapter 2, two homeopaths, Doctors George and Annie Kelso, not only competed as practitioners specializing respectively in surgery and obstetrics, but also mounted institutional competition to early allopathic hospitals by opening the proprietary Kelso Sanitarium in 1894. It is uncertain whether the Kelsos ever became full members of the medical society, although they rated entries in the 1934 edition of the Society's *Biographical History*—but not, it should be said, in the 1904 edition.[23]

The society was also active in allopaths' state-wide efforts to block regulation of the new practice of osteopathy.[24] At the June 1897 meeting, members discussed the governor's veto of a recent bill on the grounds that it would open the door in Illinois "to incompetent, dishonest, and unscrupulous adventurers calling themselves practitioners of osteopathy and there would be no remedy." The society was still opposing passage of a similar law in 1909.[25] Nonetheless, an osteopath, Dr. Boyle, began practicing in Bloomington in 1898, where he was joined by a number of colleagues in the early twentieth century.[26]

Chiropractors also appeared in the county soon after the establishment of their craft at the turn of the century. In addition, a Christian Science practitioner, Mrs. Della Rigby, arrived in Bloomington in about 1887 and, by 1908, had been joined by six full-time and as many as twelve part-time colleagues. Furthermore, according to local historian Jacob Hasbrouck, "The City has also had its proportion of eclectic physicians. It has been a favorite resort for visiting specialists, and if McLean County has not been healthy, it has not been from lack in the multitude of its medical counselors."[27]

In an era when allopathic medicine had by no means won a monopoly over medical practice and public trust, the McLean County Medical Society focused on supporting its members' competitive advantage, starting with defense of their ethical image. For example, the society lined up to protect medicine's professional reputation in light of mounting public concern about abortion.[28] The object of its February 1909 meeting was

> that the citizens of LeRoy claimed that Dr. L. A. Burr of Bloomington, now under indictment for performing criminal abortion, was about to leave Bloomington, and urged members of this society to take some action regarding it. Discussed freely and motion was made and prevailed that the Judiciary Committee of this Society with the President and Secretary see the authorities and ask them to increase the amount of Dr. Burr's bond if possible and to urge that he be given a prompt and impartial trial.

The society took this action even though it is not clear that Burr was a member in good standing at the time, since Burr's reputation threatened its own. Clearly, LeRoy residents viewed the medical society as responsible for the actions of physicians and influential with local government. The outcome of Burr's case is not known.[29]

Although the society reserved membership exclusively for allopaths and was overwhelmingly male and white, it admitted a few women. For example, Rhoda Galloway Yolton, who practiced in Bloomington between 1888 and 1932, specializing in gynecology, served as both secretary (1890 and 1891) and president (1894 and 1895) of the society. Eliza Hyndman, who located in Bloomington in 1897, served as secretary in 1899.[30] Nonetheless, between 1854 and 1954, only sixteen women physicians became members—4 percent of the organization's 384 total members during that period.

Even fewer African American doctors joined. E. G. Covington (1872–1929), the son of former slaves who graduated from Howard University's Medical College in 1899, was admitted to the McLean County Medical Society in 1901, and practiced in Bloomington until his death. He mainly treated black patients and, in February 1908, complained to the society that some white doctors were unfairly competing with him by charging "colored families who are able to pay the regulation fee of $2 per call . . . but $1.50 per visit. This, he says, works a hardship on him as he is dependent mainly on the colored people for his living." The society found in Dr. Covington's favor, considering "it an infraction of professional honor to regularly make calls for less than $2."[31] Nonetheless, Covington became disaffected from the organization, being suspended from membership in 1910 when he had failed to pay his dues for two years.[32] Only one other African American doctor, W. B. Hatcher, briefly worked in McLean County before 1954, his Depression-era practice suffering because "many patients had no money."[33] In addition, according to Lucinda Brent Posey, an African American born in 1914, although Dr. Covington had full privileges at all of the Bloomington hospitals, Dr. Hatcher, who had graduated from Meharry Medical College in 1923, "Practiced at hospitals, but without full privileges, meaning that a full-privilege physician had to okay his orders."[34]

Participation in the McLean County Medical Society could be extremely useful to members. They had access to professional development activities and developed relationships supporting consultations and referrals. Society membership opened the door to hospital privileges. For newcomers, membership validated qualifications and facilitated development of clienteles. Finally, the society performed for physicians many of the functions labor unions offered to manual and craft workers, protecting members in malpractice suits, defending their incomes, discouraging competition from nonmembers, offering social activities that included members' families, and providing financial assistance and personal support in times of illness and death.

Lectures delivered at monthly meetings allowed new members to demonstrate their abilities; gave established members a forum for their ideas; and offered updates on changes in medical science, public health, and organized medicine. Lectures exposed local practitioners to developments elsewhere. For instance, on May 6, 1897, John L. White "gave a very interesting talk on sanitary conditions in California cities Oakland and Alameda."[35] In February 1899, T. W. Bath, acting assistant surgeon with the U.S. Army, offered, "Some Observations on the Medical Conditions of Camp Life" in Cuba.[36] In May 1907, reflecting a longstanding educational pattern among elite physicians, R. A. Noble discussed the question, "Is a Trip to Europe Worth Its Cost to A Medical Man," speaking favorably on the emphasis placed on scientific research in Germany.[37]

Lectures encouraged members to talk about contemporary medical and surgical controversies. For example, in July 1897, after a presentation on "Conservatism in Surgery," there was heated discussion of appendectomy—a procedure introduced in the 1880s.[38] The speaker, Dr. White, contended that appendicitis was the fashionable disease of the day, and that many needless operations were performed. Rhoda Galloway Yolton broadened the discussion by urging conservatism in the treatment of fibroid uterine tumors. Lee Smith "facetiously remarked that it was rather an unusual thing that two surgeons should at one time get together to give surgery a general scouring." Ernest Mammen contended that conservatism was sometimes fatal to the patient, and that the surgeon's duty was "to properly educate the public when surgery was necessary." Dr. Taylor argued that the future would demand higher quality work, and Jehu Little said, "Too much eagerness to operate brings odium on the profession."[39]

Lectures introduced scientific and technological innovations in medicine. For instance, Eliza Hyndman's January 1898 paper advocated a closer union of laboratory and clinical methods.[40] Along the same lines, in February 1907, Ezra R. Larned of the Experimental Department of Parke, Davis & Company offered a presentation, illustrated with stereopticon slides, on "The Practical Application of Bacteriology to the Cure of Disease."[41] In June 1903 a lecture on the "Use of the X-Ray for Diagnostic Purposes" first decried the widespread, inappropriate, and lucrative use of X-rays by quacks, then concluded that "This form of electricity . . . is of inestimable use in diagnosing fractures, dislocations and in locating foreign bodies."[42]

Medical society records indicate physicians' leadership in public health matters. For example, an 1897 society discussion of Bloomington's sanitary condition linked filth and disease, members advising the city government "that all garbage, offal, and rubbish should be taken beyond the City limits and burned" and that "a garbage and offal crematory should be purchased and put in operation as soon as possible."[43] Because the society was still campaigning for the crematory in April 1906, it is apparent that the city was less enthusiastic than its doctors about this project.[44] Marking local transition to germ theory, in May 1908 the society called attention to the role of the common housefly in spreading disease.[45] Franklin Vandervort said,

> The season of the fly is approaching. Two things are necessary for the propagation and sustenance of the fly . . . hot weather and filth. The first we cannot prevent and the latter we should fight against with all our might. As much garbage as possible should be burned by the housekeepers. Then the refuse should be carted away as soon as possible. The chief weapon that suggests itself against the fly evil is absolute cleanliness in the streets and houses and wherever there can be breeding places for the fly and the general use of screens. A careful housewife will never let a fly remain in the house. The experiences with typhoid fever in the camps of our soldiers during the Spanish American War demonstrated in a most forcible manner that the fly must be taken into consideration in fighting typhoid fever.[46]

Physicians campaigned for pure public water supplies, particularly when epidemics threatened. In January 1903 the society traced a 1902 outbreak of typhoid fever in Bloomington to the use of well water and advocated the use of city rather than private water supplies.[47] Doctors also offered advice about management of infectious diseases. For example, in early 1907 the medical society formed a committee to confer with the school board regarding the length of time a child who had suffered an infectious disease should be kept at home. "It was the opinion of the Committee that two weeks should be the minimum length of time at which the patient or other members of the family should be allowed to return to school after the discharge of said patient by his physician."[48] The society also supported the campaign to control tuberculosis.[49]

Society members were eager to be involved in disease prevention and control, but opposed nonphysicians undertaking public health responsibilities involving direct contact with sufferers, because authority in medical matters and personal relationships with patients comprised the basis of doctors' professional status and incomes.[50] In May 1891 Dr. Hill read the following resolutions at the society's monthly meeting:

> Whereas: the city Council of Bloomington making it obligatory for practicing physicians to report all cases of diphtheria to the health officer, therefore be it resolved that this Society deprecates the practice of this City in sending its emissaries to the sick chamber to examine the case and decide as to its nature, prescribe and proscribe as suits him best in the absence of the attending physician. Also resolved that while we are willing to aid in all proper means to prevent the spread of contagious diseases, we as practicing physicians of this City and County protest against such undue interference with our private patients and practice.[51]

In April 1897 the society formed a committee to advocate the appointment of a "medical man" as chief of the Bloomington Health Department.[52] After such an appointment was made in the following year, the society and the health department worked more amicably together.

The society undertook the responsibility of supporting physicians in malpractice cases. In the early twentieth century, the State Medical Society established a fund to help members pay legal fees, and in October 1907 the McLean County Medical Society discussed this fund and malpractice accusations in general. According to the speaker, suits could be categorized as follows: "Fifty percent are pure blackmail; 25 percent sue for malpractice to beat a just bill; 15 percent believe they have been aggrieved or injured; 10 percent are very close to malpractice. Blackmailers are generally charity patients." The speaker said that physicians "are loose in their methods of keeping books, frequently omitting dates and failing to make charges or record in their books of work done." He advised members to "keep a record of all cases."[53] We will see that this early discussion foreshadowed later developments, but malpractice litigation was actually almost unheard-of in McLean County before the 1970s.

From its earliest days the society regulated medical charges. Its fee bills, updated and renegotiated every few years, helped to control competition and patient stealing among physicians. Although according to its presidential address in May 1903, the society's standard fee bill was not to be considered in the same light as an official wage scale, but merely as a guide for medical charges, it was accepted as the basis for routine fees and doctors complained to the society if their colleagues undercharged.

In addition, the society consistently opposed members accepting the paid position of physician to any organization or agreeing "to do any medical or surgical work for any club, society, or organization at a less rate than the regular customary charges for like services rendered by other physicians for patients not members of such a club, society, or organization."[54] In October 1907 Dr. F. H. Godfrey in his presidential address discussed the "degrading effect of contract practice, citing . . . certain fraternal societies in which whole families receive medical treatment for 12 cents per week."[55] This resistance to contract practice was consistent with the AMA's sturdy emphasis on in-dividual fee-for-service practice. However, in fact the society turned a blind eye to members who worked as company doctors for large local employers such as the Chicago and Alton Shops.[56]

The early twentieth century was a watershed for professional and organized medicine in the United States. The most obvious initial changes came in medi-cal education.[57] Under pressure from the AMA, state licensing authorities, and university-based educational reformers, between 1906 and 1910 almost one-fifth of the nation's weaker medical schools closed and apprentice-style preparation for practice disappeared.[58] This transition affected the socio-economic, gender, and ethnic composition of professional medicine, which in the late nineteenth-century had included rising numbers of immigrants, African Americans, and women. However, by 1910 only three medical colleges for women and two for African Americans remained open.[59] After that date, medical schools became increasingly exclusive, limiting admission of blacks, women, Jews, and other "socially undesirable" groups; thus, the composition and outlook of the profession grew more uniform. Medical graduates, who had navigated increasingly lengthy and rigorous curricula, were imbued with a homogenous *esprit de corps* and worldview. From the beginning of their careers, they assumed a high degree of authority with patients as well as social status and financial rewards that rose dramatically after World War II.

In McLean County, where the profession had always been dominantly white and male, the impact of national changes in medical education came very slowly. Credentials of McLean County Medical Society presidents between 1910 and 1940 reveal that they were middle-aged men who had been educated long before reform began. For example, Ernest Mammen, president in 1909 and 1910, was born in Germany in 1855 and graduated from Rush Medical College in 1884, when there were no standard admission requirements and Rush's three-year curriculum depended almost entirely on lectures. There was no laboratory-based instruction until the 1890s, and the school suffered from chronic difficulties in obtaining cadavers for dissection. A contemporary of Mammen's "recalled that in his class of 1888 only seven of 135 men entering the school boasted a college diploma of any description."[60] Following the nineteenth-century pattern, Mammen augmented his medical school training by spending a year studying with surgical specialists in Berlin.

William M. Young, president of the society in 1920, also belonged to an older medical generation. Born in 1867, he received his diploma in 1897 from the Eclectic Medical Institute (Chicago), which closed shortly thereafter, and later studied at the New York Post Graduate School. He practiced as a general practitioner and anesthetist in Bloomington until his death in 1939.[61]

Joseph Price Noble, president in 1930, was born in 1868 and graduated from Northwestern University Medical School in 1893. At that time, the school had "only three full-time men on its staff: the registrar, janitor, and professor of chemistry."[62] Only after 1911 did Northwestern require applicants to have two years of college preparation before beginning medical training.[63] Noble practiced general medicine in McLean, Illinois.

Daniel Raber (born in 1878), president of the society in 1940, received his medical diploma from Bennett Medical College of Eclectic Medicine and Surgery in 1908, two years before the school merged with several others to form the medical department of Loyola University.[64] His medical education straddled changes in national standards; in 1909 Raber did an internship at Rapid City Hospital, Rapid City, South Dakota. He practiced in Bloomington as a general practitioner, was on the staffs of all of the county's hospitals, and taught at the nursing schools at Brokaw and St. Joseph's hospitals.[65]

Change in preparation for practice among McLean County's medical leaders began to show in the interwar period. For example, Frank Deneen, president of the medical society in 1927, represented a newer generation of physicians. Born in 1890, he received his undergraduate education at Illinois Wesleyan University and the University of Chicago. He received his M.D. from Northwestern University Medical School in 1915, then took internships at St. Louis City Hospital and the Children's Free Hospital in Detroit. Deneen specialized in internal medicine; his training was typical for McLean County physicians educated after 1910.

In addition to educational preparation, another significant change in medicine during the early twentieth century was in work environment. Although here there was also overlap with earlier work patterns, with general practitioners continuing to provide personal services to individual sufferers in their homes, physicians saw growing numbers of patients in their offices. In Bloomington, many doctors rented space in the downtown Greishiem Building, attracting patients to a central location and developing professional relationships that nurtured budding specialization.[66] "Going to the doctor's office" began to replace "calling the doctor" in community residents' vocabularies, and physicians increased expenditure on medical equipment, while also increasing their incomes with higher volume business.

In a related development, hospital affiliation, which had been unimportant for most McLean County doctors in 1910, became increasingly central to medical careers and finances after about 1920. Surgeons including Ernest Mammen, E. P. Sloane, William Guthrie, and Joseph P. Hawks were both stars and beneficiaries of local hospitals. They led the way for other practitioners to depend on hospitals for facilities, nursing care, and professional consultation networks that generated business and fees.

In Living Memory

What has it been like to practice medicine in McLean County during the twentieth century? Although there are useful accounts written by local doctors, this study benefits greatly from oral history interviews conducted with six physicians and one dentist who was also a physician's son.[67] All but one practiced in McLean County; four were located in Bloomington. One physician, James Welch, practiced in Cuba, Illinois, a small community in Fulton County about sixty miles west of McLean County. Welch's experience, together with that of Loren Boon of Danvers, Russell Oyer of Chenoa, and Harold Shinall, who practiced in Gibson City during the mid-1930s, provides information about rural practice. (See Table 6.)

To some extent, these informants represent continuity in professional health care. All of them were trained after the reform of medical education. Thus, they had premedical undergraduate university educations before embarking on four-year professional training programs. They all took internships; medical specialists completed residencies. These practitioners began their careers after the establishment of biomedicine as the single theory dominating medical practice and after professional medicine had achieved a legally protected monopoly over the provision of medical care. Therefore, they expected and assumed the physician's enormous mid-twentieth-century position of authority and were more likely to remark on the relatively recent perceived decline in that authority than to marvel at how popular perception of the physician's expertise had grown during their years in practice.

Table 6: Oral History Informants: Medical Practitioners

Informant	Birthdate	Occupation	Professional Training	Practice Location
Harold Shinall	1909	General Practitioner and Radiologist	University of Illinois, 1935; Residency, St. Louis, 1941–43	Gibson City and Bloomington
James Welch	1915	General Practitioner	St Louis University, 1941	Cuba, Illinois
Loren Boon	1917	General Practitioner	University of Illinois, 1942	Danvers
W. L. Dillman	1920	Dentist	University of Illinois and Loyola University (Chicago), 1946	Bloomington
Russell Oyer	1920	General Practitioner	University of Illinois, 1948	Chenoa
Paul Theobald	1922	General Practitioner	University of Illinois, 1951	Bloomington
Albert VanNess	1926	Internist	Indiana University, 1950; Residency, University of Chicago, 1957	Bloomington

Nonetheless, the practitioners interviewed also witnessed tremendous changes in medical practice. Their lives spanned the transition from a profession dominated by general practitioners to one led by specialists. They witnessed the shift from home-based to office- and hospital-based health care. They also experienced a transformation of medical economics from the comparatively small direct payment (or barter) for services to the huge inflation of medical costs that brought health insurance with it.

These informants also participated in dramatic changes in the efficacy of medical interventions. Those trained before the 1940s experienced the impact on medical and surgical practice of the introduction of antibiotics. All of the informants became accustomed to using an increasing range of technology, which enhanced diagnostic, monitoring, and therapeutic processes. They also experienced the inflation of patients' expectations that both increased the status and earnings of physicians and stimulated the growth in malpractice litigation after the 1960s.

Career Choice

By the second quarter of the twentieth century when most of the practitioners interviewed were making career decisions, medicine was a well established profession—like law or the ministry, a respectable occupation. However, it was not an easy or lucrative option. W. L. Dillman, born in 1920, who had planned to go into medicine, opted for dentistry because of his father's experience of medical practice in Louisville, Kentucky. Dillman remembered,

> He [my father] worked so hard. Have you ever seen any of these wall telephones with a crank on the side and you take the receiver off the other side? I can hear that thing ringing in the night. . . . They didn't have "no night calls" or "no house calls" in those days. He had house calls, night calls; I've gone with him down the railroad tracks at night in the wintertime after a train would go through to clear a path in the snow. I'd walk and carry his medical bag and we'd walk down the tracks somewhere, and maybe someone would meet us with a wagon. I'd go to sleep in the kitchen, and maybe he'd deliver a child or something.[68]

Dillman decided to become a dentist just as he was finishing his premedical education, when his father suddenly died.

Dillman's experience was apparently typical for doctors' sons. However, in contrast to his decision, many men followed their fathers into medicine. Indeed, the *Biographical History of the McLean County Medical Society for 1854–1954* listed seventeen father-son pairs among its members; this list does not include members whose fathers practiced medicine somewhere other than McLean County.[69] Three of the seven practitioners interviewed for this study were doctor's sons.

Like Dillman, James Welch, the son and grandson of physicians who, like himself, had practiced in Cuba, Illinois, remembered traveling with his father on house calls, saying, "I guess that's the way I got interested."[70] Like other informants, Welch was impressed by the special status of doctors in small towns. Of the 1919 flu epidemic, he said,

> Every doctor in [Fulton] County was sick except two, and Dad was one of them. He'd see his patients and then at night he would drive to [the larger neighboring community of] Canton and just go around and knock on the doors, "Do you need a doctor?" one door to the next. Well, in those days the car didn't have antifreeze, and if you stopped you had to leave the motor running or drain her out and refill her again. Well, . . . he went down checking in the square and parked his car. He wanted some medicine and he wanted to get a cigar, so he left the motor running. But Canton had just passed an ordinance. It was a high crime misdemeanor to leave the motor running. Some of these cars would take off! So he came out, and here were a couple of cops. He left his motor running and they caught him. They were taking him down the street, fussing him all the way: "you're going to the pokey!" So, as they were going along, this one cop said, "Who are you anyway?" "Well," he says, "I'm Dr. Welch from Cuba." And they stopped and they said, "You the one that's been going around town?" They were really frightened! They said, "Do you know that they would lynch us,

the townspeople would, if they knew we arrested you?" So they got him back, got his car going, and sent him home. Dad always laughed at how frightened those policemen were.[71]

This story, obviously told—or performed—many times, revealed the speaker's nostalgia regarding the position of community doctors of the past.

Loren Boon, also a physician's son, grew up expecting to go into medicine. He remembered, "I kind of liked science and things like that. And . . . I kind of thought that [medicine] would be the place to go. . . . I remember one incident . . . in high school . . . they were having a ball game and a man got hit in the head . . . and had some bleeding or something. Somebody asked me if that didn't bother me, and I said, 'Nope.' 'You must gonna be a doctor then.' No, I didn't faint or anything."[72]

Albert Van Ness did not come from a medical family; his father worked for State Farm Insurance Company and his mother worked as a receptionist in a doctor's office. However, "My mother was involved with medicine and . . . I knew doctors. . . . I met them through going up to the Griesheim Building to see my mother." He remembered admiring doctors: "I was brought up that my folks taught me . . . and I don't recollect them talking about money. It was . . . that doctors are honored, revered people who are well educated. I can still remember Howard Sloan [a surgeon] telling me one Christmas when I was home from the navy, 'The interesting thing is that . . . the vocabulary of a physician is five times that of the average person.'"[73]

Harold Shinall, whose father was an insurance agent, also said that he knew "several doctors, and just sort of approved of them. . . . I was impressed that even though they didn't have antibiotics they seemed to be able to make you well again." He had had diphtheria as a child and was cured with "shots of antitoxin." Further examining his career choice, Shinall said, "I would like to be able to reduce it to helping people, but I don't know that that was primarily the thing in those days. I think it was part of it. I liked to see the favorable outcomes I had observed."[74]

Like the nurses interviewed for this study, some informants chose medicine because of its dramatic image. Russel Oyer grew up on a farm. He remembered visiting his sister, who was eight years older than himself, during her training at Mennonite School of Nursing, "She would take me to the hospital and the floors would be polished and you would . . . have those smells of ether and that sort of stuff. . . . The nurses walking up and down in their stiffly starched uniforms . . . taking care of people. I think maybe that was the early kind of fantasy . . . about medicine that sort of grew and impressed me, I guess. It continued. When I started at Bluffton [College], I decided to take a few medicine courses."[75]

Finally, in some cases medicine was simply a "natural" career option for a bright young man. Paul Theobald did not remember making a definite decision to go to medical school:

> I never planned on being a doctor until the day I graduated and thought, "That's it." I used to have a lot of infections as a kid, and everyone kept saying, "Oh, you ought to be a doctor and save some money." It never sunk into me, and basically I didn't make a decision, but it just seemed that I kept going. Premedicine, [I] still wasn't sure I wanted to go to medical school, but when I finished, it was like, "Well, I got to go to medical school. . . ." It was just one of those things: I went along until finally I graduated and I thought, "Well, I'm a doctor."[76]

Financial considerations were not significant in informants' decisions to go into medicine. Of course, several were making these decisions during the Depression. As A. Edward Livingston, who practiced in Bloomington from 1945 to 1985, commented in his history of medicine in McLean County, "Doctors were [the Depression's] victims as was almost everyone else. Some lost their savings in the ruin of the stock market. Many of these succeeded in retrieving these losses by continuing their hard work."[77] Physicians earned less during the Depression than they had in earlier years. James Welch remembered that during the 1930s, "The banks were all closed. . . . [My father] would go on a house call and he'd come back with a basket of turnips or chickens or eggs, or what-not."[78] Thus, status and the perceived drama of medical practice were more important factors than prospective incomes in motivating young men to go into medicine during the interwar period.

Medical Education

Although changes in medical education were well established by the time they began their training, practitioners interviewed for this study remembered resistance on the part of established physicians and some patients to the innovations introduced by young doctors. James Welch's father began practicing in Cuba in about 1909 after having taken postgraduate training at a Minneapolis hospital:

> When he came back . . . he was one of the first in his trade in aseptic surgery. . . . A lot of the old-timers were pretty skeptical of this new-fangled stuff. A lot of deliveries were done at home then. . . . He came back to his home town here, and he insisted on wearing rubber gloves and boiling his instruments. At that time, they used lard. Can you imagine that? . . . These women thought if they greased themselves with lard, it would make the baby come out easier. I don't know what it did about that, but it sure increased infection. . . . So the

talk went around among the ladies that he was pretty persnickety and he didn't want to get his hands dirty![79]

This comment illustrates the contested territory of expertise between older and younger practitioners, as well as that between doctors and traditional community authorities regarding childbearing—women themselves. It also reveals enduring attitudes about laywomen on the part of this informant, who was interviewed in the mid-1990s. Finally, it suggests the influence of newly trained physicians on changes in community health culture among both practitioners and patients.

Physician informants conformed to the educational path that became standard after publication of the Flexner Report. They finished high school, then did university premedical courses before going to medical school. Not all interviewees took undergraduate degrees. Harold Shinall spent only three years (1927–30) at the University of Illinois in Urbana-Champaign before starting medical school at the University of Illinois in Chicago. He explained, "At that time you could go on at the end of three years to medical school if your grades were okay."[80] Although it became usual for premedical students to finish bachelor's degrees during the 1930s, World War II temporarily shortened medical education. Loren Boon spent two years at the University of Illinois before going on to medical school; he received his M.D. in 1942.[81] Russell Oyer, who also went to medical school in the early 1940s, said, "At that time, still during the national emergency of World War II, at the medical school, you did . . . four academic years in three calendar years. You went to school all the time."[82]

Doctors trained before 1950 remembered that medical school tuition charges were low, and that cost, although important, was not a barrier to obtaining college and medical educations. James Welch took his bachelor's degree at Knox College, a private school that was expensive compared to public institutions at the time. He remembered paying $150 to $200 per semester beginning in 1933, and that his father borrowed money to send him to school. However, he was able to give up his part-time job as a busboy in a cafeteria in order to "devote myself to football" fairly early in his college career.[83]

Harold Shinall said that he chose the University of Illinois's undergraduate program for financial reasons:

INTERVIEWER: Did you ever consider going anywhere else?
INFORMANT: I didn't have the money. That [U. of I.] was only 32 miles away from [his home in] Danville. My first year, I worked while going to school. I would go home on weekends, hitch-hiked, and I would work in that Penney's store on Saturdays. My sophomore year I got a job as a waiter on the

campus. The third year I was in a premedical fraternity and was named the treasurer, and if you had that job as sort of a manager, you got your room and board provided.[84]

At $25 per semester, his undergraduate tuition was less of a challenge than food and accommodation. Shinall got a scholarship for medical school in 1930, "I made the acquaintance of the senator's daughter. She was the girlfriend of a man that I knew of my age. He brought the subject up. Maybe I could get it. Maybe the daughter could help you get a scholarship. So she did. A big boon. . . . You'll be shattered to think of how little it was in those days. . . . The tuition at the medical school was $100 per semester. But a dollar was worth more then too, so it's relative."[85]

Paul Theobald, whose father had died when he was child, had a partial scholarship to attend Illinois Wesleyan University as an undergraduate. In addition, he worked part-time jobs:

> Starting in high school days I was a *Pantagraph* [newspaper] carrier, and I carried papers up through the freshman year at Illinois Wesleyan, and I was an usher at the Irvin Theater and became Assistant Manager over at the Castle Theater, and then during the war years, I worked at Eureka Williams [factory] as a First Aid Attendant on the night shift between 11 at night and 7 in the morning. At the same time, I attended Illinois Wesleyan, carried a full course, and also had a date every night. I was busy.[86]

Russell Oyer's father was a tenant farmer who "farmed with horses." He said, "We didn't have indoor plumbing at all during my growing up. There was no running water inside, no indoor toilet. A very simple home. We were really poor. Then the Depression hit, of course, the crash in 1929 and the early years of the 1930s. But I don't think you thought so much about that in those days because everyone else was sort of in the same boat. . . . We always had enough to eat, and we had a house to live in. But there was no money." Oyer got a small scholarship and borrowed money to attend undergraduate school at Bluffton College in Ohio. "I was able to borrow some money, my sister helped me quite a bit, and my mother helped a little bit during college, but I also borrowed some money from a couple of relatives and some friends for college expenses. . . . Of course, college expenses were small, but it was a lot of money in those days." The money he borrowed went for housing, tuition, and equipment. "It seems to me that several hundred dollars might have been tuition. I remember I bought a microscope. . . . You could buy a binocular scope for $7.50 per month. . . . I finally got that paid off."[87]

Several informants received all or part of their medical training through the armed forces or the G.I. Bill. Having paid for his undergraduate education himself, Oyer remembered:

The class was about 180 with five or six women. . . . Practically all of the males went to either the Navy Program or the Army Specialized Training Program which were professional programs paid for by the government. . . . If you wanted to stay out of the draft, you had to sign up for Second Lieutenant status in the Reserves. Then you were permitted to finish medical school and in exchange for that you were committed then to two years of service after you graduated. You went from internship then directly to an assignment.[88]

After graduating from high school in 1944, Albert Van Ness was drafted into the U.S. Navy, which sent him to John Carroll University in Cleveland, Ohio:

In the so-called Navy B-12 Program . . . you got $21 a month, room, board, and you went to school. . . . I was in John Carroll for 17 months and I had almost 90 hours when I left there. . . . I was thinking about medicine and . . . that was fortified by my experience at John Carroll. At John Carroll, they really taught you how to study. If you didn't cooperate with that, you found yourself in Great Lakes [naval training center] one week and about six weeks later out in the Pacific.[89]

After the war ended, the G.I. Bill supported the rest of Van Ness's under-graduate education and medical training at Indiana University.

None of the informants worried about admission to medical school. In 1930, according to Harold Shinall, "The competition was there. You had to maintain a 3.5 [grade average] to be eligible to go to med school. That would be one-half Bs and one-half Cs as they listed it then."[90] However, competition increased after World War II because of wartime interruptions to profes-sional educations, large numbers of returning servicemen, G.I. Bill support, and growing perception of medicine as a high-status, well-paid occupation. Speaking of when he applied to Indiana University Medical School, Albert Van Ness said that:

INFORMANT: There were 5,000 applications and 141 were accepted. One hun-dred went to Indianapolis [for the final three years of training]. Eventually, though, I think 102 or 103 graduated, because in those years at least two to four medical students per class had to drop out because of tuberculosis or some illness. . . .

INTERVIEWER: What would have been the make-up of your class? How many women were there?

INFORMANT: Two. . . . Two out of 100. Two blacks. At the end of our sophomore year, Indiana always took two people from Mississippi, and two people from Alabama in the clinic years because those schools were two-year schools at the time. . . . We had two foreign students. . . . The class average age was 27. . . . Some fellows in our class had started out in night school in the '30s and working and trying to get their pre-med together so they could eventually go to medical school. Some of those fellows got drafted. . . . One fellow was 44 or 45, who had been the Dean of Men at Butler University before the war. But see, the G.I. Bill of Rights changed all that. . . . It was a varied and sundry group of people. . . . [91]

Other informants also remembered medical school classes that were overwhelmingly white and male, although some had a few more female classmates. Harold Shinall said, "In fact, my lab partner was a woman. . . . She later became a pediatrician in Danville. I think it was only a small number, about one-half dozen [women in the class]. My granddaughter [who recently began medical school] has about one-third. So that's been a big change." Shinall indicated that, although most of his medical colleagues were men, a somewhat older medical generation actually included more women. During his medical training he had a part-time job working on the switchboard at Chicago's Women's and Children's Hospital, which had "almost entirely women on the staff. . . . there were some prominent women surgeons and I think they were pretty self-sufficient. Occasionally they would have some man come in as a patient, but I don't think they really had any men listed on staff."[92]

The U.S. medical school curriculum was standardized in the early twentieth century.[93] Thus, all physicians interviewed for this study received very similar training. The oldest informant, Harold Shinall, described his 1928–32 medical school curriculum at the University of Illinois as follows:

The medical training was four years. They described the first two years as preclinical and the second two years as clinical because the first two years you had anatomy, histology, endocrinology, neurology, and all that, with microscopic and gross anatomy, physiology, and you don't have a stethoscope. The latter part of your second year you continue on pre-clinical courses. You get into a little surgical instruction in classroom and so forth. You started in on physical diagnosis at that time and you got a stethoscope. Then the last two years, you still continued courses in surgery and internal medicine and the other little smaller practices, but in addition to that, there were a lot of visits to the operating room and outpatient clinics and deliveries.[94]

At the younger end, Russell Oyer, trained in the 1940s, remembered that his preclinical courses were also concentrated during the first two years of medical school, although he participated in what was then a novel attempt to integrate the scientific preparation for medical practice:

Dr. Otto Kentmeyer had the vision that medicine ought to be well correlated so that really students would study, not human anatomy, histology, genetics, . . . chemistry, but they would study medicine. . . . So he wrote his own laboratory textbook on the human anatomy which did, indeed, correlate and incorporate, integrate the gross anatomy, histology; so actually you were in the lab dissecting part of the time, studying histology part of the time, you know, it was really an attempt to correlate the whole approach to human medicine. . . . I think patient contact started, well, physical diagnosis I think was taught in the second year. You started getting some patients after that, but basically clinical contact was the Junior year.[95]

Albert Van Ness remembered that his first year of medical training, conducted on the Bloomington campus of Indiana University, was made deliberately difficult in order to reduce from 141 to 100 the number of students who would go on to the medical school campus in Indianapolis. "It was a very nerve-wracking year. They really put the pressure on you. They literally drove some people right out of there that didn't seem to have what it takes. . . . It wasn't nearly as difficult as I thought it was going to be to make the Indianapolis cut because it [the first year] was terrible on some people."[96]

W. L. Dillman remembered that dental school was similar to medical school:

In those days we had a lot of the same courses and instructors that the medical students did. We were right across the street from Cook County Hospital. We'd go over and watch the operations and a lot of the work. . . . Some of the fellows did not see why we should have to work on cadavers, go to autopsies, until a professor finally explained to us how each part of the body can affect another part of the body. We were taught to observe any pathology in any way. Why do you think they look down your throat and say, "Stick out your tongue?" That's one of the first places you look for pathology.[97]

Clinical training, which occurred during the last two years of medical school and continued during internship and residency, involved exposure to a range of medical conditions, introduction to therapeutic techniques, and progressive degrees of responsibility taken by the student. Unlike apprenticeship training of the nineteenth century, which involved shadowing a practicing physician and visiting patients in their homes, twentieth-century medical education was, like medical practice itself, institutionalized—inextricably linked to hospitals. It was here that the urban locations of medical schools, with their associated hospitals, made their most significant contributions to medical training, since large city populations provided inexhaustible material for observation and practice.[98] Many of the "guinea-pigs" for medical students' early diagnostic and therapeutic efforts were drawn from among the urban poor, who went to public and teaching hospitals because they could not afford private hospital charges; tended to come from lower social class and, increasingly, minority backgrounds; and were in no position to either deny students access to their bodies or complain about the treatment they received. Status and power differences between hospital patients and medical students helped pave the way for the authoritative relationship between graduate physicians and their clients.

It is ironic, since hospital birth was becoming the norm in the Midwest during the interwar years, that the clinical experience most physicians interviewed for this study highlighted was attending home deliveries, which were arranged through the hospitals at which they trained. Accounts generally suggest the medical students' lack of confidence, the social gap between students and patients, and the continuing importance of maternity care to the family doctor's practice. James Welch recalled his experiences in St. Louis during the 1930s:

> Well, in our senior year, after we had lectures and been over at the university hospital in OB and so forth, we were sent out in groups of three . . . into the . . . tenements, the district along the river, you know, and worked with the poor. . . . We had delivered babies in the hospital, but when we had to go out by ourselves, we were three: one to give the anesthesia, one to take care of the baby . . . and one to deliver the baby. And then they had residents, nurses, in these vans that went around and kept close contact, you know. . . . We went to this first one and . . . we had a resident. He thought all medical students were idiots, which is probably true. . . . We went in this one, this was a big lady. She was lying on a feather tick. . . . We came in like gangbusters, you know. All of us scared to death. She laughed at us all the way through everything. Which didn't help. . . . But anyway, the baby was precipitated just as we came in the door. In other words, baby, placenta, everything came out—whoosh! She'd had eleven children! . . . But there was a big rip in this old feather tick. And it all went down. We were really frightened then because we thought the baby [would smother]. We go to get him out. We cut the cord, took him to the kitchen, and he was covered with vernix, you know, the cold cream-like stuff. . . . And we were standing there looking at him, and I swear, maybe it's exaggerated now, but he was covered with feathers from head to toe. . . . Just then, this resident walked in the back door of the kitchen. And he stared. He said, "What are you goddamn idiots doing now?" This one idiot said, "Well, we're picking the feathers off the baby!"[99]

By reference to the presence of an "anesthetist," this account reveals contemporary expectation of a medically managed birth. However, here the official authority (and nervous inexperience) of the medical students, resident, and nurses are contrasted with the unofficial authority (and laughing experience) of the mother. Furthermore, the students are at a disadvantage in the patient's home compared to the more familiar, convenient, and appropriate environment of the teaching hospital. Albert Van Ness had similar memories of postwar Indianapolis:

> In those days, they had no way to get all the women into the hospital to give birth. So, if a woman had one . . . uneventful birth, when she got pregnant the second time, she went on the outdoor service, and the hospital gave you an automobile, two students, a medical bag, and they . . . went out and delivered the child in the home. . . . I could fill up three tapes about what happened on that because, of course, you end up delivering prostitutes and people living in garages. See, during the war, there was a tremendous movement of people into Indianapolis. . . . so there were a lot of people that were relatively destitute and there was no housing for them, and nobody was building anything during the war. So people'd fix up their garages and people would move into their garage and pay rent for this and have no sanitation.[100]

In both accounts of experiences that, like dissection of cadavers, were part of the ritualized initiation of medical students, there is the unspoken subtext of race. Both physicians were white, middle-class males, whereas many of the patients they dealt with as students were poor, African American women.

All of the physicians interviewed did internships. Harold Shinall explained, "The U. of I., in those days, along with two other medical schools in the Midwest, did not actually give you your M.D. degree until the completion of your internship. Theoretically, you couldn't be called a doctor yet, but at the graduation ceremony, we were handed a little certificate that said we had completed the four years of medical training."[101] Most informants were married by this stage. The pattern was for wives to continue in full-time employment while husbands worked demanding call schedules and earned nominal stipends of between ten and twenty-five dollars a month. As Russell Oyer remembered:

> INFORMANT: Each of us had a room at the hospital where we stayed when we were on call. . . . I think every three or four nights I was in the hospital. . . .
> INTERVIEWER: What were those days like? What was an on-call day?
> INFORMANT: Well, history and physical on new patients and a conference with the attending physician. You would . . . make rounds with the attending physician. You did an obstetrical kind of thing, and you did a medical thing, and you did a surgical thing. Surgery, then you'd be scrubbing for cases that you were on.[102]

Albert Van Ness said of his internship at the university of Chicago:

> It was forever! It was around the clock, weekends, holidays, the whole business. You were just on call every other day and worked every day of course for 12 hours. It was brutal. . . . We'd have some services that have 30 or 40 people on

them, and you'd run that by yourself and most of the attendants up there would just turn you loose if they didn't think you needed much supervision. You'd get on the hematology service, and you'd give 25 transfusions in the morning and admit people in the afternoon and scrub and do bone marrows.[103]

Several interviewees did their internships during military service.

Both World War II and family responsibilities affected informants' decisions about whether to take a residency to qualify as a specialist. Doctors Welch, Boon, and Oyer had considered specializing in internal medicine. Welch explained that military service interrupted his plans; when he finished his four-year army service, he went into practice with his father in order to support his family.[104] Loren Boon recalled, "I went right from internship and got married. I thought I was going to come back for residency there at Ravenswood Hospital in Chicago. I came back from getting married, a honeymoon, and there was a . . . letter in a brown envelope telling me to report for service on July 1st.[105] When he finished military service, he did one year of general residency at Lutheran Deaconess Hospital in Milwaukee. Then, in 1947, he went into practice, where he developed an informal specialty in anesthesiology.

Russell Oyer remembered,

When I was about ready to be separated from the service, I guess I was really interested in internal medicine and did check out at least a couple places in Chicago. . . . At that point, there was a lot of competition for the best spots in residency because of everybody getting out of the service at that time [1946]. . . . I did think about that, and retrospectively, as I have thought about my career, I think I would have been much happier in a specialty practice. . . . But our three kids came along and I started deferring decisions about getting going with training.[106]

By the 1930s the trend toward formal specialization was under way.[107] Harold Shinall, who started his career as a general practitioner, decided to take a residency in radiology in 1940. He explained,

I put an X-ray machine in my office. . . . Early on, I realized my shortcomings [in reading X-rays] because I would be saying things that I wasn't sure of. I had a brother-in-law who was a radiologist, practicing in East St. Louis. The cases I was not sure about, I would send him the films for interpretation. I visited him a few times and decided that maybe I'd like to do that. He knew the doctor that was in charge at the city hospital, and so he arranged for me to go down for an interview. . . . I was there at the city hospital for two years and then I went into the military. I was associated with the army general hospital. When I finished up my period of time, I was able to apply for the [specialty] board examination.

Shinall decided to specialize, in part, because of the lack of hospital facilities in Gibson City where he had practiced as a GP. However, he reflected that his experience in general practice "helped me after I got established because I was able to handle patients a little bit better than people who had not had that prior experience."[108]

Albert Van Ness decided to specialize in internal medicine during his internship at the University of Chicago:

> I was interested in everything. I started out thinking I was going to become an E.N.T. man, but that I'm sure was because of Dr. Watkins' influence and my mother working for him. But I realized I didn't like that. Then I thought of some other things, even OB-GYN. And then, later on in my internship, when you had to start scrubbing up and being there for hours, then I lost enthusiasm for surgical procedures and that's when I began to think about medicine.[109]

After spending two years in the military during the Korean War, he finished his residency at the University of Chicago between 1954 and 1957.

Going into Practice

In the mid-twentieth century, most new graduate physicians expected to set themselves up as independent businessmen, either in a new office or by buying or joining the practice of an established practitioner. Each doctor needed an office and a car for house calls and hospital visits. Many installed X-ray and laboratory equipment in their offices; some dispensed medications.[110] The initial outlay required to begin a medical practice was an expensive prospect for a young man, often with a growing family, who had earned very little during his lengthy training. Doctors also needed hospital privileges. The key to all of these resources was the network of local physicians—both official, in the form of medical societies, and unofficial, shaped by family relationships, medical school connections, and affinity. Gender and class norms and roles—conversations in the doctor's lounge, rounds of golf, church membership, wives' relationships—nurtured what, until the 1970s, remained an exclusive men's club.

Most of the physicians interviewed for this study chose practice locations because of personal contacts. James Welch went into practice with his father in Cuba. Paul Theobald worked briefly with a physician in a resort area in Wisconsin; then, "We went out to California and I looked things over out there, and I thought we had no money, and I knew this was no place for a practitioner because when hard times come we'd be hit. So . . . we decided we would come back to Bloomington where we knew some people that if we needed some money we could borrow some."[111] Albert Van Ness also located in Bloomington because of social contacts, which were especially important to a new specialist dependent on referrals:

> We came to Bloomington for Mac Stevenson's wedding . . . at the Country Club, I think it was. . . . I got to talking to Ed Stevenson [a prominent physician] and at the time I knew that it was time for me to leave. I wanted to go somewhere else than the University of Chicago. We had great training up there. It was wonderful and I had a good experience, but I wanted to move on and the ethnic neighborhoods were changing very rapidly. Judy was pregnant and we had two children. We were trying to decide what to do. Ed Stevenson was the one that persuaded me to come to Bloomington. . . . He said that he would fix me up—that we would kind of practice in parallel if I accepted, and that he would contribute to getting me off the ground.[112]

Harold Shinall discovered an opportunity in Gibson City through a friend who was practicing in nearby Piper City. "We learned that there was an elderly physician in Gibson City who was suffering from cancer of the stomach and was not expected to live very long. I went to see him, and I took his office over. . . . During the remainder of his life, I had to pay him a certain percentage of what my income was. I took over his equipment; a lot of it was antiquated. He died within a year; so then I took over."[113]

Loren Boon had been raised in Washburn, Illinois, where his father had practiced. He decided not to locate there because the community was positioned midway between the hospitals in Peoria and Spring Valley; thus, doctors did a great deal of traveling to visit hospitalized patients. However, he wanted to return to central Illinois, and selected Danvers, partly because its residents used only the hospitals in Bloomington.[114]

As indicated above, the composition of professional medicine in McLean County was dominantly white, male, and middle class. The same social networks that created opportunities for the right young men undermined the success of physicians who, for whatever reason, were outsiders. Richard Finfgeld, who lived in Lexington (rural McLean County) during the 1910s and 1920s, talked about the only woman doctor in town:

> INFORMANT: I'll tell you about the medical situation. We had two M.D.s in Lexington: one was Dr. Hammers and one was Dr. Scott. A little later, Dr. Scott's son graduated and was an M.D. and he came there and they practiced together, and we had three at one time. That was three men and we had one woman. Her name was Dr. Bull. . . .
> INTERVIEWER: Did this woman have her own practice?
> INFORMANT: In her home. The other two had offices downtown.
> INTERVIEWER: Do you know how she was educated?

INFORMANT: No, I don't know anything about her. I knew who she was and where she lived, but I didn't know anything about her. The others were licensed M.D.s.

INTERVIEWER: Do you suppose she was licensed also?

INFORMANT: I think she must have been.

INTERVIEWER: She wasn't considered a quack?

INFORMANT: No, I don't think so, but I don't think she was very popular.[115]

According to the McLean County Medical Society, Dr. E. Martha Bull was born in 1867 in Lexington and graduated from Northwestern University Woman's College in 1895. "She was in active practice until 1928 in Lexington, when because of serious illness was able to resume practice only in a modest way."[116] She apparently suffered from not being part of the group of male doctors with downtown offices; she was also at a disadvantage with patients because of her sex:

INTERVIEWER: Why probably was the female physician not well accepted?

INFORMANT: I think maybe they didn't regard her as an authority. I don't really know what the adults thought about it. I knew she was just kind of off on the side there, and didn't seem to be in the loop. But why they would come to that conclusion, I wouldn't know.

INTERVIEWER: Were there specific types of patients that might go to her?

INFORMANT: Certain kinds of people, maybe, rather than certain kinds of patients. People that maybe were not in the ordinary flow of the community. People who would be a little odd or something. . . . I don't know. But she just didn't have a wide practice that I knew of.[117]

The rare women physicians of the early and mid-twentieth century were more likely to work in isolation than their male colleagues. One can only speculate about the work environments of non-Caucasian or non-Christian doctors in McLean County, as elsewhere in the United States, during the Jim Crow era when racism, anti-Semitism, and xenophobia were both usual and socially acceptable.

Regardless of gender or ethnicity, the working conditions of physicians settling in rural communities during the early twentieth century had changed radically by the end of their careers. For one thing, in early years there were many more doctors in small towns.[118] When James Welch's father began practicing in Cuba, Illinois, in 1908 or 1909, there were seven doctors serving a population of fewer than two thousand residents.[119] As we have seen, in the 1920s, Lexington, with a population of approximately 1,500, had four doctors.[120] Although rural practitioners maintained offices and visited hospitals, the majority of their time was spent attending patients in their own homes.

Harold Shinall recalled that when he started practicing in Gibson City in 1935, there were three other doctors working there. At that time, the community had a population of 2,200, and physicians treated many patients who lived in the surrounding countryside. Suggesting both competition and collegiality among medical practitioners, Shinall said, "I went in to see one of them [local doctors] before I started, and he said, 'I don't care how well you do here, just so I keep my share.'"[121]

Shinall took over an established practice, so he was spared the expense of building and decorating a new office. However, he also had to deal with conditions that seemed old-fashioned even at the time: "Well, he had a hard coal stove in the office. After the winter of 1935–36, they still speak of how cold it was, and I had to lug the coal up from the back outside, up the steps to the office and bank it at night to keep it warm enough. Then I could just stoke it up a little bit in the morning. There was a waiting room and a larger room."[122] Shinall dispensed medications, administered ultraviolet treatments, and eventually had a diathermy machine (which, according to the *Oxford English Dictionary*, "passed high frequency electric currents through the body by means of external electrodes.") He divided his time between making house calls, many to patients some miles distant from town; visiting hospital patients in Bloomington and Paxton; and seeing patients in his office.

To some extent, Shinall inherited his clientele. However, he was also eager to develop a good reputation so word of mouth would bring him new customers. He said, "In those days, physicians didn't place ads. That was sort of frowned upon, and so you did the best that you can as far as work is concerned and let that speak for itself." He encountered health problems ranging from farm injuries to contagious diseases to childbirth:

> INTERVIEWER: What kinds of things were you mainly dealing with?
> INFORMANT: The skin and its contents, I guess. Well, there were a lot of infections in those days, and we did not have antibiotics. So a lot of things that are controlled in a brief period with antibiotics now had complications a lot of times. . . . You don't hear about a quinsy throat or a pair of tonsillar abscesses any more, but I had a few of those. A lot of infectious diseases, I think, would make up a lot of my clients.[123]

James Welch also remembered initially dealing with illnesses not commonly encountered in the second half of the twentieth century. His first patient when he began practicing in 1946 had typhoid fever. He also remembered,

> Well, I had this cousin. . . . He was a surgeon, a good surgeon. Dad and I were up there making rounds with him one morning at the hospital and he says, "You know, I've got this patient with the strangest damn rash, and I can't diagnose

it." "Well, let's go take a look at it." We went in, "Oh, my God!" [my father] said. We went outside and he [cousin] said, "What's the matter?" He [father] says, "It's smallpox." . . . They had never seen it.[124]

The transition from home- to institutional-based practice was slow. It remained usual in the mid-twentieth-century for doctors to make house calls. Shinall recalled,

> You had to have a car because you had a lot of calls in the country in those days. House calls are not too prevalent these days. One reason is emergency rooms and so forth, but I've had people call me after a snow storm and say they planned to come in, but the snow was pretty deep, and wondered if I'd mind coming out! . . . I had a friend that was a patient. He and I went on some trips when we took shovels and were able to get to places they couldn't get through.[125]

Richard Finfgeld, had similar memories of Lexington in the 1920s:

> The doctors . . . had their offices there in town, and they made house calls. Not only house calls in Lexington, but they had all the rural territory. My older brother Cliff, he was chauffeur for Dr. Hammers, and they had a Hudson car. He [Cliff] was responsible for keeping that car ready to go, and he would drive that doctor all over the country, and that was a problem because there were no paved roads and there were no gravel roads to speak of. There might have been a little gravel around, but most of them were just mud roads. And he had a problem to get to see some of these people.[126]

Rural physicians' work schedules were grueling. Shinall remembered,

> The doctors who were there when I went there were having evening office hours as well as daytime office hours, so I had office hours in the morning, daytime, and evening, but I tried to get as many of my office patients in the afternoon and evening, because in the morning you could make calls. I came over here to see my patients if they were hospitalized in Bloomington. There was also a hospital about 15 miles to the east of Gibson City, Paxton, Illinois; they had a hospital there, and I did use that some. Some days I'd drive here and Paxton both, which was about 100 miles. I had made on unusual days three or four trips to Bloomington. . . . Because you might be over here for a surgical case in the morning, have an accident case in the evening, and an OB case at night. You were late a lot of times.[127]

Shinall did not take appointments, but saw patients on a first come, first-served basis. During the early years of his practice, his wife worked in his office; later, he hired a Mennonite Hospital Nursing School graduate to serve as nurse, receptionist, and medical records manager.

In the late 1930s, patients grew accustomed to traveling to doctors' offices and hospitals. Younger physicians encouraged this trend, particularly for childbirth. As Shinall reported:

> INFORMANT: I think when I first started over there about two [deliveries] out of three would be in the home. By the time I left, I was encouraging them to go to the hospital and I had reversed that so there were two out of three in the hospital.
>
> INTERVIEWER: What was the reason that you encouraged them to go in: greater safety?
>
> INFORMANT: I think so. . . . I think we were becoming educated to the fact about that time that this was a good idea.[128]

By the time Loren Boon went into practice in 1947, although house calls were still common for rural practitioners, office practice and hospital deliveries were the rule:

> Especially out here, when people wanted a house call, why they were sick enough to need a house call. That was just not always the case . . . in a larger city. But, yeah, I was making house calls up until the time I retired. . . . There were fewer because of the good roads and they probably realized I was able to give them better treatment at the office . . . than with what I was carrying in my medical bag. I even made a few deliveries at home. Not too many, . . . because that changed during World War II . . . and I think more of them got used to going to the hospita1.[129]

It is noteworthy that by encouraging mothers to deliver in the hospital, young general practitioners unintentionally fostered the normative consultation of obstetricians that ultimately drove GPs out of maternity practice. The same argument can be made about the decline of home visits and increase in office consultations—particularly in "medical buildings," where specialists were visible and accessible.

When Paul Theobald started general practice in Bloomington in 1953, urban medicine was organized around office- and hospital-based practice. Many doctors rented space in the Griesheim, Unity, and Peoples Bank buildings. Indicating the importance of personal relationships and professional networks, Theobald remembered,

> [My wife] Jill saw Mr. Impson in the Unity Building, and he had an office space which previously had been a dentist's office. . . . We rented the office from him, and Jill told him, "We don't have any money. If he [Theobald] doesn't make any money the first month, we won't be able to pay you." And he said, "I have no worry about that. He'll make a go of it. You just pay me the rent whenever you can." And so we hooked up the office, and there was a salesman by the

name of Robinson from Gibson City. Robbie came over to visit me. He'd heard I'd set up in practice, and told me I could have whatever equipment I wanted and I could pay it off no interest or anything. We got the office waiting-room furniture from chairs from the altar—big straight chairs that had been in the church there for years and years. . . . I hired a nurse who had been working for Dr. Ed Stevenson. He was going to have to let her go, and I told her that I might not be able to pay her at the end of the week because I didn't have any money at all. . . . Dr. Nord called me up (he's a second cousin of my wife's). Stan called and said, "Paul, I want to take a vacation. Would you take calls for me?" I said, sure! And that's how I got started.[130]

Theobald's schedule revolved around office and hospital patients:

Most doctors took Thursday afternoon off, but I found out that I was so busy taking calls for the other doctors on Thursday that I changed my afternoon off to Wednesday, and then I'd work Thursday afternoon. I'd go to the hospitals in the morning, and . . . I think I'd get in [to the office] around 10:00 in the morning and see patients from 10 to 12 and then I'd take lunch and be back from 1 till 5. And then I was making hospital calls at all three hospitals: Brokaw, St. Joe, and Mennonite, every morning and every evening. I would also have office calls on Saturday morning.[131]

Having started practice in a downtown medical office building, in 1955, Theobald led the local trend for physicians to move out of the city center, following new suburban development. He said,

In fact, the first person who moved out . . . from downtown was actually Dr. Parker, and he moved out about the same time I did. . . . I remember Reverend Loydall, minister at the First Baptist Church . . . [who] was on the Planning Commission and he heard I was going to move out on East Oakland. He came to me one day and said, "Paul, don't move out. You will ruin your practice. You won't make it out there." Well, I went ahead and moved out and actually the first month I was out there, my business doubled. My auditor, when he saw it, he just said there'd been a lot of business. He told me not to think that moving out had anything to do with it. In the second month it went up three times, and about the fourth month my auditor said, "Well, it's quite evident that the move did do you a lot of good." My business really went up when I moved out. . . . Well, uptown you'd see one member of a family. . . . When I moved out on East Oakland, they'd come out in the car and you'd see the whole family. There'd be five or six instead of just one person. . . . I thought that had more to do with it than anything.[132]

Theobald also made house calls. However, as patients became increasingly mobile, office- and hospital-based practice became more feasible and physicians' time was organized more cost-efficiently.[133] At the height of his practice, Dr. Theobald remembered seeing "upwards of one hundred patients a day in my office."[134] His comments reveal the extent to which McLean County physicians viewed their work as business activity and, despite their interdependence, continued to compete for patients.

Professional Relationships

A key change in medical practice in twentieth-century McLean County was the shift from general practice to specialization. Although this trend was already apparent during the interwar period, it became established only after World War II. Thus, general practitioners who qualified during the 1930s and 1940s continued to follow older practice patterns by working as generalists and developing informal part-time specialties. For example, Loren Boon was trained to administer anesthesia during his general residency at Lutheran Deaconess Hospital, Milwaukee. He recalled that when he started practice in 1947, "Here I was . . . before the hospitals had their own anesthesia schools. . . . All they had were about two or three nurse anesthetists and then one M.D. anesthesiologist. . . . so I got busy right away with that too."[135] General practitioners continued to deliver babies and do surgery. Paul Theobald remembered, "I was assisting in surgery, I would say probably four days out of the week. And I was delivering as many babies as any of the obstetricians in town."[136]

In the mid-twentieth century, it was unclear whether—and which—specialties would be viable in McLean County. After all, the foremost local specialist of the interwar period, Edwin Palmer Sloan (1876–1935), who was a goiter surgeon, realized by the end of his career, "Future thyroid control is the province of preventive medicine . . . [which] properly applied to the goiter problem can save immeasurably more lives than can the surgeon's art."[137] Sloan's specialty disappeared when iodization of table salt became routine. When Harold Shinall announced his intention to leave general practice and do a residency in radiology in 1940, "One of the older doctors who was here as I was leaving Gibson City, when I told him what I was going to do, he said, 'Harold, you're making a mistake. That specialty is going to be out the window. Doctors are putting in their own [X-ray] equipment and they'll be taking care of it. You won't have anything to do.'"[138] Furthermore, it was by no means certain that small urban areas could support many and diverse specialists. Albert Van Ness, who finished his residency in internal medicine in 1957, reflected that at that time, "Specialists didn't go to a town [of] less than one million. . . . There weren't any [formally qualified] specialists in Bloomington on the medical side. They were all generalists. There were just a couple of them and everybody else was a general practitioner and primary care doctor."[139]

Like new GPs, new specialists depended on personal and professional networks. As we have seen, Albert Van Ness started practice with the support of a local doctor who "really wanted me to give him some time off." Van Ness's career was far more strongly linked to hospital work than careers of his GP contemporaries. He built his practice by doing emergency room call for established physicians, "We were out there at night because people like Ed Stevenson and Bob Price and Ray Baxter, and all those people would . . . their names were on the rotation call, but if they could get a substitute, the substitute's name was out there. . . . It was a heck of a good way to start up a practice, but you were spending your entire night at the emergency room just at the hospital."[140] He also cultivated relationships with general practitioners:

> As an internist, you would tie onto a couple of practitioners, and they didn't vary, they sent you the business. . . . Even the nurses would call you up and say, "There's a patient of Dr. [So-and-so's] here in the emergency room and you ought to see it because it had this or that" . . . You know, [doctors] that lived out in the country . . . if one of their patients . . . [was] in the hospital emergency room and you were their known consultant, you just went over there. You didn't even bother them [the senior physician] until the next morning. They didn't want to come in from Danvers or any place like that in the middle of the night.[141]

General practitioners also developed relationships with specialists. Paul Theobald recalled,

> [For] OB work, I used Dr. O. H. Ball. Almost entirely until Dr. Calhoun came into town. Cal and I became very good friends, and a high percentage of my work went to Calhoun. Ball was just very busy, and although he was very courteous and treated me well, . . . Cal and I just became very close friends and I . . . referred a lot to him. With surgery, I used Dr. Wilbur Ball until Dr. John Frisch came to town. . . . John and I became friends, and so I started referring a lot of patients to John. . . . The medical problems . . . were referred to Dr. Ed Livingston, and then eventually to Owen [Deneen]. . . . Pediatrics? . . . I used Dew a lot. In fact, I don't remember using Dr. Cline. He was a pediatrician in town. I don't recall using him very much.[142]

Theobald's account reveals that social relationships were as important as professional respect in generating referrals. Russell Oyer discussed the way he made referrals:

I think that I had fairly good relationships with the people I referred to. In those days, you had basically general internists. The general internist was your primary source of referral, and he was the person who saw the patient with you and was able to make suggestions. Then you had the surgeon. . . . You had dermatologists, and some allergists, and some endocrinologists . . . and some neurologists . . . but basically the first source of referral was a general internist. . . . In OB, for example, . . . Jim Brown would help me a lot in OB. He's just a great guy and was able to help. . . . I tried never to refer the patient unless I had done a good deal of work-up. I always felt that I needed to send a letter of referral.[143]

Specialists' careers depended not only on referrals, but on hospital staff affiliation. When Harold Shinall began practicing radiology in Bloomington in 1946, he benefited from relationships he had developed as a GP sending patients to the Bloomington hospitals. During his search for a practice location, "I made inquiry up here and found out that St. Joseph's had learned that I was looking. They invited me to come up. I said, "Well, I'd like to talk to the administrator at Mennonite and if I can come to both places, I'll come." And that worked out. . . . They knew me and I knew the hospitals and people. That certainly didn't hurt a bit."[144] Albert Van Ness made it clear that hospital and collegial relationships were governed by unofficial rules:

In those days it was pretty much split between . . . three hospitals. And although you went to all three . . . you were either a Brokaw doctor, a Mennonite doctor, or a St. Joe doctor . . . Everybody was friendly and nobody stabbed anybody in the back, but you took care of your own. If I had a patient who developed appendicitis or something, I'd refer him to Ben Huff, because he was the surgeon at Brokaw. You didn't send him to the surgeons over at St. Joe, and vice versa. . . . When you did go to the other hospitals as a consultant, it was because the family insisted on it. It wasn't a doctor referral, it was a family referral.[145]

These allegiances nurtured rivalries among hospitals. Russell Oyer commented, "A doctor would sort of . . . place the hospitals in kind of an adversarial position by where they sent their patients, or they threatened to do this or do that, and somebody was admitting a lot of people and he'd get mad about something. . . . It was difficult for physicians to agree on anything. . . . Physicians had favorites. . . . Then you had the whole business of when one hospital added a new diagnostic thing, the other hospital had to get it."[146] Since hospitals depended on physicians to admit patients, this situation increased the power of individual doctors and hospital medical staffs until the advent and proliferation of professional hospital administrators, beginning in the 1950s, challenged that dominance.

Before the 1950s, relationships between general practitioners and surgeons were nurtured by the custom of splitting fees.[147] According to A. Edward Livingston, who practiced internal medicine in Bloomington between 1945 and 1985,

> It was customary for the referring doctor to assist the surgeon. He would be paid by the surgeon for this help directly from the money received by him from the patient. The referring doctor would not have to send a bill, but would receive a contracted part of the fee charged, hence the term "split fee." In itself, this does not seem to be a grave problem, but the difficulty in this method of payment lay in the fact that the referring doctors had the opportunity of selling their surgical patients to the highest bidder, not necessarily the best qualified surgeon. The referring doctor acting as a paid assistant was often unable to perform any part of the operation involved, and so would not be able to take over the procedure should the need arise. Frequently the surgeon would operate on the referred patient without actually examining the patient to determine if there was definite need for an operation.[148]

When in the early 1950s the American College of Surgeons' accreditation of hospitals became conditional upon commitment to stop fee splitting, there was local resistance. Although medical staff members at Brokaw and Mennonite hospitals accepted the new requirement, St. Joseph's physicians refused to comply. "It was then announced to the staff by the governing body of the Order of St. Francis in Peoria that the staff was disbanded and all former members had to reapply. Acceptance of their applications hinged on their signatures to suitable documents. . . . Thusly was the split-fee situation resolved."[149]

Fee splitting highlighted the widening gap between the status and incomes of specialists and GPs. Paul Theobald commented, "I enjoyed practicing medicine. I got very discouraged with . . . all the changes. I don't think that I would become a general practitioner again because I think GPs are about at the bottom of the totem pole as far as anyone else is concerned. . . ." At one point, he considered doing a residency in surgery. Although he decided against this step, he continued to do a lot of surgery:

> I gradually worked up just on my own by assisting. I got to the place where I had major surgical privileges and that was fine up until, oh, probably ten years ago [early 1980s] when some of the younger doctors in town started coming, and they had gone back to this where GPs shouldn't be in the surgical department. I had a good reputation, and Dr. Frisch often said that he'd rather have me help him in surgery than anyone else, and he would call me on a lot of cases. The new young doctors wouldn't call me to assist on any of the patients. You could

just tell by their attitude that "surgery is no place for a general practitioner to be." Which wasn't true in the old days. That's changed.[150]

Theobald suffered from rising expectation of specialty board certification to do work traditionally performed by general practitioners. Adding insult to injury, Theobald perceived a lack of respect that was both generational and related to the rising specialist elite in McLean County medicine.

Increasing numbers of specialists and their control of hospital staff privileges, as well as general practitioners' perception of their own skill limitations, limited GPs' activities—particularly in maternity care and surgery. Loren Boon stopped delivering babies in the 1950s: "I think they were getting quite a few OB-GYN men in Bloomington there. And about that time . . . when more people were taking the pill then too, the pregnancies did drop off in other words. So I figured because I wasn't able to keep up by taking care of enough of them a year, why, better to have them see somebody that was seeing more patients a year." Initially, he had had full surgical privileges in local hospitals: later, these privileges were limited. "I hadn't done too much surgery in internships . . . except for minor surgery and that. Instead, why, I gave the anesthetics. It worked out pretty well that way. That I knew and helped the other surgeons."[151] Dr. Oyer also stopped taking obstetrical cases in the 1950s, partly because of the popularity of some well-known obstetricians.[152] Dr. Theobald stopped delivering babies in the 1960s.[153]

Some informants felt that specialists' rising status caused differential treatment by hospital staff members and nurses. Paul Theobald recalled a situation when a patient he had recommended for sterilization was admitted to Mennonite hospital on a Sunday afternoon, with the procedure scheduled for Monday morning. On Sunday evening, he was informed by the Sterilization Committee, which was required to approve all such procedures:

> [that] I couldn't do the sterilization Monday morning. I got a little irritated and I found out that one of the . . . obstetricians got permission to do a sterilization on a patient who did not have near the requirements that my patient did. And so it was very embarrassing for me. That made me mad. I was making my rounds a couple weeks later and I remember walking in on the second floor by the nurses' desk . . . and I went up to the desk like doctors do. Most days, the nurses would stand up at attention when the doctor came in . . . and say, "What can I do for you, Doctor?" I went up there and the girl working right at the desk looked at me, looked back down, and kept writing. . . . I just stood there five or ten minutes, and finally all the girls jumped up at attention. . . . I looked down the corridor and half-way down . . . was Dr. Crowley [an ophthalmologist] coming down it. That's why they stood up at attention. I went down, saw the nursing supervisor, and I told her, "No one has shown me any

courtesy, but if they're going to show one doctor courtesy, then they should show it to all of them." So I got mad, figured I didn't need Mennonite, so I quit Mennonite then. Then gradually I just went over to St. Joe. I don't know why. . . . Well, the Sisters were very nice, and I am Protestant, and it wasn't a religious factor or anything like that, but it was just easier for me to get my work done. I had such a high admission out there that they catered after my business. I could get almost anything I wanted done out there.[154]

Theobald's perception of disrespect from other physicians was exacerbated by what he perceived as a decline in courtesy from traditionally deferential nurses. It is possible that the sister nurses at St. Joseph's Hospital maintained an old-fashioned demeanor toward physicians, which Dr. Theobald found comforting as well as making it "easier for him to get his work done." Sister Theonilla, who was running St. Joseph's surgical department at the time, supports this interpretation, saying about nurses' disagreements with physicians, "Yes, but then you just kind of talked, you know. There is a nice way of putting things, just like when you have something to say to your husband. It's the same thing. It's a family affair. You do the right thing. The patient has to be taken care of. The doctor is the one that is responsible and you put what you think you should do aside."[155] Dr. Theobald and Sr. Theonilla reflected traditional perspectives that, by the 1960s, were no longer normative.

Relationships among physicians were fostered by professional organizations, which also were central in informing practitioners about new theories and procedures. Dr. Boon remembered, "Shortly . . . after I started here . . . the American Academy of General Practice started, and so I joined it. . . . and I was able to go to national meetings and . . . over at Peoria they eventually . . . developed some postgraduate courses . . . that were held throughout the state. . . . so we managed to keep up pretty well."[156] In addition, McLean County Medical Society membership offered educational and social activities, as well as fostering referral networks.

The society also policed its members' behavior and ethics—a responsibility fraught with conflict of interest. Russell Oyer recalled,

I think it was very difficult to get a hold of things like that. I do remember once, we had a doctor who was quite popular in Bloomington. . . . He was doing a lot of OB. . . . I think he was doing more OB really than some of the obstetricians in town at that point, but he also gave some anesthesia. The medical society at one point . . . wrote a letter to him critical of his [decisions]. . . . Complaints had come that his nurses were making decisions. They were seeing the patient and giving medication and he was not seeing the patient. He was an extremely busy guy. Then, I remember another physician who was turned in once for advertising because he was doing something that seemed to the society as advertising.[157]

Physicians tended to handle in private issues of competence, for example, supervising the hospital orders of an aging doctor whose judgment was suspect. According to Dr. Livingston, "When a distinguished staff member suffered from a decline in his ability to direct the care of his patients, attempts were made to have him relinquish his practice, but this was almost always futile. So two charts were kept on his hospital admissions, unknown to him. A volunteer staff member would attend his patients to render the necessary care." Even more challenging were physicians' substance abuse problems. Livingston wrote,

> There were certain practitioners who were definite problems to the medical community. Efforts to support them were made, but were frequently ill-advised. This especially concerned those addicted to alcohol. Unfortunately, most such efforts were wasted, the situation usually resolving itself in the untimely death of the doctor. The patients of these practitioners would have been better served if their doctor was forced to stop practicing, but even now that is not an easy step to take.[158]

Physicians, both individually and collectively, continued to struggle with the contradictory pressures to serve the public interest, defend the reputation of professional medicine, and support their friends and colleagues.

Medicine and Money

None of the physicians interviewed for this study expected medical incomes to rise as they did in the second half of the twentieth century. Their initial earnings expectations were low, as were fees in their early years of practice. Harold Shinall remembered that in 1935, "We attempted to keep a fee schedule and in the county and in the City of Gibson, our house calls were $3, office visits were $1.50, and calls in the country were $5. . . . Deliveries were $25."[159] At that time, a five pound bag of flour cost just over 25 cents.[160] Twenty years later, Russell Oyer's charges were still moderate:

> I came in 1954. I took everybody, whether they could pay or not. I didn't ask anybody any credit things. And, of course, not so many people had insurance at that time either. You just took everybody, whether they paid or not. I started off with office calls at $3. We were delivering babies in Ohio [his first practice location] for $35 and driving ten miles to the hospital. I think I started with a fee of $50 here. I'm not sure, surgeons here got around $50 to $60. And, of course, here you drove twenty-five miles to the hospital. . . . I grew up in the Depression years, and we had no money. I always had a lot of problem with fees and charging people to do things.[161]

In his first month in practice, he earned $400. At the same time, the average manufacturing wage in the United States was about $282 a month.[162]

Even in the years immediately following World War II, specialists earned considerably more than general practitioners.[163] Albert Van Ness recalls that in his first year of practice, 1958, he "netted somewhere between $10,000 and $12,000."[164] He discussed the rising importance of hospitalization and third-party reimbursement to physicians' incomes:

> So much of your money you made on hospitalizations. Back in those days, it was $5 a day, but that added up because sometimes you'd have all those women in the hospital for three weeks and Blue Cross Blue Shield thinking they'd have pneumonia and a little congestive failure and the son-in-law and daughter would go to Florida for two weeks while Grandma was in the hospital recovering from this congestive failure and it was legitimate. . . . Some little eighty-four-year-old woman who got pneumonia or congestive failure would be expected to be in the hospital for four weeks.[165]

Thus, all doctors had a financial interest in hospital admission and long stays, but specialists, with their comparatively greater dependence on technology and hospital facilities, benefited most from the trend toward hospitalization. As Van Ness's account indicates, that trend was fostered by the extent to which hospitalization had become a part of community health culture—expected, accepted, and even welcomed as an alternative to home care.

Physicians interviewed for this study were in mid-career when Medicare and Medicaid were introduced in the 1960s. Many McLean County doctors opposed what they viewed as government interference with physicians' independence.[166] Medicare introduced both opportunities and challenges, particularly for rural practitioners. Russell Oyer remembered,

> Your people get older with you, so I was seeing . . . by the time I quit, a lot of the people were Medicare age—probably 60 percent. I had to stop doing OB, and was doing some pediatrics, but I wasn't in the nursery any more for the last ten or fifteen years. So my pediatric population began dwindling. So I was . . . in a sense doing mostly geriatrics at the time I quit. That became a financial problem a little bit. Medicare never pays for what you [do]—even though you follow the guidelines in charging, they never pay you. And cash flow began to be a little bit of a problem for me.[167]

According to Albert Van Ness, in cities surgeons benefited most from the introduction of Medicare. "When Medicare came through, the individual who had worked his life out here on the railroad or something . . . he then decided he could get his hernia repaired . . . or take out the gallbladder. This is the first time they ever had the where-with-all to do anything like that."[168] However, other specialists also found that Medicare added to their incomes. Dr. Livingston, an internist who had opposed the Medicare legislation, commented, "So it came to pass that doctors' incomes increased markedly due to the pay received from all the elderly patients on Medicare."[169]

Means-tested Medicaid reduced pressure on physicians to provide charitable care to the poor, but did not cover all services. Paul Theobald remembered,

> The patients I had, I had an awful lot that were on Public Aid. . . . A lot of the Public Aid patients didn't have to pay anything. We got paid for two calls a month. My first office calls were $3 and for a house call it was something like $3. . . . They would only pay for two house calls a month. I had one lady who was on Public Aid, lived out at Holton Homes, and I used to have to go out and see her every week. She wanted to talk, really. I knew her sons in high school, and really I would go out and give her a B12 shot once a week. Once time I remember I tried to get her to let me send the nurse out for this shot. "No, Dr. Theobald, I've got to see you." So, I would go out and sit there and talk with her for half-hour or so, but I only got paid for two calls out of the four I would make.[170]

The proportion of medical costs paid by third-party payers (both public and private) rose after World War II, between 1960 and 1975 rising from 45 to 67 percent.[171] Since virtually all insurance packages paid on the basis of fee-for-service, physicians had a significant incentive to increase both services and charges. With payers determining rates of reimbursement from usual, customary, or prevailing rates, according to Paul Starr, "Fees began to soar when some young doctors, who had no record of charges, billed at unprecedented levels and were paid. When their older colleagues saw what was possible, they, too, raised their fees, and soon what was customary was higher than ever before."[172] Inflation of medical charges was also stimulated by the rising cost of medical education and a newly significant expense, medical malpractice insurance. Nonetheless, it is clear that medicine's increasing reputation as a highly paid occupation also was a growing factor in occupational choice for a new generation of doctors.

Physicians interviewed for this study—particularly general practitioners—viewed younger doctors as more mercenary than they had been themselves. Paul Theobald said, "They're good doctors, technically and all this. I hate to say it, but I think a lot of them are in it for the . . . money."[173] Russell Oyer amplified on this theme:

When I went into medicine, you hung up your shingle and you did it on your own. You were it! You were not going to be paid a salary. You were not going to have any benefits. You were a private and solo practice. Solo practice, of course, is going by the board now. Maybe that's good, I think. . . . Solo practice is probably a poor way to practice medicine from the point of view of stress and all that sort of thing. But I think that young physicians . . . are asking questions . . . these days—you know, "How much time will I have with my family? How much can I earn? How much vacation will I get? How many nights a week can I be off and away from the telephone?" I think these kinds of questions . . . didn't occur to us. Whether we were just naïve . . . you expected that you were going to be . . . tied to your patients and that was your first loyalty and family or whatever came after that.[174]

Oyer's statement reveals both disapproval of self-interest and greed among younger practitioners and what he perceived as the drift toward contract practice—anathema to the organized medicine of his own youth. Both Oyer and Theobald straddled a moral divide—on the one hand, viewing themselves as businessmen and, on the other, perceiving the physician's role as essentially and appropriately altruistic, rather than profit driven.

Relationships with Patients

The physicians informing this study experienced the absolute historical zenith of patient dependence on doctors. Unlike their nineteenth-century forebears, they did not have to compete with a host of alternative or amateur healers. They also did not face the challenge, encountered by their early twentieth-century colleagues, of having their knowledge outstrip their ability to intervene effectively. They agreed that patients tended to follow doctors' orders. Indeed, Paul Theobald said, "Most of my patients were very good. If I told them to sit down and drop dead, they would sit down and drop dead."[175]

Informants agreed that the relationship between general practitioners and their patients was more satisfying than between specialists and their patients. According to Harold Shinall, when he was a GP, "I liked the people and the community, and I really liked the practice. I missed it a great deal after I got into my residency. It was not impersonal, yet you just saw patients that were referred to you, and then you'd see some others. That was it."[176] Russell Oyer commented about increasing specialization:

I guess one of my chief concerns has been the human part of medicine, the personal part of medicine and how much does that mean to a patient? How much importance is it to a patient? Do we lose something if medicine becomes much more impersonal? I think some specialization, I think the way we manage patients with computers and numbers and all sorts of stuff . . . I think . . . as we learn more and as we do more, and as we fragment all the approaches to patients, somebody does this and somebody does that, I think the approach becomes less personal. The patient, I think, does get the impression, "Hey, I'm really just kind of a number here." I always used to have a strong feeling that the GP was the kind of person who needed to keep all that put together for the patient.[177]

These accounts sketch the image of the normative family doctor, which was shared by lay informants. That kindly physician knew the family well, dealt with the individual patient holistically, and was different from the specialist, for whom scientific knowledge, technical competence, and efficiency were of primary importance.

That family doctor deserved the complete trust of his patients—a trust that was betrayed, from the physician's perspective, by the threat of malpractice litigation. Harold Shinall remembered of his early days in practice in the mid-1930s, "I was practicing several months in Gibson City without any insurance at all. Even at that time, I wouldn't drive my car around the block without insurance. There was a salesman from the Medical Protection Organization who drove through from Springfield one day and stopped in my office and asked if I would be interested in any insurance. I talked to him awhile and he sold me a policy. That was my first insurance plan."[178] According to other informants, malpractice litigation came to McLean County late, compared to other areas. Loren Boon recalled, "When I first started, why . . . no lawyer would take a malpractice suit here in McLean County. Patients had to go over to Peoria."[179] Nonetheless, after the 1960s, the threat of a malpractice charge hovered over doctors and affected the way they practiced medicine. As Russell Oyer said:

INFORMANT: I definitely worried about malpractice suits. I think that stimulated my effort to really make good notes in the office. . . . I became more concerned about being sure that any contact I had with a patient was recorded.

INTERVIEWER: So, not necessarily any particular event, just the whole climate.

INFORMANT: Well, knowing colleagues for example who were sued, and being very dismayed when a colleague that I respected was sued for causes that I thought were totally unjust. Things that had no bearing on competency at all. That's one of the problems that you have. You know, an obstetrician getting sued for a very difficult breach delivery, for example.[180]

Nurses also perceived a change in the atmosphere of care after the increase of malpractice litigation. Alice Swift said, "I thought it was terrible. I felt like you couldn't be yourself. You couldn't be relaxed like you once were. . . . The thing that directed your care-giving was whether or not there would be a lawsuit, not whether the patient was getting the kind of care he should get."[181]

From the physician's perspective, the litigious atmosphere introduced an element of suspicion that had not been previously present in the doctor-patient relationship. A. Edward Livingston attributed this to popular "health advisors":

> It is truly unfortunate . . . that the physician's greatest weapon against illness, whether organic or functional, namely, belief in the healing power possessed by the practitioner, has been greatly diminished by the continuous encouragement of so-called popular "health advisers" for patients to challenge all decisions made for their treatment. Various medical mistakes are cited by these advisers to emphasize their position. Certainly errors do occur, but these incidences are now magnified by publicity so that it would appear that most medical activities are fraught with improper care.[182]

These lay "advisers," speaking to the public from the popular media, by the 1970s arguably took over the traditional role of "old wives," challenging physicians' authority and costing them both respect and money. Alternatively, Loren Boon suggested that lawyers stimulated malpractice suits for financial reasons, saying, "I think they probably got more trial lawyers here [in McLean County], and then they decided to keep some of the money themselves [rather] than refer them [the patients to lawyers in Peoria]."[183] It is noteworthy that physician informants commented neither on rising costs nor rising expectations of health care as stimuli for malpractice suits. It is also significant that lay informants did not mention medical malpractice at all. Although malpractice has become a dominant element of community health culture for practitioners, it is less important to consumers than cost, quality, and relationship issues.

Conclusions

The most significant change in twentieth-century Western health culture was the inflation of expectations regarding health and medicine on the part of both practitioners and the general public. In the years following World War II, dazzling new biomedical discoveries and interventions were so frequent that they became commonplace. In the 1950s, 1960s, and 1970s, there seemed to be no obstacle that could not be overcome—no killer that could not be vanquished. New drugs undermined the powers of infection and mental illness; new surgical techniques and technologies redrew the boundaries of possibility between survival and mortality. Biomedicine made the covers of glossy magazines, headlined major newspapers and national television news programs, and comprised an ever-expanding portion of federal and private grant funding.

As the agents, gatekeepers, and interpreters of these changes, physicians represented them. The white lab coats or surgical greens, firm hands, and incisive decisions of media doctors including Kildare, Ben Casey, and Hawkeye Pierce merged science with altruism and attributed to physicians the heroic, yet human, (white male) face of Western progress. Sufferers eagerly relinquished traditional responsibility for health-care decision making, relying on doctors to solve their problems. No intervention has been too radical, no price too high, if the life of the premature baby, the sick child, the injured spouse, or the failing parent could be saved. Laypeople have demanded the impossible of physicians; physicians have expected the impossible of themselves. At the same time, in McLean County as elsewhere in the United States, doctors accepted the rewards and demanded the trust attending their new image. Thus, they became both eager participants in the transformations described by Paul Starr and targets of a new shift in health culture that has discovered the physician's feet of clay without being able satisfactorily to replace him.

This chapter has not discussed the broad-based critique of physicians and biomedicine that began with works such as the Boston Women's Health Book Collective's *Our Bodies, Ourselves* (1971) and Ivan Illich's *Medical Nemesis* (1976) largely because none of the oral history informants for this research referred to it.[184] In their 1990s interviews for this book, McLean County physicians expressed regret about changes in the doctor-patient relationship and nostalgia for by-gone medical authority, but did not express concern about biomedicine, in general, or either the American or the local health-care delivery systems, in particular. Similarly, nurses observed physicians' dominance of health care and deplored increasing specialization and bureaucratization, but were uncritical of biomedicine. Consumers expressed growing dependence on doctors, while displaying both greater sophistication about medical theories and therapies and concern about access to and cost of services for which they felt an ongoing need. All informants contributed to a collective discourse viewing biomedical progress as axiomatic and developments including rising health-care prices and erosion of what is latterly viewed as the traditional relationship between physicians and patients as inevitable byproducts of an otherwise positive history.

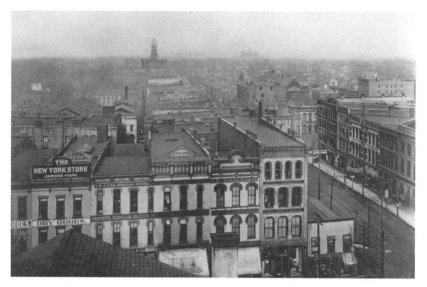

Bloomington, Illinois, 1896. By the end of the twentieth century, Bloomington was a prosperous, growing Midwestern city, which required—and was represented by—its organized medical profession and new hospitals. (Martin A. Wyckoff and Greg Koos, ed. *The Illustrated History of McLean County,* McLean County Historical Society, 1982, p. 227. Courtesy of the McLean County Historical Society.)

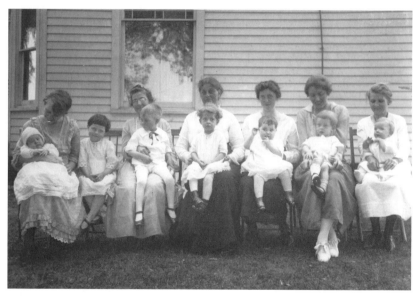

McLean County mothers and children, ca. 1920. The Home Bureau brought university-based information about home management to McLean County's women beginning in 1918. Particularly eager for this information were farm wives, photographed here with their clean, well-fed and well-dressed children. (Courtesy of the Clara Brian Collection, McLean County Historical Society.)

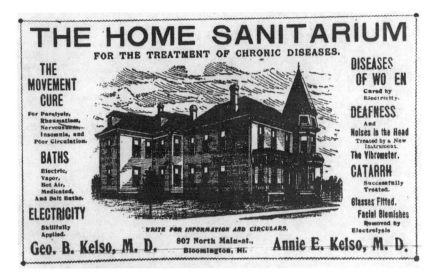

Advertisement for the Kelso Sanitarium, 1897. Catering to McLean County's prosperous residents, the private Home Sanitarium offered both medical and spa treatments for those willing to pay. Barred from privileges in the county's nonprofit hospitals, homeopaths George and Annie Kelso were also able to exercise their surgical and obstetrical specialties in their own facility. (*Pantagraph,* February 8, 1897, p. 4. Courtesy of the McLean County Historical Society.)

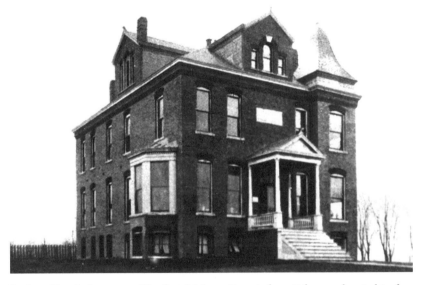

Brokaw Hospital, ca. 1900. The first McLean County hospitals were located in former private homes. Although inconvenient and often inappropriate for their new functions, these "domestic era" facilities offered patients comforting homelike atmospheres and dispelled traditional fear of hospitalization. (Courtesy of the McLean County Historical Society.)

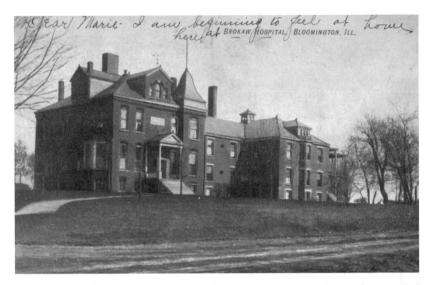

Brokaw Hospital, 1907. With repeated additions, Bloomington hospitals expanded beyond their original domestic structures and became more institutional in form, functions, and culture. It is thus ironic that, with long average lengths of stay, patients came to "feel at home" in them. (Courtesy of the McLean County Historical Society.)

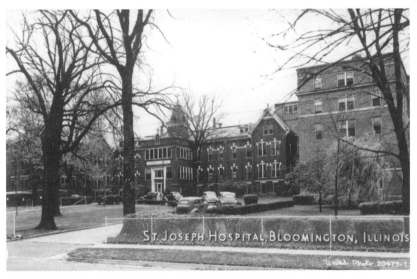

St. Joseph's Hospital, ca. 1940. By World War II, McLean County's hospitals had become large, specialized institutions providing medical intervention for the sick rather than the charitable room, board, and nursing care offered by their pre–World War I forbears. (Courtesy of the McLean County Historical Society.)

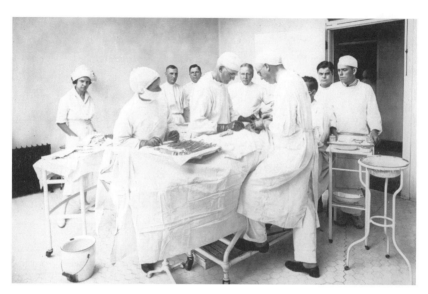

Surgery, Brokaw Hospital, ca. 1922. This photograph illustrates the long transition between antiseptic and aseptic surgery. Note the inconsistent use of masks and gloves, as well as the open door and transom in Brokaw Hospital's operating room. (Courtesy of the McLean County Historical Society.)

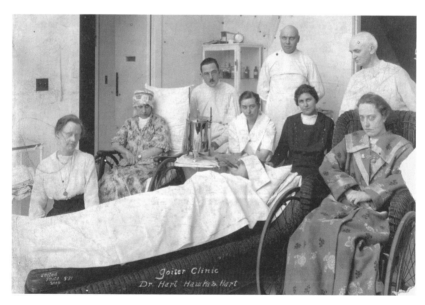

Goiter patients, doctors, and nurses, 1922–23. During the interwar years, Bloomington became a center for surgical treatment of goiter, attracting both patients and new surgical specialists and winning an international reputation for a procedure that declined in use once iodization of salt became routine. (Courtesy of the McLean County Historical Society.)

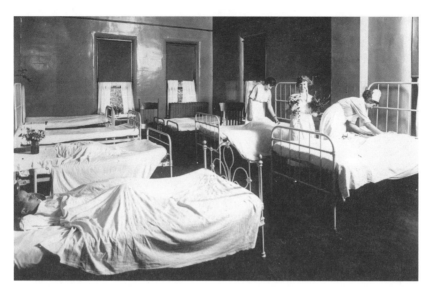

Brokaw Hospital children's ward, ca. 1922. After World War I, McLean County's hospitals expanded to serve populations that had previously been cared for and treated at home, including children. The new practice of removing tonsils for preventative purposes swelled the numbers of children who were hospitalized. (Courtesy of the McLean County Historical Society.)

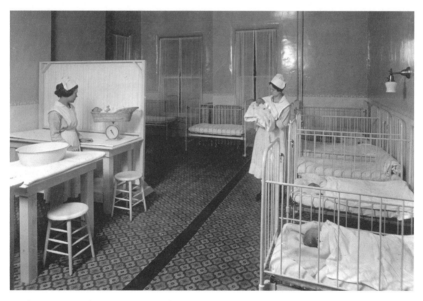

Brokaw Hospital maternity ward, ca. 1922. Increasing numbers of McLean County mothers chose to deliver in hospitals after about 1920. Brokaw Hospital's nursery included both a traditional homelike atmosphere and attention to new concerns, such as the weights of newborns. (Courtesy of the McLean County Historical Society.)

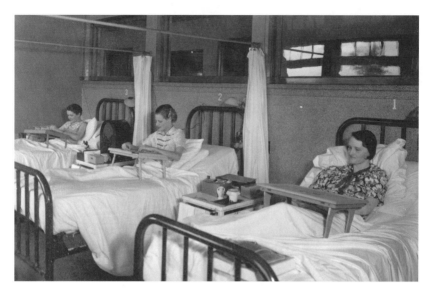

Patients, McLean County Tuberculosis Sanitarium, ca. 1930s. Sanitation treatment involved stays sometimes lasting for several years, extended bed rest, inculcation of healthy personal habits, and exposure to fresh air. (Courtesy of the McLean County Historical Society.)

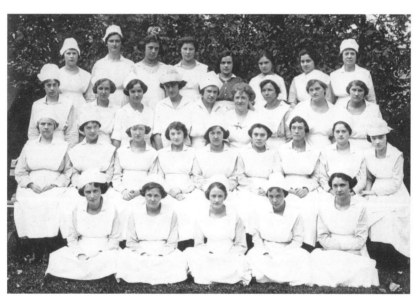

Brokaw Hospital Nursing School class, 1915. By the second decade of the twentieth century, McLean County's hospital nursing schools attracted large numbers of local young women who performed the daily work of the hospitals, as graduates did private duty nursing in homes and hospital rooms, and spread the "gospel" of biomedicine to patients throughout the County. (Courtesy of the McLean County Historical Society.)

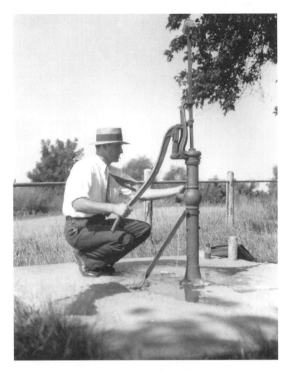

Illinois Department of Public Health water inspection, ca. 1925. County health departments undertook an increasing range of inspection tasks in the mid-twentieth century. This McLean County official is testing the quality of well water. (Courtesy of the Clara Brian Collection, McLean County Historical Society.)

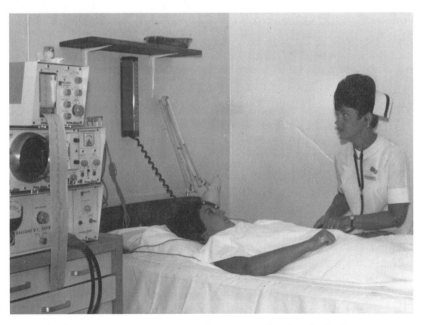

Nurse checking monitors, ca. 1970s. By the 1970s, technology had taken over many of the tasks previously performed by nurses, whereas nursing had changed to include expertise in the use of medical technology. (Courtesy of BroMenn Healthcare.)

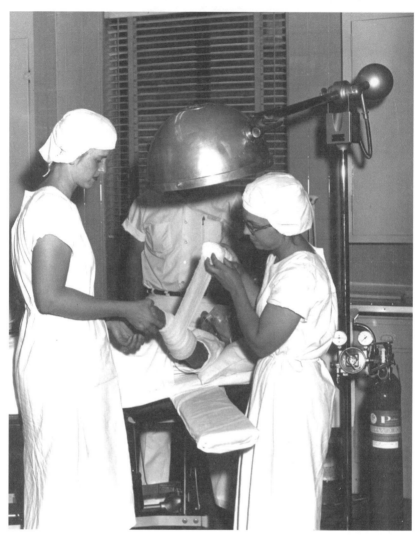

Emergency room care, ca. 1970s. Emergency rooms were new in McLean County after World War II. Here, the patient receives both hands-on treatment from multiple attendants and oxygen in a care environment increasingly set up to respond to diverse injuries and other health crises. (Courtesy of BroMenn Healthcare.)

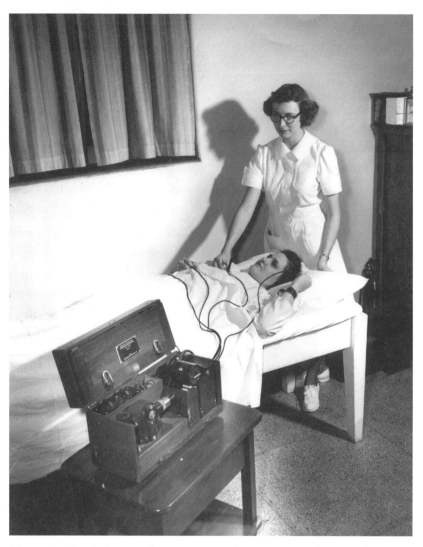

Mennonite Hospital nurse administering EKG test, 1950s. Mid-twentieth century McLean County hospitals housed both the growing range of medical technologies and new occupations supporting their use. (Courtesy of BroMenn Healthcare.)

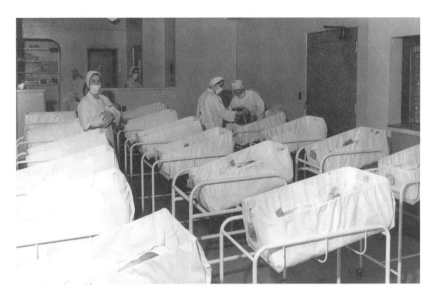

Post–World War II nursery. Rising choice of hospital delivery coupled with the baby boom led to bulging maternity wards and nurseries in McLean County, as elsewhere. This photograph also illustrates increasing attempts to limit newborns' exposure to germs. (Courtesy of BroMenn Healthcare.)

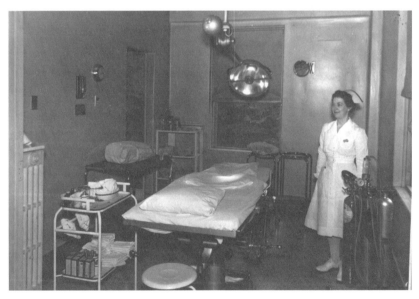

Hospital delivery room, ca. 1940s. By the 1940s, hospital births were becoming the norm in McLean County, for reasons including physician convenience, quick response to emergency complications, and concentrated access to technology. Hospital delivery rooms contrasted dramatically with traditional birth environments in mothers' homes. (Courtesy of BroMenn Healthcare.)

5. An Ounce of Prevention

Public Health Services

The history of public health is underscored by tension between individual rights and needs and actions leaders determine to be in the public interest. Mid-twentieth-century historians told a story of sanitation and other prevention activities defeating contagious diseases, but more recent scholars have questioned the ways state, professional, gender, and class power have been used to control the less powerful.[1] Although it cannot be denied that in the United States during the past century average lifespan has lengthened and some ailments have become less common, it is also arguable that organized public health and professional medicine have followed the old community developers' adage to shoot anything that flies and claim anything that falls— taking wholesale credit for changes they may or may not have influenced. Tuberculosis was declining in incidence and severity before communities built sanitariums to isolate sufferers and streptomycin offered a cure; infant mortality was dropping before women started having prenatal checkups and giving birth in hospitals. Furthermore, it is legitimate to question the means toward "progress" and the outcomes for both advocates of those means and the general public.

What Dorothy Porter calls "collective action in relation to the health of populations" has always been determined by theories of disease causation and ideas about the ways human beings relate to the natural environment.[2] As we have seen, nineteenth-century McLean County residents attempted to prevent disease with approaches ranging from isolation or exclusion of sufferers to development of urban public water and sewerage systems. At the turn of the twentieth century, germ theories subsumed and reinterpreted miasmatic explanations for disease causation, stimulating shifting social and individual responses to a newly dangerous environment, whose worst dangers were detectible only in a laboratory—a world where the handshake of a stranger, a mother's breath, or a glass of fresh well water could carry lethal infection.[3] Thus, public health initiatives, which in the late nineteenth century took the form of public works, in the twentieth century had as much to do with changing individual and household hygiene practices as they did with continuing collective approaches to disease prevention.

Progressive Era public health activities also radiated both a new sense of human power over natural and social forces and concern about morbidity and mortality exemplified by statistics that were kept in increasing quantity and quality at federal, state, and local levels. As Lynne Curry observes, whereas early health reformers had focused on cities, with their concentrations of industry and new immigrants, in the twentieth century awareness grew that rural areas, previously considered havens of physical and moral strength, were actually less healthy, according to many indicators, than cities.[4] McLean County, with its mixture of agriculture, heavy industry, educational institutions, and prosperous leadership, developed health and social services addressing both urban and rural challenges. As was true of public health initiatives elsewhere, these efforts were class related, recognizing both the relationship between poverty and disease and the responsibility of social elites to improve matters. They were also gendered, emphasizing the role of mothers in maintaining child health and reducing infant mortality—the touchstone of local and national progress.[5] In addition, they projected a growing local consensus that government should provide some health and human services, at the same time revealing the tension created by official public health enforcement powers.

This chapter considers selected twentieth-century McLean County public health activities, including the battle against tuberculosis; the establishment of a Cooperative Extension Service Home Bureau that concentrated its efforts on the health of rural women and children; and the expansion of county public health infrastructure and administration. In addition to evidence provided by local records, the chapter is informed by the memories of four oral history interviewees: Dr. W. L. Dillman (born in 1920), a dentist who worked for the McLean County Health Department between 1948 and 1956; Margaret Esposito (born in 1923), who served as McLean County's home bureau adviser for twenty-seven years; Jane Tinsley (born in 1924), who worked as a public health nurse in the county for thirty-five years; and Ben Boyd (born in 1927), who was director of environmental health for the McLean County Health Department between 1966 and 1989. The advantage of these perspectives is that they offer firsthand accounts of local public health activities and relationships; the disadvantage is that they present only the views of convinced advocates.

Fighting Tuberculosis

At the turn of the twentieth century, awareness that tuberculosis was contagious was new; after Robert Koch's discovery of the tubercle bacillus in 1882, there was widespread determination to convince the public that the disease was transmitted from person to person and to develop community responses to TB. The antituberculosis movement, in the United States initiated with foundation of the Pennsylvania Society for the Prevention of Tuberculosis, spread quickly to Illinois, where the disease remained a leading cause of death.[6] Advocates used "the new visual culture of advertising to sell their gospel of prevention," making theirs "the first mass health education campaign in American history."[7] Success of the movement was reflected in the hugely popular annual Christmas Seals campaigns, started in 1908, which raised an enormous amount of money to fight TB. It also stimulated local initiatives, including development of sites for administration of the open-air cure, then thought to be the best treatment for the disease. For example, in 1906 the Chicago Tuberculosis Institute established an open-air camp for poor sufferers living in congested areas of the city, and the Illinois Homeopathic Medical Association founded an open-air sanitarium at Buffalo Rock in LaSalle County.[8] The movement also stimulated policies, ranging from local antispitting ordinances to state legislation funding community sanatoria.

In addition to the positive influence of fresh air, sanatoria optimized separation of the sick from the well and control of sufferers' behavior. The 1900 Illinois State Board of Health's recommendation for sanatoria to the governor emphasized this aspect of institutional care:

> A patient outside the sanatorium is disinclined to accept the yoke of a rigid and severe discipline. In the sanatorium nothing is left to his caprice, he never receives recommendations more or less vague, but rest, exercise and alimentation are measured and even the cough is disciplined. This almost military education creates an influence very favorable to the evolution of recovery and assures success of therapeutic means, and the patients rapidly acquire habits of hygienic discipline which they continue in their homes.[9]

The interest of McLean County's medical community in the battle against tuberculosis was stimulated at the 1904 annual meeting of the Illinois State Medical Society in Bloomington.[10] In March 1907 the McLean County Medical Society called a public meeting, where Dr. J. W. Pettit of the Ottawa Tent Colony argued,

> Much harm is done by calling tuberculosis a contagious disease. It is not conta-
> gious as smallpox, etc., but is communicable. It is only feebly contagious under
> certain conditions which can easily be avoided, i.e., by destruction of all sputa.
> The uncontrolled patient only is a menace. Sanatoria, properly conducted, are
> the safest places possible because of control had over patients. Physicians and
> nurses at Sanatoria are practically free from disease. The great work of Sanatoria
> is in what they teach the patient, and through him the public, towards limiting
> the spread of disease.[11]

Concerned citizens formed the McLean County Anti-tuberculosis Society, which supported passage of a state law permitting counties to levy a tax to maintain local sanatoria.[12] Such a law, named the Glackin Act after the state senator who proposed it, was enacted in 1908.[13]

McLean County was among the first in Illinois to take advantage of this law, passing a referendum in 1916 to build a sanitarium. Meanwhile, the Anti-tuberculosis Society hired a visiting nurse, provided free advice, and carried on a public education campaign.[14] Constructed on a "pleasant rise" north of Normal at a cost of $125,000, Fairview Sanitarium opened in August 1919. From its original thirty-four beds, it was enlarged to accommodate a total of forty-nine within the main building. During the 1920s, "three new rooms, six beds, and a cottage for colored people" were added.[15] A nurses' residence and superintendent's apartment were also built.[16] These facilities were justi-fied by continued incidence of tuberculosis (revealed through increasingly systematic screening), with Bloomington reporting 100 new cases in 1920, 111 in 1921, 109 in 1922, and 131 in 1923. Incidence dropped to 93 in 1924 and 82 in 1925, but rose again to 202 in 1926 and 199 in 1927.[17]

In addition to inpatient treatment, a free clinic for TB sufferers opened in 1918 in downtown Bloomington. Medical Director Dr. Bernice Curry, who also served as sanitarium director, and the tuberculosis nurse, Mrs. Brett, saw 333 cases in 1918 alone. The TB nurse also made home visits; her travel expenses were paid by the County's Anti-tuberculosis Society.[18] In addition to offering outpatient treatment, the clinic, which moved to Fairview in 1932, diagnosed new cases and provided follow-up care to patients discharged from the Sanitarium. A 1954 account indicated both continuation of clinic services and changes in diagnostic techniques: "With increasing emphasis on chest X-rays as a means of case finding, attendance at the clinics gradually increased until in 1946 it was decided to again hold the clinic downtown. This was made possible by the purchase of X-ray equipment by the McLean

County Tuberculosis Association with funds obtained by the sale of Christmas Seals. . . . In the last year, 1952–53, 4,914 x-rays were taken."[19]

Sanitarium treatment changed over time. Initially, Fairview patients occupied unheated rooms with open windows throughout the year. "The fresh air treatment as it was practiced in those early years brought much hardship to both patients and nurses in the winter weather. In 1930–31, heat was installed in the wards, and since that time windows have been kept open only in rest hours and at night, making it possible to give much better care to the patients and adding much to their comfort."[20] Sanitarium care was free to McLean County residents. However, because it often lasted for several years, inpatient treatment had a huge impact on people's lives—regardless of whether they were cured, continued to suffer, or died from TB. A sanitarium stay was a public announcement of a diagnosis of tuberculosis. This affected workers' ability to get and keep jobs, because employers were concerned about both the worker's productivity and his or her potential danger to other employees. Jane Tinsley, who began work as a public health nurse in the 1950s, commented, "There were people who hid the fact that they had [tuberculosis] or thought they had it, because they could hardly give up their jobs . . . to go into the sanitarium."[21] Indeed, even the possibility of TB influenced people's employment opportunities. Ruth Carpenter worked as a nurse at Bloomington's General Electric plant between the 1950s and 1970s. She handled accidents and health screening, reporting, "We took chest X-rays in those days. Everybody got a chest X-ray."[22] Public acknowledgement of infection affected marriage opportunities, because the belief that TB was inherited lingered and women sufferers were thought unable safely to bear children. Indeed, TB was one of the few legal justifications for therapeutic abortion.[23] During the interwar years, sanitarium treatment marginalized African Americans, who were segregated in the "cottage" out back. A sanitarium stay was analogous to a prison sentence; sufferers were held for a term determined by medical authorities and, as we have seen, required to follow rigorous discipline in uncomfortable conditions. Perhaps most importantly, it stigmatized sufferers even after effective treatments were developed.

Declining from the early years of the century, mortality from tuberculosis plummeted after the introduction of streptomycin in the late 1940s. Nonetheless, Fairview Sanitarium received county tax funds until 1965, when it closed due to lack of patients.[24] According to Ben Boyd, who was appointed director of environmental health for the McLean County Health Department in 1966, "We still had TB patients . . . The TB treatment occurred prior to 1966, so we were not hospitalizing but very, very few TB patients at the time. . . . Oh yeah, but they were under treatment though. TB was there. TB has always been there."[25] After this time, county residents needing inpatient treatment for tuberculosis received tax support for care in other institutions in Illinois.

Home Bureau

Progressive Era belief in germs as enemies to individual and public health, on the one hand, and science as the solution to most problems, on the other, influenced the ways reformers thought about homes and homemakers. It was no longer possible to leave science to men in the public arena, because germs did not discriminate between public and private.[26] People became ill and received treatment and care at home; infants were born—and too often died—at home. And mothers, as primary caregivers and health-care decision makers, were the pivotal figures on whom outcomes—illness prevention, recovery, or death—depended. However, because mothers were also women whose rationality and knowledge were questioned, a variety of approaches were developed to teach science-based health information and middle-class home management and childcare techniques to women from diverse backgrounds. The domestic science movement offered academic preparation to middle-class white women.[27] The settlement house and visiting nurse movements provided health advice to poor, often foreign, urban women.[28] And the home extension services, sparked by the Country Life movement and funded by the 1914 Smith-Lever Act, took university home economics information to rural homemakers.[29] Run by and for women, the Cooperative Extension Service Home Bureau constituted both a gendered approach to reform and uplift and, as a voluntary club-based activity, an interesting contrast to male-dominated antituberculosis and public health services, which were prescriptive and enforcement oriented.

Extension came early to McLean County—in part, because of food shortages during World War I. A local heiress and McLean County's food chairman, Mrs. Spencer Ewing, observed "the lack of rural organization through which to accomplish the food conservation work."[30] She met with Isabel Bevier, founding head of the University of Illinois' Department of Household Science, and embraced the idea of bringing a trained home economist to the county to work with area families. At the same time, in the long tradition of Midwestern women's reform organizations, she spearheaded the development of the voluntary Home Improvement Association of McLean County.[31] The association, organized on a township basis, required members to pay annual dues of one dollar; by 1918 there were both 1,500 members eager to participate in educational activities and a local match for the $1,500 that the

University of Illinois Cooperative Extension Service was prepared to pay a home adviser.[32] That June, Clara R. Brian (1876–1970) began the work she would continue, with a brief interruption, until she retired in 1945.[33] Like most other Illinois home advisers, Brian was single and had a college degree in home economics. She also exemplified the modern woman who could both bake bread and drive a car, demonstrate new labor-saving household devices and cuddle a toddler.[34]

Appealing to mainly rural, educated, socially aspiring women, home bureau programming emphasized practical training based on principles of modern science and efficiency. It presumed that women, "once they were properly instructed in the fundamentals of preventive health care and household hygiene, stood ready and able to take whatever steps were necessary to elevate their own health standards as well as those of their communities."[35] In 1926 Brian wrote, "Home Bureau Work in McLean County is getting on a good basis. The women are beginning to believe in the organization and to see its possibilities. The social side of Home Bureau work to them is worth all its costs, as it is the only organization financed by Federal Funds for women; and, next to the church, the Adviser considers it the most important organization for women that has ever been organized."[36]

By 1919 McLean County's home bureau was offering programs in five areas of study: conservation and consumption; health and sanitation; accounting; equipment and household management; and textiles. Information on home nursing was provided to individuals on demand.[37] Brian and her secretary, Agnes Huth, offered practical demonstrations to groups of women in small communities distributed around the geographically largest county in Illinois, traveling its 125 miles of paved roads, 350 miles of gravel roads, and 1,542 miles of dirt roads in a car donated by Bloomington's Rotary Club. A new driver, Brian had more to contend with than her lack of familiarity with the Ford's starting mechanism, as her account of her first journey indicates:

Monday, July 15, [1918,] was a memorable day. The meeting place was Bellflower—thirty-five miles away. There were no paved roads—just dirt. The County tuberculosis nurse, Mrs. Earl Cooper went with me. The car was a Ford Coupe, 1918 model. With fear and trembling, we started on our journey to the southeast corner of the County. We hadn't gone far until it started to rain. The top was down. It had to come up. The shower was soon over; then we came to a part of the road under construction and a bridge was not there. It was necessary to drive down a steep embankment and up on the other side. Impossible? How did we know until we tried. Down and up without a mishap, with perhaps a little more confidence in driving ability. A little more driving and we were at Bellflower. Meeting over, ready to start to Bloomington, but the car would not start. A man came, by request, from the garage, gave a few whirls to the handle in front and we were on our way home. Everything seemed to be going fine. When we were a mile east of Downs, the car stopped. Well, what is the matter now? Nothing except there was no gas in the tank, and even Fords in those days would not continue on their way without gas. Gas stations were not open after five o'clock that summer. A quarter mile walk and I was at the home of an obliging farmer who sold me five gallons of gas and delivered it to the tank. This was our last interruption and we arrive in Bloomington tired but with a lot of good experience out of my first day with a car.[38]

Between June 1918 and April 1919, Brian traveled 4,654 miles in the home bureau car and 1,300 miles by rail to meet with township unit members.[39]

Brian's demonstrations emphasized health education. Food preparation and canning were taught with hygiene foremost in mind. Recommendations for kitchen layout and equipment considered the health of homemakers and family members. Even textile demonstrations related to the healthfulness and comfort of clothing. For example, accompanying a recipe for laundry starch was the comment, "Since starch closes the pores of the fabric, a starched fabric is hotter in summer than an un-starched one. Young children's clothing should not be starched in hot weather."[40] However, Brian also organized programs that focused on specific contemporary health issues. Lynn Curry writes of the emphasis on fly eradication in the early twentieth century, "Although they were an inevitable presence in agrarian life, in the wake of the energetic rural public health reform efforts that were launched in this era, flies had now become a potent symbol of a farm mother's inexcusable negligence. The presence of flies in the farm home could no longer be tolerated, particularly by those women who were becoming increasingly sensitive to critiques about the apparent backwardness of country life."[41] Brian extended her concern to other vermin as well, launching a campaign in county schools in 1920 with the title, "Bat the Rat, Swat the Fly, Rouse mit the Mouse." Teachers and mothers worked with schoolchildren to present short plays on this subject, and the home bureau offered a five-dollar prize to the township reporting the largest number of rodents killed. "Twenty-three townships reported 40,372 rats and mice killed."[42]

Extension's most enduring work with children came through organization of 4-H clubs. Brian started seventeen clubs for girls in McLean County in 1918 that emphasized normative feminine roles. The girls learned domestic skills used by farm wives, including sewing, canning, bread making, and poultry management. Sewing was particularly popular. In 1925 McLean County's nineteen clothing clubs had 212 members who made 815 garments, made-over 53 garments, mended 245 garments, and darned 220 stockings.[43] Club members had the opportunity to demonstrate, compete, and be recognized at county and state fairs. In the second half of the twentieth century, the county's 4–H clubs continued to mix practical domestic skills, health education, and reform. For example, its 1980s "Quilts for Infants with AIDS" project involved girls in sewing quilts, delivering the quilts to Chicago agencies, "And on the bus we had video on AIDS and mothers went with them, so there was some education there. And to do all that we put together a networking committee of home economics teachers and homemakers in the County and the Health Department."[44]

Like the home advisers who took her place, Brian worked extensively with other community groups. During the 1918 influenza epidemic, for example, Brian reported that home bureau members "joined with women of other organizations to help care for the sick":

> Monday, October 14, I began work as dietitian of the Emergency Hospital set up in the Bloomington Country Club. A fine group of women joined with me in preparing and serving food to the sick and to all the doctors, nurses, and nurses' aids who so willingly gave of their time and strength to this emergency work. The Home Improvement Association units of both farm and home organizations furnished most of the food. All kinds of vegetables, milk, butter, chickens, eggs, etc. came in abundance from all parts of the County. During the two weeks, 3,600 meals were prepared and served. One hundred and fourteen patients were cared for by the doctors and nursing staff. Four of the patients died; only two of those who worked at the hospital took the disease, and they had light cases. Again, the organization had proven to the communities the value of a rural people organized.[45]

Brian designed Fairview Sanitarium's kitchen. She also planned menus for Bloomington's Girls' Industrial Home and consulted on time and motion management for the local Young Women's Christian Association's (YWCA) food service.[46] In 1920 she worked with the public clinic and the Red Cross to provide physicals for school children.[47] She actively advocated establishment of the McLean County Health Department in 1945, the year she retired.

Brian had a hobby that offers a useful window into county quality of life during the interwar period. She was a photographer who took her camera to work. Her photographs document work, play, education, transportation, farms, and homes—both inside and out, as well as suggesting Brian's professional interests and concerns. They show household equipment—washing machines, gas stoves, built-in iceboxes, dumbwaiters, and plumbing. They depict ideal and substandard kitchen layouts. They illustrate then-modern indoor bathrooms and crumbling backyard privies. One depicts inspection of well water by a representative from the Illinois Department of Public Health. Most of all, they put human faces on ordinary McLean County residents of the time—particularly women and children who otherwise would be remembered only in family albums. Brian's photographs were collected and published by Margaret Esposito, who became McLean County's third home adviser in 1970 and was also interviewed for this study.[48]

Esposito's career development in some ways echoed Progressive Era interest in applying laboratory science to homemaking. It also illustrates challenges and choices facing middle-class women in the mid-twentieth century. Born in Bloomington in 1923, Esposito planned to go to college. In high school, "I took all the science that they offered and all the math that they offered and language. . . . It was what I was going to do was go on to school. . . . But I didn't even know there was an area of home economics, which was what I finally finished up getting my degree in. . . . I knew it was there, but that was not any part of the learning that I was going to be involved in. . . . Originally I thought I was going to be a pharmacist. Chemistry was something I enjoyed."[49] Her education was interrupted when she married a career military officer in 1942. Subsequently, she took college classes whenever the opportunity arose.

> I'd come back here and go to Illinois State Normal University. By the time my husband died [in 1960] I had only student teaching to do to finish a degree. . . . That was my bachelor's degree in home economics. And I did home economics because I knew it was going to be a segmented kind of education. I could not continue with scientific education. You have to have that consecutively. It has to be in a block and all of my science courses would transfer into home economics. And so that's where I ended up. . . . I liked the subject area. I was keeping house. It was meaningful to me. I was rearing kids, you know. And so that was a fit. But it certainly would not have been a career choice that I would have made under different . . . circumstances.[50]

She expected to teach high school, but could not find a job. Meanwhile, she took graduate courses and looked after her children.

> My daughter joined a 4–H club in town. And they called me in, saying would I volunteer to help with it. . . . and one of the things I had to do was attend a training school down at the Extension office. . . . And when the Adviser got some place in the presentation, she said, "Well, now, we will not be doing as much this year, because I don't have an assistant." And so when the class was over, I went up and said, "What is it that qualifies you for employment as an assistant?" And she said, "Home Economics degree." And I said, "You know, . . . I'm finishing my masters. Is this a possibility?" And I think within a month I had the job.[51]

Esposito began her work as an assistant to the 4–H program. Then, eight years later, "When the expanded foods and nutrition program came out, which was a federally funded program for the poor in nutrition, that was my job." When her boss retired in 1970, Esposito moved into the adviser's position.[52]

Like Clara Brian, Esposito saw extension as having an important role in health education. For example, she said that people "always had a great desire for food information. They weren't as crazy about knowing about nutrition, but you know, a good teacher doesn't have to stop with what they want. Give them what they need. It's like caster oil that Grandmother gave. . . . And then you could lead them gently over because we'd always had a specialist in health."[53] In addition to delivering their own programs, however, extension staff also worked closely with the county health department, beginning with its establishment in 1945. Esposito explained,

> There was a great feeling of need. Now, there had been some, there had been a physician who was a public health person here. There had been tuberculosis nurses. . . . But there was a strong need . . . for better sanitation, nutrition . . . that there be a health department here. And so McLean County was not the first [county] health department, but it was relatively early in the size county it was. . . . So . . . we always had that as a resource and . . . the Health Department might share with us, you see. . . . You always considered [the Director of Nurses] in program planning—what is it that she thought the community was in need of? We did a lot of work on nutrition related to health, on the nutrition related to heart disease, on epidemics when you'd have something coming out in that area. . . . [You'd] encourage immunization clinics sometimes, you know, gave them help.[54]

Extension also encouraged water inspection and testing. "We constantly networked with Health Department to know . . . where we should be sending [rural residents] to take their water supplies. And we even had the sample kits sometimes in our office early, and then transferred all that later to the Health Department to take care of."[55] The quality of extension's relationship with the health department depended on who was in charge; at one point, staff changes generated "a protective wall" that limited collaborative efforts.[56]

As home adviser, Esposito dealt with the people who came to her programs—a self-selected audience that tended to be composed of older middle-class women. Reflecting on her organization's effectiveness, she said,

> You can't just always be sure how much penetration you've got out of any one thing. But one thing I was always sure of is that they not only came to the Unit or to the open meeting, or whatever we had to do this thing, and heard it. They

talked about it with their family, with their daughters who didn't have time to go to the meetings any more, with their daughter-in-law. And so the message got out quite well in a carrier method, and as long as you always had good literature that they could carry along, this was helpful.[57]

Although her programs did not often specifically target low-income people, "Sometimes if I had a homemakers' unit in a community, they would decide to help by having some additional lessons for the disadvantaged in their community and . . . they would invite people in that were not a part of organizations, and we would have a few lessons and some of them would always be on nutrition. . . . I saw, then, some disadvantaged people, because they were people living in the small communities where they kind of get lost and are not viewed . . . as you see them in public housing."[58]

Esposito retired in 1992. Like other extension educators, she participated in an effort to mold community health culture. Like them, she represented university-trained expertise and authority, at the same time interpreting official health information for women without scientific training and, arguably, with roots in traditional health cultures. She said, "I looked at the world, and I took a look at the people, and I tried to help them understand the world they were in and tried to make the program meaningful, but also stretch it."[59]

Public Health Infrastructure, Services, and Enforcement

Until the interwar period, in McLean County public health was an urban issue. Rural residents experienced few regulations and fewer services; sanitation and hygiene depended on households' cultural backgrounds and finances. Country families relied on self-help, calling the doctor only in cases of serious illness or injury.[60] Immunizations were available only on request or when an epidemic threatened. Consequently, this discussion begins with the county's urban center. Bloomington's late nineteenth-century public health initiatives were generated by elite consensus about disease causation, commitment to public service, and desire to join other progressive modern communities in appearance, amenities, and safety. As we have seen, by the turn of the twentieth century, Bloomington had begun to pave its streets and develop public water and sewerage systems. Beginning in the second decade of the twentieth century, Normal followed Bloomington's lead, initiating paving, sewer and water works.[61] In 1919 the communities collaborated to form the Bloomington and Normal Sanitary District.

Of course, public works do not automatically dictate popular use. Houses that had been built before installation of the water and sewer systems had to be connected at the owner's expense. Thus, many households continued to use private wells and outhouses. Only approximately 85 percent of Bloomington homes were using city water in 1925.[62] Similarly, outhouses were cheap, and people were accustomed to them. Indeed, some felt that it was more hygienic for people to void their waste outside of their homes than in them. As late as 1925 only an estimated 80 percent of Bloomington's households had flush toilets connected to the public sewers.[63] However, new residential construction and pressure from public health authorities pushed the trend toward domestic utilization of water and sewerage services.

It is noteworthy that the sewerage system did not completely prevent pollution from human waste and resulting disease, because the system continued to dump untreated sewage into Sugar Creek. In 1919 two lawsuits were filed on behalf of rural landowners against the City of Bloomington, Town of Normal, and several factories located along Sugar Creek. One of the plaintiffs "Represented that the water which flowed over his farm for quite a distance so poisoned the crops that they were unfit to feed the stock and that the water created an unsanitary condition about his premises causing he [sic] and his family to become ill." In 1925, the case was decided in favor of the plaintiffs. Bloomington and Normal's sewage treatment facility began operating in 1928.[64]

Despite slow public utilization of city water and sewer connections, it is fair to observe that by the interwar period, Bloomington-Normal residents had traversed the cultural distance between backyard outhouses and pumps to indoor bathrooms and potable tap water. This distance marked the gap between city and country, and between old-fashioned and modern. Within two generations, conveniences that had been luxuries became necessities structuring normative expectations for domestic and personal hygiene.

In addition to its public works, Bloomington had a health committee, which in the late nineteenth century supervised the work of a part-time medical officer and a sanitary policeman. This organization's staff and functions expanded as time went on. In 1901 the health commissioner began to keep vital statistics for the city—a task that had previously been done by the county clerk. After 1915 the health department began to employ two inspectors—one for foods, one for sanitation—who worked under the supervision of three physicians. At about the same time a small laboratory was set up to run tests of food and milk and for certain contagious diseases (diphtheria and gonorrhea in particular). Other types of tests were conducted in Springfield.

Beginning early in the twentieth century, the department employed three nurses, who dealt mainly with schoolchildren. They weighed and measured students and tested vision and hearing. They conducted tonsil clinics that referred children for surgery. They also taught health and hygiene in public schools and to mothers' clubs at Bloomington's Day Nursery, which was also operated by a public health nurse.[65] Thus, like the home adviser and the tuberculosis nurse, public health nurses were agents and translators of science, medicine, and demeanor. Waging a battle against contagious disease, they also sought to influence childrearing practices, personal hygiene, diet, and other behaviors—as Barbara Melosh argues, teaching the public the "laws" of health from their own social class and disciplinary perspective.[66] Operating largely without the immediate supervision of physicians, public health nurses also had considerable independent authority.

Although the home bureau and tuberculosis clinic extended the reach of public health information and services to rural McLean County, the health department served the City of Bloomington. As indicated previously, by the mid-twentieth century, there was increasing perception of a need for the county's diverse public health functions to be more closely coordinated. In addition, with expanding state regulation of water, milk, and food quality, there was growing need for county-level inspection, enforcement, and administration. The McLean County Health Department, established in 1945, operated on a combination of state and county funding.

According to Ben Boyd, who began his career as a sanitarian in Oklahoma in 1952 and joined the McLean County Health Department in 1966, the powers of the new department were enhanced by 1946 state legislation providing that "If the County Board passed a law, a public health law, it was applicable to everyone in the County. . . . In McLean County, the Public Health Department has jurisdiction for the entire County, including Bloomington-Normal."[67] The Department tested water and milk, and inspected restaurants and nursing homes. It provided immunizations and treatment and contact-tracing for infections including tuberculosis and venereal diseases. Its nurses offered health education and screening examinations.

The department's services fluctuated with changes in science and pressure from advocacy groups. For example, W. L. Dillman, a dentist who practiced first in the military during World War II, remembered,

> When I got out of the service, the McLean County Health Department was just getting organized. They were looking for somebody to do that [dentistry] end of it, so I said, sure, I'll try it. I worked there for eight years, working on the fluoride program. We had all of our studies, but the extent of oral health was terrible. There was no way that we could catch up. We had to work to try to prevent it. There was a study out west where these people had some little stains on their teeth, and they tried to find out what was causing it. At that time they did not have the methods of testing for elements in water or anything that they have

today. . . . They finally found a way to test, and found fluoride in four or five parts per million in the drinking water, and these people had excellent teeth. They found out that water filtered through some rocks that had some fluoride out west and down in Texas . . . and one part per million or 1.2 fluoride is ideal. It helps prevent a lot of oral disease, and it would still not mottle the teeth, so they wouldn't get any spots on them. So that was my main push—prevention. Public health is prevention. . . . I worked there until 1956.[68]

Dillman remembered opposition from some local dentists, who worried about losing business, and also from chiropractors, "but they just wanted to advertise." He said, "So, like a knight on a white charger in my shining armor, I wanted to see what I could do with it. . . . I talked to a lot of schools, a lot of the municipals . . ."[69] Dillman commented that opposition to the program faded: "You don't hear too much about it now. Some people check the chlorination of water. . . . Well, you know what they do if they stop chlorination of water, all kinds of illness."[70]

Jane Tinsley, who worked as a public health nurse for thirty-five years beginning in the mid-1950s, also remembered program changes:

I started out as a field nurse, everybody had their own area. I did that eight or nine years, and then I was made what they called an assistant supervisor. Over those years, it kept evolving and doing different things. And any time something new came along, they used to send you off to four- or five- or six-day seminar things. . . . Shortly after I started vision and hearing evaluations, I went to Jacksonville to the School for the Deaf to receive training. . . . When they started the spinal exam for scoliosis, they sent us for training. The same when they started the lead poisoning program and rehabilitation.[71]

Ben Boyd recalled the introduction of Medicare:

The Medicare-approved health department was a whole gimmy-gammy of . . . we would be supported by Medicare when we did home health visits, etc., that were identified by the Medicare system, about 1965–66. Because we had a home health activity in McLean County. . . . But there was an opportunity right in the mid '60s to become a Medicare-approved health department. That means that their home health services will be Medicare subsidized. They began the program . . . just before I came here. That became so administratively stressful. It was a terrible program, in terms of keeping track of everything. Your records . . . at that time they were not geared to take care of that kind of thing. It got far worse later, but at that time they were not geared to bill. . . . Health promotion didn't bill anybody for anything. You just did your projects and put it down and told the County government how much you did, and they got County funds. So it was a very simplistic sort of thing. But when this Medicare thing hit, the record-keeping was so difficult to do. We had people who we wanted to serve and we felt needed visitation, but they were not on the Medicare program. And because of Medicare regulations, it was felt that we could not do these people. . . . In about 1968, the Medicare program was abandoned in McLean County as far as public health was concerned. What that meant was, we would do everybody, Medicare or not. If they needed home visitation, we would take care of it for free. The Board of Health said we do not want to charge our homebound anything. That's a public health service McLean County is going to do. And we did it.[72]

He also remembered the late 1970s when, "There was a host of state-mandated programs that had money attached, state and federal. The big one in 1977, 1978 was called W.I.C., that was the first one: Women, Infant, and Children. . . . This was an attempt . . . to improve the health of stressed women, infants, and children. Low income, pregnant teens. . . . W.I.C. was only an example of one. It goes on and on and on."[73]

When Boyd was hired in 1966, the health department had about thirty employees working in three main areas: environmental health, nursing, and administration. As director of environmental health, he was responsible for food, water, nuisances, and insect control. This involved inspection and enforcement—sometimes in response to residents' complaints. He offered as typical examples of nuisance situations:

It's a situation where somebody is living in an apartment house and they look out and the garbage is overflowing their dumpster and it has been doing that for weeks! And all of a sudden, they get to the end of their rope and they'll call the health department just madder than hell, which I don't blame them at all: "Why don't you guys do something?" Well, we can, but we didn't know about it. We don't inspect all the garbage dump sites in McLean County. That's the basics. Another one would be from a farmer with the same thing . . ."Hey, you guys! Come out and look at this corner of my property. There's somebody dumping out there." We'll go out there and there is garbage all over everywhere in that little spot. Well, the first thing we do is start looking for magazines, which . . . I don't know, when you throw garbage out, never put anything out which has got your name on it![74]

Boyd's staff regularly inspected food establishments—restaurants and grocery stores. However, again, violations tended to be caught as a result of complaints—in this case, incidence of illness. Boyd said, "The physicians may observe an illness that they suspect is a food-borne illness, that could have come from improper food. If they let you know right quick so you can get back and do interviews and find out where these people are coming from

. . . in other words, where did they eat, what was their last food . . . But you
have to have the cooperation of everybody to do that."[75]

According to Boyd, tension between McLean County's physicians and its
health officials, evident in the 1890s, continued in the following century:

> The physicians really . . . we didn't relate to them. The public was our real source.
> The problem became that occasionally the physician would find a food-borne
> illness, but they wouldn't report it. Either because they didn't think about it,
> or they were more interested in solving the person's illness. I'm not quite sure
> why. But that's a problem country-wide. The physicians get narrowed in on their
> individual patients and they don't think about the community as a patient. Of
> course, that's our focus. The community is our patient, not the individual. I don't
> want to say that the physicians didn't do their job as far as their public health
> responsibility, but we found out that the younger, the new physicians coming on
> and some of the old ones, had never had any public health training: very, very
> little. So it was very difficult for them. It didn't help the community much.[76]

This situation revealed the physicians' emphasis on maintaining relationships with individual patients without interference from other—particularly
government—entities. It also indicated the status difference between doctors
and public health officials, which had widened since the late 19th century.
That status difference was also expressed in the prices of services delivered
by doctors and health officials, which also occasionally created competition.
For example, Boyd remembered that in 1966, whooping cough vaccinations
had been done in doctor's offices: "Now, the vaccine was made free to the
physicians, but his cost kept going up to the point that . . . I think probably
the majority of the vaccines done today are done at the Health Department.
Just because of costs."[77]

Public health officials depended on cooperation from both doctors and
members of the public to do mandated venereal disease enforcement activities. Boyd remembered,

> In 1966, the environmental health division, one of the things we did was do
> field work for syphilis and gonorrhea. . . . That's because it's men. If a man had
> . . . well, this was because of the Director [of Nursing] at the time. She didn't
> want to send her people out to contact men who had venereal diseases. So we
> went. Just a gender problem with her. After she left, then that no longer ap-
> plied. The disease people handled it all. But we had some interesting stories
> . . . Well, we'd get a case . . . now see, the physician was [mandated to report if
> they treated someone for VD]. We'd get a copy of the report. We'd do a follow-
> up on it and find out what happened. Did they get their follow-up treatment?
> And more importantly, what we were after is contacts . . . A lady would come

in and get treated for gonorrhea. She would then say who her contacts were to somebody. Sometimes the physician, most generally not. . . . The physician would say, "Jane Doe has gonorrhea. Here's her address." Well, half the time that would not be the right address, so we lost a lot . . . What we preferred was people to come into the Health Department to be treated. We'd give them the same treatment as their doctors. . . . We even had a physician on staff, clinician or the Health Department Physician would be responsible for the Communicable Disease Program.[78]

He discussed challenges with following up on sexual contacts:

Our problems were, you know, we'd get in to knock on this door where this guy lived, and the wife would answer the door or the phone. What do you say? "I'm the health department and I'm looking for John, where's he at?" So all sorts of devices you learned to try to find a guy without . . . you try to go to his business. I had one, he refused to answer. I made contact with him. He said, yeah, come on out, so I went on out. We went and had coffee. I said, "You know, John," and I'll just use John, "Why aren't you letting us know who these people are?" He said, "Well, the problem is, I'll be real frank with you. I got gonorrhea in Lincoln. I went down there last" whatever day it was "and had sexual contact with this beautiful blonde at this tavern. Well, she had gonorrhea. Which is not really my problem. The problem is, I don't know who she is. She's Jane and that's all I know. She's in this tavern at this place." Well, what we would do is take that information, send it to state. They would take it and run it back to the county if there's not a local health department, and they actually go to that tavern and look for Jane. Sometimes they found her. They were pretty good at that.[79]

Venereal disease enforcement highlights tension between individual rights to privacy and choice, on the one hand, and the welfare of the general public, on the other. It is an arena, like services provided to TB sufferers or poor women with children, which is highly gendered and riddled with power relationships. It also exemplifies the tension within public health between enforcement and service.

Conclusions

Public health information, infrastructure, services, and legislation have both reflected and caused changes in community health culture. The installation of flush toilets, hot and cold running water, bathtubs, and showers in people's homes has revolutionized domestic and personal hygiene. Behaviors intended to prevent germ transmission—covering faces when sneezing and coughing, avoiding public expectoration, washing hands before eating and after toileting—have become expected tokens of civility. Immunization of young children is both a sign of responsible parenting and legally required for public school admission. These developments have occurred in different places at different times. In McLean County, they happened mainly during the first half of the twentieth century—within living memory.

6. Matters of Life and Death

Experience and Expectations
of Health, Illness, and Medical Care
in the Twentieth Century

In living memory, the experience of suffering has been transformed. The diseases people most feared and those they most frequently died of were very different at the beginning than they were at the end of the twentieth century. The experience of care and treatment also changed as the power—perceived and actual—of biomedicine to alter the course of disease and delay death permeated twentieth-century culture, shaping expectations and experiences. As we have seen, during the brief span of one or two generations, management of birth, injury, illness, and death moved from homes to medical institutions, and from the responsibility of mainly female lay caregivers to that of formally qualified experts. At the same time, conceptualization, interpretation, and maintenance of health became increasingly complex and challenging; although people lived longer, they feared more.[1] This chapter explores these changes from the perspective of McLean County residents who lived through them.

It is largely based on oral history interviews with forty-one people born between 1894 and 1966. Twenty-nine interviews were conducted specifically for this study; nine were collected for the Bloomington-Normal Black History Project; and three were done by a graduate student for a class project. Nearly three-quarters of these informants were women; just over one-quarter were African American (see Table 7). Twenty-seven informants had spent most of their lives in Bloomington-Normal, and fourteen had lived mainly in rural Central Illinois communities, ten of which are in McLean County.

Informants were chosen within three broad occupational categories to provide information about ill-health and health care from the perspectives of medical practitioners, nurses, and laypeople. Eight nurses, six physicians, and one dentist were interviewed, as were twenty-six people whose occupa-

Table 7: Oral History Informants: Age, Sex, and Race

Birthdate	Males	Females	African American	White
1890–1900	0	4	0	4
1901–1910	2	3	1	4
1911–1920	6	10	5	11
1921–1930	4	8	4	8
1931–1940	0	2	1	1
1941–1950	0	1	0	1
1951–1960	0	0	0	0
1961–1970	0	1	0	1
Total	12	29	11	30

tions included domestic service, teaching, factory work, journalism, farming, insurance, medical records management, public health, and homemaking. Because health-care providers talked about their own experiences of ill-health and childbearing in addition to their occupational activities, their memories are discussed in this chapter along with those of laypeople. (See the appendix for a brief profile list of the oral history informants.)

The educational attainment of informants ranged from three years of high school to graduate degrees. Although no information about respondents' current income was elicited, interviews reveal that whereas many informants experienced poverty as children and young adults, at the time of their interviews most had moderate or high incomes and comfortable lifestyles.

Informants came from a range of socioeconomic, ethnic, and religious backgrounds. They represented both rural and urban experience. Their memories covered almost a century. The preponderance of females among them is appropriate because of women's traditional and normative roles as health-care decision makers and caregivers in most households. Most informants had lived in McLean County all their lives; their experience was arguably typical of residents of small cities and rural communities throughout the Midwest. As the development of the county's health-care delivery system conformed, generally speaking, to the national model, changes in informants' beliefs, behavior, and experience regarding health, illness, birth, and medical care also exemplified broad cultural trends.

Fear, Self-Defense, and Resignation: Infections and People before World War II

When asked the question, "As a child, were you healthy or frequently ill?" oral history informants often responded in a way that seemed strange to 1990s interviewers. Grace Allman, born in 1896, said, "Oh, I was healthy. I always had tonsillitis every winter. Of course, we had the mumps and the measles, all the catching [diseases]—chickenpox, everything that went around."[2] Marie Bostic, born in 1897, said, "Oh, I never was sick. I had every kid disease, but I was not sick, and haven't been. . . . I had the whooping cough the first year I went to school, and I had the measles in high school. . . . And I had scarlet fever. I caught that from a kid at school."[3] And Ethel Cherry, born in 1911, who had diphtheria and pneumonia as a child, described herself as having been healthy: "We had the normal amount of diseases, like measles and all of them, but never anything else."[4] At least in retrospect, these informants defined child health as the usual absence of illness, and also regarded as "healthy"—or, at least, expected—experience of short-term acute infectious ailments. Martha Ferguson, born in 1916, explained that her children got sick, "But they was the things you recover from. They weren't ongoing. . . . Glenn [her son] fell and cut his tongue. Jim [another son] had polio. Just stuff like that."[5]

These comments reveal, not lack of concern about the threat posed by these health problems, but the expectation that illness and injury were "normal" parts of childhood experience—hurdles that, like birth itself, might maim or kill the child. There was little systematic effort, at either community or household level, to prevent specific diseases. Thus, for example, although smallpox vaccination was readily available in the early twentieth century, informants remembered immunization being given only when an epidemic threatened.[6] Grace Allman recalled that during the years between 1910 and 1920, "Everybody had to get vaccinated for smallpox. That was a bad experience for me too, because when I got vaccinated my arm swelled up and it was that big . . . It was just sore. I was teaching, and to go to school, I carried my arm, I fastened my thumb in my belt so that I had no weight on this."[7] Caribel Washington, born in 1914, said, "When I was in the eighth grade . . . there was quite an epidemic of smallpox. Our teacher had it, so then everybody had to be vaccinated."[8] Perhaps, in part, because of the fear of the immunization process, there were 140 reported cases of smallpox in Bloomington in 1925.[9] Ruth Carpenter was vaccinated only when she started nurse training in 1928. She said about vaccination, "We just didn't do stuff like that when I grew up."[10]

Other contagious diseases routinely sickened McLean County children and could not be prevented. Measles was epidemic in some years and dormant in others; in 1925, 771 cases were reported in Bloomington, but in 1922 there were only seven cases in the community. Whooping cough and scarlet fever were also endemic, more virulent in some years than in others. Both of these ailments were bad in 1921, with 751 cases of scarlet fever and 135 whooping cough cases reported, whereas in 1924, there were only 62 and 68 cases respectively.[11] New to Illinois in 1917, poliomyelitis, also referred to as infantile paralysis, began to visit McLean County on a regular basis; twenty-two cases and two deaths were reported to the state health department in 1927; twenty cases and two deaths in 1931. Mainly striking otherwise healthy children and crippling victims it did not kill, polio was feared out of all proportion to its incidence. Unique among the major childhood infections because it could be prevented and cured by the use of antitoxin, developed in 1890, diphtheria sickened twenty-one children in 1921 and killed three. In a 1925 outbreak, there were 374 cases and one fatality reported.[12] Although informants did not mention it specifically, preventive immunization for diphtheria became common during the interwar period.

In addition to infections mainly threatening children, there were contagious diseases that were less discriminating. Although the number of cases declined steadily in the early twentieth century, as we have seen, tuberculosis remained a constant threat until the 1950s. Pneumonia also continued to claim lives, particularly as a complication of other diseases. For example, during the influenza epidemic of 1918, in addition to eighty-three deaths in Bloomington from flu, fifty-seven people—more than twice the number reported the following year—died of pneumonia.[13] Typhoid was also a regular visitor to the county, as were syphilis and gonorrhea.[14]

Except for TB sufferers admitted to the Fairview Sanitarium, victims of the 1918–19 influenza epidemic nursed in temporary wards at Bloomington Country Club, and polio patients hospitalized first at St. Francis Hospital in Peoria and later at St. Joseph's Hospital in Bloomington, sufferers from infectious diseases were cared for at home.[15] An early twentieth-century public health official explained, "Toward the end of the nineteenth century, in common with forward-looking citizens all over the country, the people in Bloomington began to regard scarlet fever, diphtheria, typhoid fever, and other infections as communicable from person to person and therefore subject to prevention by quarantine. Accordingly the practice of case notification and the placarding of infected premises came into vogue about that time."[16] Visited by physicians and nursed by mothers, other female relatives, or servants, the sick either recovered or died in their own beds. Diphtheria and tetanus could be treated with antitoxin; beginning in the late 1930s, some pneumonia cases could be cured by sulfonamide drugs. Paul Erlich's "magic bullet," Salvarsan, released in 1911, made syphilis curable.[17] Otherwise, no effective treatments were available for most infections. Sufferers were comforted and watched during the often lengthy course of illness. The healthy were protected from contagion by quarantine of the sick and fumigation of "infected rooms," and personal hygiene procedures intended to limit the spread of germs increasingly became part of household routines and the general education of children.[18]

A booklet used in McLean County, *Home Care of Communicable Diseases,* published in 1942 by the John Hancock Mutual Life Insurance Company, offers a glimpse of contemporary management of infectious illnesses before the introduction of penicillin and effective immunization campaigns. Directed at mothers of young children, it provided information in simple language about symptoms of major "childhood diseases," the ways infections were spread, and development of immunity to some diseases. It debunked outdated ideas about disease transmission, including miasma and fomite theories, for example.[19] It also indicates how quickly "modern" ideas can become passé, maintaining, for example, that German Measles (or rubella) had no common complications.[20]

The booklet recommended that contagious sufferers be put to bed in a room by themselves, partly to speed recovery and partly to protect other members of the household. Patients were to be completely isolated until all danger of infection had passed; thus, they were to use a bedpan rather than the bathroom and to eat all their meals in bed. The booklet stressed the importance of keeping babies and preschoolers away from the patient, because "communicable diseases go especially hard for youngsters between the ages of six months and three or four years. Most deaths from these diseases occur among babies and toddlers."[21]

Regardless of the diagnosis, the "nurse" was instructed to "Wear a large apron while caring for the patient and leave the apron always in the sickroom; wash hands thoroughly after caring for the patient; turn away from the patient when he coughs or sneezes and keep own hands away from mouth." Additional special precautions were necessary in nursing people suffering from diphtheria, polio, scarlet fever, and smallpox: "All articles used by the patient must be kept in the sickroom or until they can be burned, boiled, soaked in disinfectant solution, or aired. Soiled linen should be washed in soap and hot water apart from the family wash and unnecessary handling avoided. Dishes should be boiled for fifteen minutes before being washed with the household dishes. Partly eaten scraps of food should be burned." Special procedures were also recommended for disposal of the excrement of sufferers from ailments, such as polio and typhoid, known to be transmitted by fecal matter. After the patient had recovered, the sickroom was to be thoroughly cleaned and aired. In addition, "All articles such as mattresses, blankets, or books should be put in the sun for at least six hours. Articles badly soiled, of course, should be cleaned or destroyed if they cannot be cleaned."[22]

Although the booklet prescribed an ideal that may not have been achieved in many households, it also indicated the "terrible and exhausting struggle" of home caregivers.[23] Female relatives and maids carried specially prepared food, washed soiled linen, scrubbed bedpans, and watched sufferers through long nights. They took ultimate responsibility for care of the ailing person—either according to traditional knowledge or experts' instructions; they also suffered the grief and guilt when infections killed.

Oral history informants remembered the impact of contagious diseases on families and communities. Reginald Whitaker, born in 1925, said that his mother had been married as a young woman to John Duff, who died of typhoid:

> INFORMANT: He died, I think, he died in 1907. My mother was carrying John; he never saw his father. She was seven months pregnant, or something like that. He died . . . John was born in 1907. . . .
>
> INTERVIEWER: He must have been quite a young man, Mr. Duff.
>
> INFORMANT: Twenty-one. . . . they had a typhoid fever epidemic, you understand, going through the Twin Cities [Bloomington-Normal] at that time.[24]

Grace Allman recalled that her husband's family was decimated by influenza. "His mother and a sister died with the flu. My husband was so ill they thought he was going to die. They were buried the same day, his sister and his mother."[25]

Informants also described the communal dread of lethal infections. Ruth Carpenter, born in 1909, recalled the following:

> INFORMANT: We had a neighbor down the road . . . and the family got diphtheria and one of the little girls died, and that [household] was quarantined. And when she died, they brought the body outside. . . . They brought it from the funeral home and . . . set it out in the front yard.
>
> INTERVIEWER: Did people come, and . . . ?
>
> INFORMANT: Yeah, they did. Oh, everybody was so kind and they brought stuff. Of course, they didn't go in the house. . . . but I can remember the quarantine signs. . . .
>
> INTERVIEWER: And who put them up?
>
> INFORMANT: The doctor, I guess the doctor that took care of 'em and reported it. As far as I know, it was when the doctor reported it, then they hung the sign on. And they treated you like you had the plague. . . . Oh, yes. They was scared to death of you.[26]

Martha Ferguson remembered fear of epidemic diseases in the interwar period:

INFORMANT: Scarlet fever was terrifying, you know. Anything like that was really pretty dangerous. They didn't really have good cures for anything.

INTERVIEWER: How did you and your family and the community deal with these problems?

INFORMANT: Well, we were just taken care of at home. They quarantined . . . for a lot of things in those days. Scarlet fever was always quarantined. I think chickenpox was. I think whooping cough was. . . . Well, we were scared of scarlet fever; yeah, you could get pretty ill from that and people did die.[27]

Both fear of diseases known to be transmitted by personal contact and the isolation imposed by quarantine undermined traditional mutual aid that provided practical support as well as the comfort of the social bedside.

Even when contagious diseases did not kill, they disrupted people's lives. Marie Bostic, born in 1897, taught in a one-room school as a young woman and caught scarlet fever from one of her students. "They sent that kid to school that morning with a terrible sore throat. He was just a little boy and was just a-crying. I had him on my lap most of the day. I'd rather hold him as to have him cry. That was on Friday. Sunday morning, I had scarlet fever. I caught it from him. We were quarantined five weeks. There was no school for six weeks."[28] Bostic's account indicates that people understood that scarlet fever was communicable and that the child's parents were irresponsible to send him to school when he was ill.

Most families took seriously the obligation to separate the sick from the well. Mary Finfgeld remembered being quarantined with influenza at about age twelve during the 1918 epidemic. "[I was in] that bedroom in the house and nobody came in there, and I mean *nobody* came in there, excepting my mother to look after me and bring me my meals. Nobody even stuck their head in the door. It was . . . well, I haven't ever seen anything like it since, because people, they were just dropping dead like flies."[29] Isolation was also thought to benefit the sufferer. Ralph Spencer recalled being quarantined:

If you were sick, you stayed in bed. That was the understanding. . . . I stayed in bed one time by myself for a school term with the measles. Folks were going to the last day of school, which was always a picnic deal, but I couldn't go. I had measles. "And you don't get out of that bed!" I stayed in the bed by myself. . . . That was the reason you stayed in bed when you got them. They were contagious diseases. You stayed in bed because if you didn't, then you didn't get over them. Plus the fact that if you didn't stay in bed . . . it would have an effect on you later on, you know.[30]

After a quarantine was lifted, according to Ruth Carpenter, disinfection was done by "burning sulfur in the house."[31]

Polio was especially feared because it attacked young, healthy children and maimed those it did not kill. Reginald Whitaker remembered a playmate having the disease:

> It seems like it went through their family. They lived a couple blocks north of us on Poplar Street. Just about all of those kids had it. . . . There was Marjory, she had it. Wound up kind of walking with a slight limp. Then Paul . . . he fell on his bicycle or something and had lots of trouble. . . . He walked with that limp for, I don't know, a year or so. Then she [oldest sister] took him up there [Chicago] and he had an operation on his hip. I think they replaced . . . took a piece of bone from somewhere, out of his back or some place, and put in his hip. He was out of school. . . . We were in the same grade. When he got back in school, he was a year behind me. He was in a cast for about a year. . . . That would have been in . . . 1937 or 8.[32]

Polio also attracted media attention unrivalled except by tuberculosis. McLean County's main daily newspaper, *The Daily Pantagraph,* tracked national and local outbreaks, provided information about changing theories about disease transmission and appropriate treatments, and stimulated support for area services and sufferers.[33]

Infections affected lifestyles and decisions. Roberta Holman's husband had TB when he was discharged from the army in 1946:

> Well, we tried farming, working for my folks. . . . We lived in the tenant house on the Gravitt farm. Because of his tuberculosis, he was sick all the time. The minute he'd get on that tractor to get out in the field, he was sick. Pneumonia—one fall he had pneumonia six times. He knew he had to change. Of course, he had been in the army 17 years, and he had an eighth-grade education. He was one of nine children and his father died. They were farmed out. Anyway, this station right over here where I'm parked, Shell station, was displayed. He said, "I think I could do that because it's outside work and has fresh air." So we bought the station and he had that for . . . probably 37 or 38 [years] . . . but he was sick all the time too.[34]

According to Dr. Harold Shinall, who worked as a general practitioner in Gibson City during the 1930s, most of his patients had infections.[35] Correspondingly, laypeople interviewed for this study most frequently recalled consulting physicians for acute infectious diseases, although they also remembered being treated at home. For example, Richard Finfgeld, born in 1906, described his brother Ray's experience with a serious upper respiratory infection in the 1920s:

They didn't think he was going to live. Dr. Hammers was his doctor. He was coming to our house to see and take care of him [Ray]. As I remember it, he had pneumonia or something. He had a high temperature. They put a plaster on his chest. I think they called it antiphlogistine or something like that . . . This wasn't a mustard plaster. This was something milder. It was supposed to be something good. They were so concerned they called in Dr. Scott. The two doctors came to our house and had a consultation. Dr. Scott suggested or ordered that they change to put on a mustard plaster. . . . That was the second plaster. . . . He was really afflicted. They didn't think he was going to live, but he recovered.[36]

This account reveals lay awareness and longevity of medical theories and therapies (antiphlogistic and counterirritant treatments) that, by the 1920s, were out of date in elite professional circles.[37]

As important as the doctor's advice was the support of friends and relatives during times of illness. Lavada Hunter, born in 1913, said,

What I can remember about death was, the first time I was ten years of age. My father died then. . . . In 1923, he had the influenza. He was at home, and the family doctor would come and attend him before death came. During those days, people used to sit up with the sick. They would come and help my mother with him, you know, in many many ways. They helped cook, wash, and iron. I was ten years old, and I counted twenty people at our home when my father was so very ill. Then was when my mother found out that she thought that he was dying. He was in a delirious state. Then he died; he finally died at home.[38]

Marie Snyder had similar memories, saying that when people got sick, "Your neighbors come in and helped you when you needed some assistance."[39] This kind of community mutual aid decreased only when hospitalization of birth, serious illness, and injury became usual in the 1930s.

Tuberculosis was endemic in McLean County. Despite declining mortality from this cause, awareness of its bacterial cause heightened public concern about TB. Ferne Hensley, born in 1894, talked about TB in her family. Her aunt had died of the disease at age fourteen. "She was a tiny little girl. She died of what they called consumption—TB, you know. . . . Well, I guess it sort of just consumed them. One of my father's next to the oldest brother—he also died with it. A number of people. Of course, there were no sanitariums or anything like that. They just—you had it and that was it. You didn't get well from it then."[40] Caribel Washington's middle sister was frequently ill as a child: "I can remember at one time we had a doctor that said she had tuberculosis. Now whether she did or not was always a little doubtful, but I can remember that we had put two front porches in our house because it was in two sections. My dad screened in one of the porches and she slept on the porch, even in the wintertime."[41] This approach reflected the officially approved open air cure for tuberculosis and, arguably, served as the parents' way of preventing the need for sanitarium treatment for their daughter—a prospect that was particularly dreadful to this African American family.

Tuberculosis was one of the first diseases for which people accepted institutional care. Younger people interviewed for this study remembered friends and relatives undergoing the long course of treatment at the Fairview Sanitarium (opened in 1919) during the interwar period. Reginald Whitaker recalled family friends—a brother and sister from Bloomington—who suffered from TB:

> INFORMANT: They were both out there at McLean County Tuberculosis Center. Her brother got along real well, came out, and I guess didn't do what he was supposed to and he died. Got very infected. Didn't follow the doctor's orders, as far as I can remember. She's still living. This would have been back in the '30s, the middle '30s. She stayed out there in that Sanitarium—she had to learn to walk all over again.
>
> INTERVIEWER: Because she'd been in bed so long?
>
> INFORMANT: Yeah. Been in bed two or three years. But she finally got out. I don't know how long she was there. . . . I think back then they would collapse a lung and let that rest. . . . They collapsed the one and waited until it healed. Then they put it back in action and collapsed the other. I think that's what took so long. She had to learn to walk all over again.[42]

Whitaker's account reveals that McLean County residents internalized medical ascription of blame to TB patients who refused to "follow the rules." It also documents awareness of contemporary therapies for the disease in the 1930s. Although surgical interventions were developed for TB in the 1920s, there was no reliable drug treatment until the late 1940s when streptomycin was introduced.[43]

In addition to diseases, such as TB, that still threaten McLean County residents, oral history informants remembered suffering from ailments that virtually disappeared after 1950. Mary Finfgeld got undulant fever, also called brucellosis, as a young adult in the early 1940s. She recalled the following:

> INFORMANT: You get it from cow's milk. I had always been taught that you never use anything but pasteurized milk, but when we moved here a man out in the country had dairy cows and . . . left a quart of milk on our back porch. So I continued to take some milk from him, but I bought pasteurized milk for the children. . . . It [the brucellosis] was traced to his herd, one cow. . . .
>
> INTERVIEWER: You said you had a fever of 105?

INFORMANT: At one time when it spiked highest. They put me in the hospital then. I went to bed on December 7, 1941, Pearl Harbor Day, and I got out at Easter time. And you carry that in your system all your life. So I've never been able to give blood. But I haven't had any more trouble with it. They had no medication for it at that time. Doc Ryder consulted with Mayo's and they had nothing. Within two years, they had a vaccine. You got one shot in your hip and one in your arm. . . . There were a few cases of that around in the area, and one man had died from it, but I didn't know that at the time. But I guess I had people plenty worried—although I never thought I was that sick.[44]

She was given fever treatment in the hospital where "Dr. Poppins and this nurse that had been looking after me and giving me these shots—how often I had to have them—several times in succession, it was an awful ordeal until they raised my temperature and then they'd drop them back, and then they'd increase them until they raised it again."[45] Undulent fever largely disappeared as pasteurization became universal among dairy farmers, and the general public stopped drinking untreated milk. However, informants' accounts indicate the overlapping use of pasteurized and unpasteurized milk and the extent to which people ignored official advice to use only treated milk.

Like doctors, sufferers became accustomed to using hospitals for inpatient and outpatient treatment during the interwar period. Caribel Washington remembered having rheumatic fever in 1939:

INFORMANT: I was quite ill. I was on crutches and I limped, and I had a cane, and all of these kind of things. It was from an infected throat. I never had any heart problems because it moved all over my body. . . . I think that's why I have such a heavy tolerance for pain. I used to sit for a half hour just making up my mind to get up. It was excruciating. . . .
INTERVIEWER: What was really done for you?
INFORMANT: I used to go out to—when St. Joseph was still up here, I'd go and they would put me in a cabinet and close it clear up to my neck up here, and then turn on these electric lights and then stand there and feed me ice water so I would sweat.
INTERVIEWER: You were lying down?
INFORMANT: No. There was a chair. And you'd just go in that cabinet and they'd just close the whole thing up and your head was out. It would close up to your neck and you were just in a cabinet. When they did that they would take me downstairs and have pans of wet salt. They'd use scrub brushes to rub that salt into my skin because they said the pores were full of this poison. Then they would—and this one I couldn't take—they'd put me in a bathtub and put electrodes in the tub, you know, but that made me sick at the stomach, so I couldn't take that at the time. . . . But this cabinet bit, oh dear.

INTERVIEWER: And there were lights, you said, so it was hot?

INFORMANT: Right. There was all different types of watts of lights that were inside. When I would get in there and they would close it up and then they would turn that on. Then heat would get in there. . . . I always felt better after that . . . because they did it until I would sweat a certain amount. The more I sweated, the more that would leave my system.[46]

This account illustrates both the association of technology with hospitals, and the degree to which patients accepted and tolerated dramatic medical interventions in search of relief.

Hospitalization, however, remained an unusual experience for McLean County residents until the second half of the twentieth century. And home care continued, even after it became expected for the seriously ill to be hospitalized. Margaret Esposito, born in 1923, nursed her husband at her mother's home during his long battle with lung cancer in the 1950s. Her grandmother also needed home nursing care at the time:

INFORMANT: So I came home and we [she and her mother] threw in together and took care of [my] two kids and the two ill people . . . My daughter had always spent summers with my mother. And she [daughter] always enjoyed sleeping with grandma. And so mother had her sleeping in bed with her and she had my son in a cot at the foot of the bed. And so I just took my old room for my husband and I, and my grandmother had her bedroom, and . . . my husband had to stay up there in bed. He didn't come down too much. And I took care of my grandmother down here on a cot in the dining room, and my husband up there during the daytime. And then when my mother came home [from work] at night, we each took our own patients and . . . we all took care of the kids.

INTERVIEWER: Did you have any support from professional nurses at all?

INFORMANT: No. We didn't need that. It didn't seem to be that kind of care. I was beginning to think at the very last that I might have to learn how to give shots, but actually Darvon took care if it all the way through for him. I was lucky.[47]

However, as Dr. Loren Boon reflected, demographic and economic change stimulated need for institutional care in the second half of the twentieth century: "Of course, when I very first started [in 1947] there were a lot of families that still had people at home there, and there was always a maiden aunt or somebody at home to help take care of them there, and then after awhile everybody had to work that was at home, and they didn't have nursing assistants and practical nurses . . . to help out in the home there so much."[48] Although two-earner families reduced the capacity to look after the ailing and disabled at home, it is equally true that home care was less expected as institutional care became usual and accepted.

Injuries and Interventions

People have always been injured in domestic and work environments.[49] In early twentieth-century McLean County, minor—and even some major—injuries were dealt with by laypeople, who used diverse methods to staunch bleeding, splint sprains and fractures, salve burns, and poultice bruises. Also, before the introduction of antibiotics, lay caregivers gained broad experience with the infection that often followed injuries.

Before the 1930s, it was usual for injury victims to be cared for at home. When Marie Snyder was four years old in about 1903,

> I was scalded. She [mother] was washing in the kitchen. We had a house and what they called a summer kitchen was off the back of the house. There was a step down. She'd just taken this pan of boiling water, soap and everything in it, off the stove and I came to the door. She told me to go back. Well, I flew around to go back, and my dress caught on that bump, and I fell in all that boiling water. We lived next door to a doctor. That was the only thing that saved me. Of course, she [mother] screamed and his sisters came running to see what was wrong, so he was right there. . . . It was a mess. I was burned from my waist to my feet. I'm still. . . . I didn't walk for almost a year. This leg is really burned. This one is spotty. Then it started infecting and they scraped it to the bone. . . . My mother wheeled me in a baby buggy for a long time. She said they used sulfur and lard after they got to where the skin was growing back, but it just came off with my clothes. . . . For years she rubbed that on my legs. But she'd massage my legs with it to keep it from growing to the bone.

The doctor visited every day; all treatments were provided in Snyder's home.[50] Similarly, as we have seen, when Richard Finfgeld broke his leg playing baseball during the 1920s, the doctor came to his home and set the leg there.[51]

Ralph Spencer said about his youth on the farm during the 1920s,

> Oh, I got hurt several times. Got a foot mashed up. . . . Jumped into an oats bin one time without any oats in it—12 feet down. Was on a hard floor with all my weight on top of it. I was pretty heavy at that time too. For a kid, you know. My dad had been hauling oats out and went up to push more oats down a hole so he could put in another load of oats, and I didn't realize he had taken the oats out of that end, and I ended up on the floor . . . so I got a foot mashed up at that time and it bothered me in high school when I was playing basketball and would use that foot to pivot on. . . . He [father] had to take me to the doctor.[52]

By contrast, when Spencer tore his biceps tendon handling hogs as an adult (ca 1930s), his family doctor sent him to a specialist, Dr. Gordon Shultz, in Bloomington:

> Dr. Shultz was a big man and he said, "What did you do?" I told him, and he said, "Okay." There was a file cabinet up against the wall. He took his hand like this, and he laid it over here on top of the file cabinet. Then he said, "You hold my arm and tend yourself." Of course, I got a hold of the arm and pulled down like this, and he said I'd have to pull harder than that. I pulled again, and he said, "Okay, that's all right. Now straighten your arms out." This is when I'd about froze and stayed right there—never moved. He said I would have to go to the hospital . . . they got this fixed. They had to go in here on this side and put it into this here muscle. They couldn't put a tendon back onto a bone, or they couldn't at that time. . . . They probably can today, but then they couldn't. So it had torn shoulder blade bone cartilages.

It took eight months for this injury to heal.[53] Spencer's use of anatomical terminology regarding the second injury provides an interesting contrast to the first account, suggesting both a change in his own role, from child patient to an adult managing his own interactions with physicians, and the degree to which, as a layperson, he shared the biomedical culture that increasingly dominated health care by the 1930s.

Care of serious injuries moved into hospitals during the interwar period, although effective ambulance service did not come to McLean County until after World War II. Ruth Carpenter was in a car accident in 1943:

> I had taken Joe [husband] to McLean [in rural McLean County] to work and was on my way back [to Bloomington, sixteen miles away]. Something happened to one of the wheels on the car and it threw me . . . Nobody else was involved. I totaled the car . . . It lifted me out on the passenger side into the road. . . . Broke nine ribs off my shoulder, and I got a floating shoulder from it. . . . There was a man come along, and you know, probably he picked me up like this and put me in the back seat of his car and drove me to Bloomington. I got to St. Joe's. That was the first place he came to, and the Sister picked me up and carried me in the same way, in her arms. It's a wonder I didn't have a punctured lung between the 3rd and the 12th vertebrae. . . . When they got me in the bed and rolled me over, I was as loose as rocks in a tin pan. That's exactly what it sounded like. I can remember that. I was only there 11 days, I had to let my ribs heal enough so that I could go home. I couldn't get out of bed for a long time. . . . They didn't have therapy in those days. . . . Bed was therapy—when I could get out of bed by myself. Joe'd get me up when he was getting ready to go to work and take me to the bathroom and that sort of thing. Then I had a neighbor girl that came over and stayed with me for a long time. [It was] seven

or eight weeks before I could get out of bed on my own power. I didn't work again for about a year.[54]

Carpenter's experience illustrates overlap between institutional and home care and continuation of informal ways of managing ill-health at home.

Home Care: Prevention, Home Remedies, and Patent Medicines

Along with home care for most health problems, oral history informants born before about 1920 remembered using both traditional methods to maintain health and home remedies made of local herbs, kitchen ingredients, and other household substances. Many families had ways of preventing illness that harked back to humoral and magical theories of disease causation. Ralph Spencer, born in 1914, said, "My mother always had a remedy for whatever it was. In the spring of the year, she had a blood thinner that she gave you, and things like that. . . . For blood thinner, we used sassafras tea and stuff like that. The mint is strong and that would thin your blood."[55] Ruth Carpenter said that a lot of older people prevented and cured illness by doing "what they called 'purging themselves'. . . . That was a regular practice."[56] Believing that colds came on "Because you got the chills or you got your feet wet," Martha Ferguson's family wore "flannel things on [our] chest sometimes; long underwear. . . . When you had a cold you always wore a flannel rag on your chest."[57] Lucinda Brent Posey and Caribel Washington, both born in 1914, remembered wearing asafetida bags around their necks as children to ward off disease.[58]

Informants remembered food being important in health and illness. Richard Finfgeld said, "I think that if we weren't feeling well, it was something we had eaten or we had abused ourselves in some way. . . . I think my mother and father learned about eating when they grew up as children and had good eating habits. I know we always had very well-balanced meals at our house. There was always a vegetable, potatoes, and meat. One big meal and soup. We used plenty of eggs."[59] Martha Ferguson remembered that stomach problems were caused if "You overate or you ate something you shouldn't have eaten. You pigged out!"[60] Similarly, Reginald Whitaker, twenty years younger, said his mother and sister agreed that if he ate better, he would not have been frequently ill as a child. "I was so finicky about my eating like a lot of children are. If I would have eaten better, maybe I wouldn't have had those problems. But I just wanted sweets all the time."[61] All of these comments suggest a culture of personal responsibility for health maintenance and disease prevention that blurred the boundaries between traditional and biomedical health cultures and affected both sufferers and healers.

The memory of home remedies and informal health authorities is particularly strong among African American informants, perhaps because of a sturdy cultural tradition, perhaps because of the difficulties blacks encountered until comparatively recently in obtaining professional medical care.[62] Lucinda Brent Posey remembered,

> Every Fall, I had to go with Grandma [half Cherokee and half Black] . . . to get her roots for bitters. A bottle and a blue granite kettle were kept on the top shelf of the pantry for this. Hickory bark from the tree, dandelion roots, plantain roots, and I don't know what other kind of roots went into the bitters. Grandma spent the next day scraping and cleaning her roots. They were put in the blue granite kettle with water and simmered all day; strained through a cheese cloth. Eventually, the brown liquid went into the tall bottle. Mother was told to bring home one-half pint of whiskey. It was poured into the bottle. If your toe hurt, you got a teaspoonful; if your head hurt, you got a teaspoonful; the same for a stomachache. I learned *never* to complain; the pain was not nearly so bad as taking the bitters.[63]

Caribel Washington recalled, "My dad's mother was a kind of herb doctor. They could go out in the yard and find several leaves that were good for sores, and good for bathing the feet or poulticing different places and that sort of thing. . . . They believed in ginseng weed and poke berries. When poke berries were ripe, they would make a kind of tonic out of that."[64]

Regardless of race, many informants remembered favorite family recipes for cough syrups. Grace Allman said her mother's contained "honey and horehound. I don't know what else was in it. She'd make it and a great big bottle would always sit up in the cupboard. If we had a cough or a cold, we had the cough medicine ready. . . . Now, my husband's mother used to use whiskey in medicine that she made, but my mother didn't believe in that."[65] Ruth Carpenter's stepmother "had an old teacup. It was still useable and she put a big onion in there and maybe sectioned it off and covered it with sugar and then set it on the back of the cookstove and made it simmer. And it made a good cough syrup."[66]

Onions were also used in poultices for congested chests and sore throats. Lucinda Brent Posey remembered the onion being "heated, put into a piece of cotton sheeting, and put on your chest when you had a chest cold."[67] Poultices were also made of other household substances. Ruth Carpenter recalled applying poultices made of bread and milk to "draw" local infections.[68] And Lucinda Brent Posey said, "The final remedy of *all* remedies was when I had the flu in 1918. A cow manure poultice was made and put on my chest. Mother went somewhere with an old kettle and got the cow manure. Grandma heated it, but it into white sheeting, and (despite my screams and hollers) put the *hot* stinky poultice on my chest. It was covered with a piece of flannel to hold in the heat. Despite all of that, I was better in the morning and the cough loosened up."[69] Many families treated chest congestion with more conventional goose grease, often covered with a flannel cloth.[70]

Caribel Washington remembered her family using home remedies for colds, "We always had coal oil glycerin that we took for a bad cold. . . . I guess they don't call it coal oil these days, do they? What do they call it? Kerosene! When we were children, they called it coal oil, but it was kerosene and glycerin. They would mix some portion of that up in a big bottle and then if you had a cold, . . . shake that bottle up and give you some of that."[71] Informants also remembered home cures for croup. Ruth Carpenter's stepmother would soak a towel in cold water, "wrap it around my neck and it [croup] would soon disappear."[72] Possibly harking back to traditional magic, Ethel Cherry, born in 1911, recalled, "My brother used to have croup all the time, and my mother put a silk thread around his neck to keep him from having croup. And it worked!"[73]

For injuries, some families used turpentine. According to Ruth Carpenter, "We had a bottle in the house for the humans and another for the horses out in the barn." When asked, "What would you do with it? You'd just rub it on the injured part?" she responded, "Well, yeah, or pour it. If it was an open wound, you just poured it on. In made it burn like crazy."[74] Martha Ferguson remembered another approach: "For the nail in my foot, they used a home remedy which consisted of burning wool in a shovel and putting my foot over the smoke."[75]

In addition to homemade remedies, many people took patent medicines, purchased from itinerant salesmen or stores. Margaret Esposito recalled that her father had had the reputation within his own family for being something of a hypochondriac:

> INFORMANT: I can remember him having a propensity for some kinds of over-the-counter drugs. I don't remember now what they were.
> INTERVIEWER: Do you remember him regularly taking tonics or laxative, say?
> INFORMANT: Yes . . . I can't say what they were or anything. I think the most ridiculous thing that happened that I can remember rather distinctly. . . . I was then grown, and he was having an upset stomach, and he went to the cabinet and got out a bottle of pink fluid, and thought it was Pepto Bismal and it was . . . Caladryl. . . . He took a swig of that and just was shocked!

Esposito's father regularly spent his summer vacations at a spa in Missouri, "Taking the baths. . . . and drinking the water and that sort of thing," in an effort to improve his health.[76] Marie Snyder's mother made a cough syrup recipe containing laudanum: "I imagine it was an opium of some kind. Some kind of drug. She used some of that. What else was in it, I don't know, but it finally got so you couldn't get that without a prescription from the doctor, and of course the doctor wasn't going to give you a prescription!"[77]

Ruth Carpenter remembered her family purchasing remedies from traveling salesmen. "In those days, we had Raleigh men and McNess men and, what was the other one . . . ? They . . . would come traveling through the countryside with their . . . big bag. . . . and they had, like, mentholatum salve and . . . carbolic salve and then he had just a little of everything. Oh, it was wonderful for that man to come!" She recalled that her father took a laxative called a "Hinkle Pill," saying, "He thought it would cure anything."[78] Marie Bostic remembered buying a tonic from a traveling peddler, saying, "We'd go to the show they had."[79] A number of informants also remember being given castor oil or cod liver oil as children to ward off illness.

As we have seen, patent and home remedies were used even for serious illnesses. Caribel Washington remembered her mother's bout with pneumonia in the 1920s:

> She was a big beautiful woman, but she got pneumonia and those were . . . the days when you didn't send people to the hospitals. We were so afraid she was going to die. . . . We would take half-gallon fruit jars and put big gobs of Vicks salve in and pour boiling water over it, you know, to set up the vapor in the room for her. In those days, they put a flannel jacket on a person, and you didn't take that off, unless for bathing or something. We just always felt that those were the things as much as anything else that helped our mother. I don't recall the medicine that she took. She must have taken some. I can just remember how religiously we would boil that water and just keep it hot to help her.[80]

Washington also recalled dosing her own son with patent remedies used when she was a child. "You see, as children, we believed a lot in quinine. . . . and castor oil was always in our house. I can't ever recall an aspirin, but back in those days it was quinine. We did a lot with it. So, whatever we gave him [for scarlet fever], he got better."[81]

Sufferers and Families: Patients and Doctors

In addition to providing treatment and care, mothers decided when to "call the doctor." Ralph Spencer recalled, "Well, my mother always said, 'I think it's time,' to my dad, 'that you take Ralph or you take Orville to see the doctor. . . . He did whatever she told him to do in regards to something like that—oh yeah."[82] Other female relatives were also involved in medical decision making. On a number of occasions, Reginald Whitaker's older sister, who lived in Chicago, took him to a doctor when he visited her as a child during the 1930s. "Now, my sister Fay had taken me to doctors downtown [in Chicago] when I was much smaller. She was always taking me to the doctor . . . You don't find many sisters that will do these things for you like she did. Like I said, she was like a second mother to me."[83]

However, older informants remembered little contact with doctors, despite repeated reference to them. Ruth Carpenter said, "My father was allergic to doctors, I think . . . 'cause he didn't believe in going to the doctor. . . . We had two doctors in town and one of 'em was about the same caliber as the other one, and then we had a veterinarian. And my father said many times that he'd rather go to the veterinarian as he would to the M.D. . . . He just said they [doctors] didn't have any good common sense."[84] Martha Ferguson said, "I know that we had a family doctor, although I don't remember him. . . . He came for my sister's birth . . . and he came when we had scarlet fever. He even came when I had pneumonia, but those were so far apart."[85] For such families, despite reference to a "family doctor," the physician was not a routine component of health management; he was called only for serious illnesses and, in this case, births. Far more important were family caregivers' knowledge and skill.

Ethel Cherry reflected on the confidence of an older generation of women to handle their children's health problems: "It's funny, but you didn't consult all that like they do now. It was sort of an instinct or something you went by. You just knew how to do it. There have been so many times that people used to have the instinct to take care of their babies, but now you have to go to all of this counseling and everything. You didn't have that then. . . . My mother I would ask questions. . . . Even the doctor, I wouldn't run to like they do nowadays."[86] Furthermore, during the early twentieth-century transition to professional institutional care, family members sometimes attended ailing loved ones even in the place most thoroughly controlled by the doctor—the hospital operating room.[87]

However, even in an era when home care was the rule, some families developed long-standing relationships with local general practitioners who delivered babies, did surgery, set bones, sutured lacerations, and dealt with internal ailments. Physicians were not expected to be able to solve all health problems, but rather to use their special expertise to diagnose, intervene, and predict outcomes. The doctor-patient relationship was built on trust, which in many cases withstood doubts about the physician's methods. For example, Grace Allman consulted a rural Stanford doctor whose office was, by some people, considered unsanitary. "In fact, the Health Department came up and inspected his office at one time and suggested that he change things." When she had a growth on her leg, Allman's adult niece, "a physical education teacher . . . [who] thought she knew quite a few of the rules" advised her against having this doctor remove it because, "I might get . . . blood poisoning or something, you know. I ought to go some place else. I did have enough faith in [my doctor] so I didn't think that would happen." She went ahead with the surgery, which was performed in the doctor's office.[88]

Allman's trust stemmed from her personal relationship with the physician and his wife, beginning when they were newlyweds and Allman was in her teens. "His wife was from Baltimore, and that was horse and buggy days of course. When he had to make a call, she was kind of timid and didn't like to stay by herself, so he would come down and get me, and I would go up and sit with her. If he didn't get home very early, they invited me to stay for supper. I was always real happy to eat supper with them."[89] Such relationships were nurtured by proximity. As Ethel Cherry, who lived out in the country, said, "You didn't go a hundred miles to see a doctor. You just went to the doctor that was close to you." In her case, a seven-mile distance was involved.[90] Informants who lived in Bloomington-Normal also consulted nearby physicians. Reginald Whitaker, born in 1925, grew up in Normal, which today shares a boundary with its larger "twin" city, Bloomington. When asked if people traveled to Bloomington to see the doctor, Whitaker answered, "No. All the doctors were doctors here. . . . Dr. Doud was here, Dr. Penniman. . . . They had doctors in Bloomington. I guess some people would go to Bloomington. . . . Dr. Doud was on North Street [in Normal]. Up over, you know, where the ice cream store is down there? Used to be Velvet Freeze, they called it. . . . He was upstairs there. Dr. McCormick, he was upstairs there too."[91]

Before World War II, despite consultation of physicians, expectations regarding outcomes of health events (e.g., illness, childbirth, injury) and medical intervention were low. Martha Ferguson remembered, "Scarlet fever was terrifying. . . . They didn't really have any good cures for anything." She also revealed general fatalism regarding childbirth: "People, women, were still dying in childbirth quite frequently when I started having my children [1930s]. There is a lot of stuff they do now to help women. Then, you either had it [the baby] or you didn't."[92] Thus, the doctor was one of a number of resources and weapons people used against ill-health.

Informants who consulted physicians had a high degree of faith in them. This was related both to some informants' sense of themselves and their families as "modern" or sensible, and their perception of medicine as scientifically valid. For example, Reginald Whitaker said, "My parents . . . didn't have a lot of foolish . . . ideas. If there was sickness and it didn't go away in a reasonable time, we'd have to get the doctor." Reflecting McLean County's links with cities in the region, as a young adult Whitaker consulted Chicago specialists for a problem with his eyes. "Dr. James Richardson was his name. I understand he was one of the finest ophthalmologists this side of the Mason/Dixon Line! He was more of a scientist than really a doctor. He didn't have any bedside manner. But he was really a wonderful eye doctor, Eye, Ear, Nose, and Throat."[93]

Informants also tended to take the physician's advice. As Grace Allman said, "If I go to the doctor and pay him money, I want to do what he says or else I wouldn't waste my money."[94] However, also important was the widening gulf between patients' and practitioners' understanding of biomedical knowledge, on the one hand, and inflation of patients' belief that doctors could solve any problem posed to them, on the other. People's trust in physicians' expertise transcended expensive and time-consuming experience with inaccurate diagnoses and ineffective treatments. For example, as children in the 1930s, Whitaker and his sister, Josephine, began to experience symptoms of the rare eye condition that eventually blinded both of them:

> INTERVIEWER: When did you find out about that?
> INFORMANT: My mother noticed. She'd tell us to pick something off the floor at night, and we'd be feeling around for it, and she knew something was wrong. So we were taken to an optometrist . . . no, an eye doctor . . .
> INTERVIEWER: A specialist, an ophthalmologist?
> INFORMANT: Yeah. They said, "Oh, it's night blindness." We were fine in the daylight or with lights on. I even used to drive at night. So we went for years thinking we had night blindness . . .

In 1948, at age twenty-three, Whitaker was examined at the Illinois Eye and Ear Infirmary in Chicago:

> I was going up there once a month or maybe twice a month, [for] about three months for different examinations. Doctors were coming in from around the state and other states; for cases like mine, they would have them come in, and those doctors would examine us. . . . but nobody ever came up with what the problem is. . . . My sister, Fay, had heard about . . . a doctor who had set up practice there in Chicago, and that he was very good. She was gonna have her eyes tested for new glasses. She went to him and told him about Josephine and I. He said, "I sure would like to see them when they're in the city again." So we were up there one Saturday, and she called him and said we were there. . . .

He was in his office on Saturdays, and then you could go at 7:00 on Saturday evening and he was there until 9:00. . . . So we went out there to his office and he examined us. Then he said, "You don't have night blindness." Boy, that sure felt good. "But! We call this retinitis pigmatosa and we don't know what to do for it. . . ." Then he wanted to know our family history. He said it's inherited, it's somewhere back in your family. . . . So he worked with us and tried different things. He would give us some kind of serum that they get from hogs. He was trying to . . . do a little experimental chemistry on Josephine. I think it did help her. She'd take about a shot a week, an injection. She spent the summer up there so she could go get some medicine orally. . . . I didn't go through it. I was working and all.[95]

Whitaker's account indicates the extent to which medical specialists were increasingly accessible in the mid-twentieth century, although it is significant that he traveled to Chicago to consult experts his sister thought superior to those available in McLean County at the time. It also reveals both the escalating belief that doctors could diagnose and find a cure for almost any condition and patients' declining confidence in their own ability to deal with what were increasingly thought of as "medical problems."

By the post–World War II era, delegation to professionals of all knowledge and authority regarding matters of health and illness had both distanced patients from their own bodies (and those of their family members) and rendered them less capable of effective participation in decision making or caregiving. Rebecca Rittenhouse, born in 1941, said, "Well, at that time people went to their family doctors, whether they were having children, stomachache or headache or whatever. The family doctor took care of it." She reflected on her dependence on experts during her pregnancies: "Ignorance is bliss. If nobody tells you that there is a problem, you don't know to ask. You know, if they don't offer a person with my background of not being told anything at home and not being told anything by the doctor, you don't know what to ask either. So you just go through."[96]

High expectations of physicians increased the frustration and disappointment of patients and their relatives when something went wrong. Margaret Esposito described her husband's experience with military physicians in 1959:

He became ill when were at Luke [Airforce Base in Arizona] and we thought it was a cold. And after a long weekend, he went in to the infirmary to get something for the cold and he never came home because they found fluid on the lung and they withdrew some of the fluid and cultured it and when the culture came back I got a call from his doctor. And his doctor said that he had carcinoma of the lung and that he had, I've forgotten how much time to live. A year, year and a half to live . . . That was in the unfortunate era when you didn't talk to the patient about all of this . . . So they sent my husband up to Letterman General, which was the major military hospital for that area, and the children were in school. This would have been February, late February by that time. The children were in school and I didn't want to disrupt that. My mother came down and stayed with me for a little bit, just while I kind of got my feet on the ground again and we could see what was happening. When he got up there, he hit a doctor that wouldn't accept that diagnosis and the fact of that culture. And that doctor decided he had tuberculosis. And they put him into a program that went quite a few weeks before the results of the testing would come back and they were treating him for tuberculosis. And when those cultures came back and all of that came back, it was not tuberculosis. And so then the surgery was almost immediate . . . I've never had really bad things happen except that, but that was so bad, so bad. Anyway, then as soon as I could I arranged to, well, he was in a week postoperatively before he could talk to me . . . And so then he had to go through all the radiation therapy. And then he had a little summer vacation time and I flew home with him here and then I took him up to his family's and he was having some reaction from radiation. We went to the beach one day. They didn't tell us not to, and that sunshine on the water . . . was really bad.

As we have seen, Esposito cared for her husband at home until his death in 1960. She said, "We had a doctor . . . I don't think he was the greatest doctor in the world, but he at least would come." He was not a specialist. "No, no, no, no, no. Oncology was only a word about that time, really, about 1959, 1960. It wasn't much of a specialization that was here."[97]

After about 1960, consultation of medical experts extended from situations where the sufferer sensed that something was wrong to monitoring of health. Reflecting on her rural childhood in the 1940s and '50s, Rebecca Rittenhouse said, "I'm sure we didn't have a pediatrician and we probably only went [to the doctor] when we got sick. So I doubt very much that we went like you would today—take your children for six-month checkups and all that."[98] Similarly, in remarking that her mother "didn't do yearly physicals. . . . She didn't do that sort of thing, we just had a family physician," Margaret Esposito was recognizing this change.[99] By the last quarter of the twentieth century, determination of health, like diagnosis of illness, was increasingly left to doctors, supported by an expanding array of specialized nurses and technicians. Aspects of experience that had previously been considered part of a normal life course (such as pregnancy and senility), personal characteristics (such as difficulty concentrating or sitting still in the classroom), and behaviors that might previously have been considered character weaknesses or vices (including substance abuse and homosexuality) were medicalized—a process led by physicians and researchers, but enthusiastically embraced and supported by laypeople.

This study's youngest informants revealed both internalization of bio-medical concepts and dependence on physicians to help them manage their own bodies and make day-to-day decisions. However, the normative good patient's role had become that of an educated health-care consumer, able to make the best possible use of the medical system. Linda Rohm, born in 1966, became pregnant with her first child in the mid-1980s. She chose to consult an obstetrician recommended by her sister-in-law. Her evaluation of her physicians indicates both mounting sophistication and expansion of patients' ability to criticize doctors' competence: "I really liked Dr. Carlson. He was a little too fast, though. He would come into the room and I would have to write the questions down and say them while I was laying down just to get . . . because he was out the door like that. And I didn't like Dr. Domingo, and he ended up delivering Daniel. I was much happier that he did it than Dr. Carlson, because he had a better bedside manner. He was calmer and not in such a rush." She began prenatal care when she was two and one-half months pregnant.

> They give you an internal examination to make sure you are pregnant. They start listening to the heartbeat at three months . . . I had to have a lot of blood work done. I had to have an alpha-feta protein test, I think that's what it is called, and that is to distinguish whether the baby has spina bifida or not. It's a proof positive test, and I didn't want to have it, because I wouldn't have had an abortion had it had that. But he convinced me to have that test by saying you could have specialists there if there is something wrong. . . . Then I had urine tests every month, and you get weighed every month to see how much weight you gained. Then they would chew you out or say you did okay. There was only one month that I gained the right amount of two pounds, the other months I gained six or ten. And then I had an ultrasound when I was about seven months pregnant, and the reason I had the ultrasound was because I thought I was having pains right above the baby, and we thought it might be gall stones. So I had a gall bladder ultrasound and then a full baby ultrasound. . . . They give you a pregnancy vitamin and that just—it gives you extra of everything you would normally take.

She also got advice about physical activity during pregnancy:

> The only advice he [doctor] gave me as far as during the pregnancy—he said you can do the same things you can do now, but don't start anything new. Like, if you never do aerobics, don't start an aerobics class. Or if you never bowled, don't start bowling. But like the question you asked earlier, it is not an illness. You do what your body can already stand. Like I was bowling at the time, and I bowled up until a month before Daniel was born. You can do the normal things, as far as they explain to you. You can have sex, and they will tell you

what you shouldn't do as far as sex . . . and they will tell you how much weight they think you should gain. Now, a long time ago, it didn't use to be a lot. But now, like when I had Daniel, they told me 30–40 pounds is normal, but now it is coming back lower again as what you should gain.[100]

Rohm, a high school graduate from a small rural community, reveals the extent to which by the 1980s biomedicine pervaded lay health culture and doctors had become authorities about every detail of pregnancy—the process that had been most central to traditional laywomen's health culture before the mid-twentieth century. However, her interview also indicates a late twentieth-century shift toward the empowerment of health-care consumers.

Paying the Doctor

Although many oral history informants remembered growing up in households where there was very little money, paying the doctor was not mentioned as a major challenge. In the first half of the twentieth century, doctor bills were very small. Caribel Washington said, "We ran across a receipt. . . . I believe it was dated 1918, 1919, something like that. It was one dollar, where the doctor had made a house call. . . . Otherwise, I don't know. We were young and not concerned with the price of it, but I don't know that they [doctors] weren't paid. I don't imagine it was an exorbitant rate. If it would have been, we couldn't have afforded them."[101] Affordability of doctor bills depended on family income. Martha Ferguson's oldest two children were born at home in 1937 and 1938. She recalled, "The doctor and the nurse came for $25 and they stayed the entire time. Jim . . . was born in the country [in 1944]. . . . The doctor came at that time too, but I'm not sure how much that cost. It was a lot more than $25."[102] Ferguson's husband was a farmer who worked for the Works Progress Administration (WPA) during some of the Depression years. Ferguson herself worked in a tomato canning factory when her children were small, where she was paid "by the bucket." Thus, medical expenses were significant for her family. Marie Snyder's son was born in the hospital in the 1920s. "When he arrived, I was in the hospital for 19 days and I think it was just a little over $200."[103] Snyder's husband worked for Illinois Bell; in 1920, average wages in telephone and telegraph work were $1,115 per year.[104] For her family, the hospital charge was probably affordable.

Before the 1950s, medical bills were paid out of pocket. When asked how people paid for their health-care services when he was young, Richard Finfgeld responded, "I suppose they sent you a bill. I don't know. My father's principal objective was to see that every bill was paid. So he would ask them what the bill was and pay it. When we came here to Henry [a rural central Illinois community north of McLean County], I went in to see Dr. Dicer down here when I had a cold or something. I asked him how much it was for the visit and he said, "A half a dollar." And I paid him. So maybe they paid that way."[105] When asked about medical insurance, Marie Snyder said, "They didn't have it then. I don't think they started that until after he [husband] died [in 1955]."[106] Only Martha Ferguson, who worked for General Electric in Morton, Illinois, for almost thirty years beginning in the 1950s, remembered employer-based group health insurance, saying, "You had to pay for the family card, which didn't cost that much, and I did pay for it."[107] Ruth Carpenter, who worked for Brokaw Hospital, had Blue Cross insurance that helped cover her care when she was injured in a car accident in 1943.[108]

Of course, some local people received health care through the Veterans Administration. In the 1940s Roberta Holman's husband, who had been a prisoner of war, was treated for tuberculosis at Fitzsimmons Hospital in Colorado.[109] And, as we have seen, Margaret Esposito's husband was a career military officer when he was diagnosed with lung cancer in 1959. When asked whether the military paid for his treatment, she said, "All the medical treatment that was done, and I could take him over to Chanute [Air Force Base, Rantoul, Illinois] any time, and then they did put him in a couple of times down at Scott for X-ray therapy to relieve the pain. . . . I could get the medications from them. But I don't think they paid the doctor bill. I think that was an insignificant amount . . . and we just paid." The family had no other medical insurance.[110] Dr. Harold Shinall said that when he started practice in the 1930s,

> Insurance was not prevalent like it is now. I mean, Blue Cross Blue Shield. I don't know what year they started, but I don't ever remember filling out any of their forms. . . . Very few of my patients had insurance, except insurance for employees of the factories or companies. That was primarily accident insurance, not health insurance. . . . Some of the poor who required surgery, for example, were required to go see the township supervisor. They just didn't have funds. I remember the fee schedule they had at that time was $40 for the surgeon, $10 for the assistant, and $10 for the anesthesiologist.[111]

With innovations and increased effectiveness in medical interventions—as well as growing patient expectations—charges climbed. Dr. Paul Theobald commented on the first shipment of penicillin he received in 1945, "It had a little box . . . a little vial with one shot of penicillin in it, and sort of a brownish powder in the bottom that you mixed with water. I think there were 24 bottles in that box. Maybe 48. . . . And I know that the supply chart of the company said that these were worth $50,000."[112] In many respects, the dramatic impact of penicillin on infection represents the post–World War II dynamic between the public love affair with biomedicine and the rise in cost of all types of medical intervention; because it was so difficult—and seemed so churlish—to put a price tag on the lives saved and pain avoided, there were virtually no limits on what Americans were prepared to pay for health care.

Several informants commented on the increase in medical expenses— particularly during the last quarter of the twentieth century. Linda Rohm, who commented that the cost of her mid-1980s deliveries increased some $200 within those two years, reflected,

> We were lucky with both of them, really. A lot of people have complications and stay in the hospital longer and have a bigger bill. [My friend] Rhonda, she was in premature labor from the time she was three or four months pregnant with Shelby. So she had a home contraction monitor, which cost. She was in the hospital two weeks before she had her. She thought she was going to have her, and they wouldn't let her have her, and then they gave her a shot to develop her lungs, and then a week and a half later she finally went and did have her. So she had a hospital stay previous to when she had her. So her bills were easily $10,000 with insurance. They are still paying on that.[113]

These observations reveal more than inflation in charges for medical services. They indicate that the services themselves have changed. Technologically dependent health care delivered in institutional settings is expensive compared to advice and service given in patients' homes.

Childbearing, Birth Control, and Abortion

Before about 1920, pregnancy, although regarded as a special condition, was a private matter, concealed if possible and rarely considered a medical condition requiring a doctor's supervision. Indeed, laboratory diagnosis of pregnancy, for which physicians were the gatekeepers, became available only in the 1920s.[114] Older oral history informants did not remember their mothers receiving prenatal care. Indeed, Grace Allman said, "I don't think she [mother] ever saw a doctor until he came to deliver the baby."[115] Regular visits to the doctor during pregnancy became common at the same time as hospital delivery—between about 1920 and 1940.[116] During the same period, the environment and management of birth also changed. Home deliveries, usual before the 1930s, occurred in the familiar domestic setting, largely controlled by the mother and her family. Although experts, including doctors, midwives, and nurses, supervised the birth process, interventions such as the use of anesthetics, instruments, and surgery were less common than they became when birth moved into hospitals.

Doctors welcomed this move for a number of reasons. As we have seen, physicians increasingly viewed childbearing as a pathological process, fraught with dangers to mother and infant. Beginning in the 1920s, use of forceps, episiotomy, and anesthetics (ether, chloroform, and scopolamine) became routine in physician-assisted births.[117] In hospitals, these interventions could be more conveniently and safely administered. In addition, the hospital environment offered resources useful in case of the complications that could arise even in apparently normal births. For example, as hospital utilization grew, the number of caesarean sections increased, as did the number of board-certified obstetricians available to perform these procedures. Although increased levels of intervention did not, in the first half of the twentieth century, reduce maternal or infant mortality, as we have seen, both physicians and laypeople became convinced that hospitals offered a kind of insurance against the hazards of childbirth.[118] Hospital deliveries were also more cost-efficient for doctors, who could often supervise several labors at the same time, rather than dealing with one patient in her own home.

After World War I, McLean County women were persuaded that hospital delivery was safer and more convenient than home birth. Hospitals were increasingly seen as germ free compared to homes, thus minimizing the risk of infection to mother and baby. Pain relief in childbirth, understandably popular among women, was more readily available in hospitals than at home. In addition, hospitals were equipped to deal with the mess of birth, whereas homes were not. Finally, in an era when people became less likely to employ servants and family support became less routinely available, a hospital stay could be regarded as a luxury enabling the new mother to rest and be relieved of household responsibilities.

With the move from home to hospital, childbirth became a medical matter. Accomplished in an environment controlled by institutional regulations and procedures, birth was separated from ordinary social and family life. In addition, experience of labor and delivery changed with routine use of a growing range of diagnostic and monitoring technologies, according to one authority, between the 1940s and the 1960s, resembling "the processing of a machine by machines and skilled technicians."[119] Not until the 1970s did McLean County parents begin to seek a more active role in the birth process and question practices and power structures that, by that time, had become culturally sanctioned components of local childbirth.

Oral history interviews document changes in the expectations and management of childbearing that have occurred in living memory. Alice Swift, born in 1927, grew up in an Amish Mennonite community that maintained social childbirth traditions.[120] She described what her mother had done before marriage:

> INFORMANT: Housework as well as taking care of mothers with new babies in their homes.
> INTERVIEWER: Was this part of a church role that was customary?
> INFORMANT: Yes. It was a customary pattern for single women to do this. Women in those days did not go to the hospital, in our particular group at least, so they always had their babies at home. . . .
> INTERVIEWER: Did she actually assist during the childbirth?
> INFORMANT: Possibly, but not as a midwife particularly; just to be there to take care of the baby.[121]

Rebecca Rittenhouse, born into a Mennonite family in 1941, remembered rendering similar services to her maternal aunts when she was a teenager. "I know as a young child or as a young teenager—real young teenager, 12 or 13—I would go to her [mother's] sisters and help after they had their children, and stay for a week or two. And just help with the chores and stuff like that."[122] Lucinda Brent Posey, an African American born in Streator, Illinois, in 1914, also remembered attending relatives' births as a young girl. "Nothing [about sex and reproduction] was explained by my mother. However, she had a book hidden in her trunk that I read. My sister-in-law taught me the facts of life, about babies, etc. Aunt Lucy Dabney had nine children, all delivered at home. My mother would be called to come. I had to go with her, so I learned a lot from listening to conversations."[123] These practices arguably served the dual functions of providing useful help to the newly delivered mother and educating girls about their future roles and experiences.

Betty Rueger, a Mennonite born in 1913, said that, in addition to a doctor, her paternal aunt and a midwife, who was also a friend of the family, were present at her own birth: "Of course then, you see, as you called the midwife, she stayed for ten days and she would do cooking and everything."[124] This informant called the same midwife when she gave birth to her own second child in the 1930s:

> INFORMANT: I . . . had her spoken for to come when the baby came. That was the way we did it. She knew and would call the doctor and say, "Well, now, you better come pretty soon."
> INTERVIEWER: So the midwife notified the doctor then. Did you have a telephone at that time?
> INFORMANT: Oh, yeah. . . . We were at Harold's parents that evening until about ten o'clock, I guess, and came home and I could not get comfortable. Pretty soon we thought that this was it. So we made the telephone call so my mom would bring out the midwife. And Bill [son] was there at eight o'clock.

INTERVIEWER: . . . During the actual labor or delivery part of it, did the doctor use any kind of instruments? Medicine?

INFORMANT: No. At one time, he thought he might need to, so he told the midwife to put on water to boil. But we didn't need it. And I had no medication.

INTERVIEWER: What would they have used the water for?

INFORMANT: Instruments—sterilize them.[125]

Before about the 1930s, it was usual for families to have voluntary or paid help during the home birth and lying-in period. Grace Allman, born in a rural community in 1896, recalled the following:

INFORMANT: All five of my mother's children were born at home.

INTERVIEWER: Do you know who delivered?

INFORMANT: Dr. Wright.

INTERVIEWER: Was anyone else present at the birth?

INFORMANT: Yes. There was a woman who came and stayed with her, kept her in bed for ten days.

INTERVIEWER: Do you know who that woman was?

INFORMANT: No . . . We all had different women. I don't know the woman who was there when my brothers were born, but I know the one who was there when my sisters were born; her name was Mrs. Morris, Alice Morris. The last . . . [nurse] was Rachel Wright, and my sister was named for that nurse—Rachel.[126]

Allman's mother also "had a hired girl that came and helped her. It was a woman who lived next door to us who came and worked there. She got $3 a week."[127] Ruth Carpenter, born on a farm in 1909, said of her own mother, "She had all of her babies at home. And we had a lady in the neighborhood that was what we'd call a midwife. Only she wasn't certified of course. But she did a lot of it, and she never had any problems."[128] As a nurse, Carpenter assisted with home births during the 1930s. She said, "And Dr. Mull told me just how to fix this stuff. We'd bake these linens in the oven and, you remember those white narrow-top tables about yea long? They were our delivery table. . . . I had Dr. O. H. Ball deliver four children out in the homes in the late '30s. This would be about from '35 to '40. I got called out into the country to go and there was a lady out there with a baby that was dead. I cleaned it, dressed it, it was a beautiful child."[129]

Dorothy Jean Stewart's 1933 birth in Bloomington suggests a transition from traditional birth practices. "I was born at home in the dining room. Dr. Brown delivered me, and I understand that Elizabeth Johnson, a native of Bloomington, also assisted in the birth. I suppose they were so busy watching the second coming of me that they almost put the ether in my mother's eyes instead of to her nose."[130] This account is noteworthy because of the use of anesthetic for a home delivery.

Although birth was regarded as the natural and expected role of women, it was also considered dangerous. Ruth Carpenter remembered that when she was young, "Mother mortality was terrific."[131] Indeed, her own mother had died shortly after giving birth to her younger brother. Margaret Esposito, remembered that her father's first wife had "died in childbirth or shortly thereafter."[132] Martha Ferguson said, "Women were still dying in childbirth quite frequently when I started having my children [in the 1930s]."[133]

The days immediately following delivery were traditionally thought to be an especially risky period, during which the new mother stayed in bed; the standard period of convalescence was between ten days and two weeks. Getting up too soon after giving birth was believed to be perilous. Ruth Carpenter remembered, "And I knew a lady . . . well, it'd be my cousin's wife, and she died from a hemorrhage from getting up postpartum."[134] Caribel Washington's son was born in Bloomington in 1935. She was hospitalized for "Thirteen days, which I felt was ridiculous! Absolutely ridiculous! But that's when they believed women ought to stay in the hospital for two weeks."[135]

As hospital deliveries became usual in McLean County, management and expectations of the birth experience and outcome changed. There was a growing presumption that birth, if properly handled, would result in a healthy baby and mother. However, even technological support and authoritative expertise could not guarantee this. Ruth Carpenter gave birth to her only child in the hospital in 1934:

> My daughter only lived 24 hours. I had a very very bad delivery. . . . I was born with a heart-shaped uterus; that's what part of the trouble was. They had to turn the baby around. . . . Well, I had a pretty good pregnancy, but the heart-shaped segment would come down into the uterus about a third of the way into the uterus, and they finally drug it out feet first. . . . Dr. O. H. Ball, he was just sick about it. When you went into labor, you just didn't do a C-section. We [she and her husband] never did have any more. We had two or three miscarriages.[136]

Margaret Esposito's daughter was born in 1947. Esposito was also attended by the obstetrician, Dr. O. H. Ball, and her complicated delivery was more managed than was typical for older respondents who gave birth at home. However, the outcome was better than Carpenter's:

> INFORMANT: I had a breech presentation with my daughter. A very difficult time. . . .
>
> INTERVIEWER: Did you have any anesthetic when you had your daughter?

INFORMANT: Only for the last little bit . . . to kind of give me some pain relief. And I had an extensive episiotomy. Because she also had the cord around the neck. And so I know I wasn't any cooperation to him [doctor]. He had to do it. . . . I was something. I'm sure he was pretty upset with me. Because I would not have a spinal. I did not have good impressions from what I had heard other people say.

This account is noteworthy because it indicates the ability of some patients to negotiate their care in the hospital situation—together with the informant's acknowledgement that such behavior meant she was not a "good" patient. It also reveals that by this time hospital stays after delivery had shortened; despite a difficult delivery, Esposito went home after five days.[137]

Hospital management of birth changed over time, with earlier practices modeling traditional home birth experiences, and later practices increasingly regulated and medicalized. These changes altered the culture of childbearing. Ruth Carpenter said that at the beginning of her career, newborns were not isolated in nurseries:

INFORMANT: In those days, we had a cart, and they had a pan around the cart about that high, and you could lay babies crosswise, and that cart would hold eight babies. Yeah. And we'd take 'em over in the middle building [at Brokaw]. And I know. . . . Especially on Saturday and Sunday, when people would flock in like bees on honey, and . . . I bet there wasn't a baby on them carts that didn't get kissed.

INTERVIEWER: So you weren't as worried about the germs then.

INFORMANT: No. We didn't worry about it.

INTERVIEWER: Well, did you let the other family members come in—you know, dads and grandparents and other children in the family?

INFORMANT: Yeah. Everybody could. Yeah. They could come in . . . and see 'em.

INTERVIEWER: So when did they change that rule, then . . . ?

INFORMANT: It got pretty strict. . . . In 1940 I had an OB case that had a C-section, and they became part of my family sort of. And I brought the baby down from surgery and the father was waiting at the elevator for him, and I let him look at that baby, and the supervisor like to had a fit.

INTERVIEWER: Really?

INFORMANT: I said, "Well, it's his baby. If he can't look at it, I don't know why."[138]

As we have seen, hospitals also dictated who could be present for the birth, often banning all family members.[139] Margaret Esposito's husband attended the births of their two children in the late 1940s, despite what the obstetrician presented as the nurses' resistance: "All he [Dr. Ball] said to him [husband] was, 'If you want to come in, and I would encourage you to do that, you just tell the nurse.' He said, 'They [nurses] will object.'"[140]

By the 1960s medical management of birth reached its zenith, and social childbirth had faded from community health culture. When Rebecca Rittenhouse's first child was born in 1961, she called her parents to tell them she and her husband were going to the hospital for her delivery. Her parents stayed at home because, "They couldn't come in anyway, so nobody came over. Bill [husband] was there, and that was it." She went on to say, "Nobody else was allowed on the delivery floor. Nobody was allowed in the delivery room. Even Bill wasn't allowed in the delivery room. He was just allowed in the labor room and the parents weren't allowed to come in anyway."[141]

However, in the 1970s, birth practices in McLean County began to change as the "natural childbirth" movement attracted local advocates.[142] Sally Wagner, an obstetrical nurse, began to teach Lamaze classes in Bloomington in 1972. She said,

> At first, . . . the doctors were real skeptical about Lamaze. They were used to heavily sedating patients and the patients were not active in their labor process. They were very passive because they were sedated heavily. The doctors were really negative—how could this possibly work? They definitely did not feel like the father belonged in the delivery room, and so that was a big battle. . . . They thought that they [fathers] would get sick, faint, or sue the doctor. . . . It took awhile to get them convinced and so forth, and now they do let them go in for C-sections and so forth, and it took a few years to convince them that it was okay to let them in for an operation. We've come a long ways, and the doctors are very positive.[143]

This statement reveals important factors of late twentieth-century health culture, including the power and authority of physicians, medicalization of birth, tension over malpractice litigation, and expectations regarding normative gendered responses to birth and surgery. It also indicates that local health-care consumers and providers (in this case, nurses) participated in shaping—and changing—health culture. By the 1980s when Linda Rohm's two children were born, although Rohm's pregnancies and deliveries were medically monitored and managed to a much greater degree than those of older respondents, she was also much more actively involved in the process than they had been. She and her husband used Lamaze techniques supported by pain-relieving drugs during her deliveries. However, harking back to traditional health culture, Rohm also depended on advice from female relatives during her pregnancies, saying, "I would ask Wendy [her sister] first, before I asked the doctor."[144]

How did McLean County residents limit family size or deal with an unwanted pregnancy? Although oral history informants were not routinely asked this question, it is clear that in McLean County, as elsewhere, people tried to control their own reproduction. Not everyone wanted children. Marie Bostic, born in 1897, said about childbearing, "That's one thing I never wanted. . . . I saw a couple of them [births], but I said I hope that never happens to me. He [husband] said, 'We'll do what we can to keep you from it.'" The Bostics remained childless.[145] Ruth Carpenter and her husband, born during the first decade of the twentieth century, planned to have two children. "He was from a family of twelve. . . . You can afford to do more for a child in a smaller family. I read in the paper nowadays that so many families have six or seven children. I don't know how in the world they can take care of them."[146] Richard and Mary Finfgeld expressed traditional fatalism about spacing their children: "There is no way that I would say you can plan a family. It just happens. We tried to have them. . . . I thought two years apart was the way it should be."[147] Since the Comstock Law, passed in 1873, outlawed provision of birth control devices and information, before the 1930s it was difficult for people to obtain condoms or diaphragms.[148] Consequently, it is likely that many couples used withdrawal or abstinence to space pregnancies.

Things had changed somewhat by the time Rebecca Rittenhouse married at age nineteen in 1960. She said there were birth control methods available: "You could go to the drug store, or I suppose you could have gone to the doctor, but the doctor I went to to get the blood test before the wedding . . . he didn't really say anything. I think he gave us a book to read or something like that, and that was about it. He didn't mention anything about contraceptives at all." After her first child was born, "We used birth control, because I didn't want one right away definitely . . . [Options available included] condoms and there was a foam. And they probably had I.U.D.s and that, but like I said, the doctor never mentioned it. So what you did for birth control was on your own or what you went to the drug store and got. I didn't ask the doctor for anything. I don't know what his opinion would have been, but he didn't offer any advice either."[149] Linda Rohm used the birth control pill in the 1980s before she had her children.[150]

Physicians were gatekeepers for birth control information and materials. The diaphragm and birth control pill—the two methods that most effectively enabled women in the second half of the twentieth century to control their fertility—were available only by prescription. As Rittenhouse's account reveals, it was sometimes difficult for even married women to ask for or obtain these prescriptions; in many communities, unmarried women lacked access to birth control information or supplies. Paul Theobald, who was a general practitioner in Bloomington for more than thirty years and delivered babies until the 1960s, said he never offered family planning or birth control services.[151]

How did McLean County residents deal with unwanted pregnancies? Certainly, pregnancy out of wedlock was traditionally considered shameful. In rural Chenoa after World War II, according to Russell Oyer, "I remember a couple of girls who had sexual encounters and were up against . . . pregnant . . . that . . . I think there would have been people in town who would have been critical of that. . . . But, a lot of that of course, was kept pretty much . . . I'm sure a lot of this stuff was never known about these people. I'm not sure how much publicity some of those things got. At the barber shop and around the filling station, you know, people talk about it."[152] There is evidence that abortions were performed in McLean County as far back as the 1890s when, as indicated in Chapter 4, a local physician was accused of this practice. In the 1950s and 1960s, it was generally known where abortion services could be obtained. Dr. Theobald said, "There was a doctor over in Peoria who was doing abortions [before it was legal]. . . . So some girls would go over there. I wouldn't recommend it or anything. If they would ask, I would say that there was an abortionist over there, but I wouldn't recommend it. And they would somehow or another find out who the guy was and go over there."[153] Dr. Oyer remembered,

> My convictions were that I did not feel ethically able to do abortions. But I also felt that patients needed to have the right to make their own decision. So basically, what I did with girls who came to me who were pregnant out of wedlock, I would talk with them in general terms and if they were willing to come with a parent . . . but I would certainly talk to them about the options. These are the options you have. In those days . . . I think Peoria was doing abortions even in the early days. . . . I would always try to be very cautious with the patients who were looking at the possibility of abortion after it became legalized. "Are you aware of the psychological, moral kinds of impact of this? Do you understand this? Have you talked with a trusted friend or have you talked to your pastor about this? Have you talked to a counselor?" I tried hard to work it all here. But by the same token, I did not feel like I could take in upon myself, in the self-righteous way you got to do. But in the early days, patients who wanted abortions. . . . I had one patient who went to Michigan. I think one patient went to New York.[154]

Doctors could legally perform abortions if the hospital's therapeutic abortion committee (composed of staff physicians) determined that the procedure was medically necessary.[155] According to Dr. Theobald,

> In town, they were very careful at the hospitals about doctors and abortions. If you wanted to do a D[ilatation] and C[urettage] on an incomplete abortion,

you had to make application or at least have two other, I think it was two other doctors say, "Yes, this is an incomplete abortion and needs to be done." At St. Joseph's Hospital you had a very difficult time doing so unless you had some tissue that a pathologist had said, "Yes, this is fetal tissue." Then you could go ahead and do a D & C on her. As far as some of these other cases, you had to be very careful. We always had to have at least a consultation with at least one other doctor to be able to do a D & C in the case of an abortion.[156]

Another option available to women who were unable or unwilling to keep an unwanted child was putting it up for adoption. According to Theobald,

I adopted out a lot of babies. I, when I say a lot, I imagine I probably adopted out 20–25 babies over the years when I was delivering babies. I used to, I didn't solicit them, but people would come to me and say they were interested in adopting a baby. Then I'd have one of the young girls who would be pregnant and didn't know what they wanted to do with the baby, and so I would tell them they could do whatever they wanted to do, but if they did want to adopt it out, I had some people who would like to adopt it, and I always made these arrangements with the mother. The people who were going to adopt the baby would always pay the hospital bill and pay my bill. There would be no exchange of information as to who the parents, adoptive parents, were, who the mother was or anything like that. In fact, I told the mother that I would never ever tell in regards to the circumstance, even if I had to go to jail.[157]

In addition, several local charities provided adoption services.[158]

Health Care and Race

There have been African American residents in the McLean County region since before the county's establishment. Always a small minority, African Americans composed just over 1 percent between 1880 and 1900 and approximately 2 percent of the county's population between 1910 and 1960.[159] Although some African American families farmed in the county during the nineteenth century, this number declined after 1900. In 1900 the small town of Normal had 253 (7 percent) African American residents out of a total population of 3,795; Bloomington had 599 (2 percent) African American residents, out of a total of 25,768. Turn-of-the-century African Americans in Normal tended to be skilled workers and homeowners, whereas those in Bloomington more often worked in laboring and domestic service jobs. During the early twentieth century, with rising racial discrimination, settlement patterns changed. The number of African Americans living in rural McLean County and Normal decreased, but new migration from the Deep South added to Bloomington's black population. In 1950 only 76 (less than

1 percent) of Normal's 9,772 residents were African American, although in the 1970s and 1980s, the town's black population increased again with the growth of Illinois State University.[160]

Although McLean County's black residents had advantages compared to African Americans living in the Jim Crow South, their opportunities and quality of life were limited by racial discrimination expressed both formally, in local policies and regulations, and informally, in attitudes, speech, and popular culture. Thus, for example, as a young man Reginald Whitaker's father had received a college degree in business. However, he was never employed in a white-collar job. "There was nothing for an Afro-American in Business Administration." Thus, Oliver Whitaker pressed pants for the Model Paris laundry for over twenty years, and finished his working life as a janitor in Bloomington's Livingston Building. When asked if his father felt frustrated by his limited career opportunities, Reginald Whitaker said, "No. He understood the period of the time, and I guess there was no point in being frustrated. Things were like they were then."[161]

Things were also "like they were then" in areas other than employment. McLean County movie theaters and swimming areas were segregated until after World War II.[162] Although African Americans were able to attend Illinois State Normal University in the mid-twentieth century, they did so under conditions different from those of their white classmates. According to Beulah Kennedy, born in the 1920s, "When I was coming up and going to school at ISNU, it was very discriminatory. You couldn't live on campus. You had to live in somebody's private home. Of course, I didn't have that problem because I was at home."[163] When African Americans began to be admitted to local nursing schools in the 1950s, they also had to find accommodation outside the residence halls.[164]

Nonetheless, African Americans were able to obtain professional medical care in McLean County. Caribel Washington remembered,

> Oh, yes. We had doctors all the time. We had Dr. Covington who was an African American doctor. A very good doctor. I can recall my mother's doctor was Dr. Greenleaf. . . . Then there was always Dr. Brown and Dr. McNutt. Those were the two doctors for the most part who doctored the African American people. There might have been others. . . . I don't say there weren't others, but I do know that those two seemed to be the main doctors back in the '20s and maybe the early '30s. Of course, with the Depression, we had another [black] doctor, but he had no business during the Depression because we had no money. But there were always doctors for the people.[165]

Oscar Waddell, born in 1917, remembered his family's relationship with its physician:

INFORMANT: And back in those days, we had a Negro doctor here.

INTERVIEWER: Was that Dr. Covington?

INFORMANT: Yes, that was Dr. Covington. But Dr. Fenelon took care of us boys. Dr. Fenelon would always call and want us to come up and get a shot. He was on the sixth floor of the Grieshiem Building. The building that burned. We would go up there; here were two little black boys come in there. And the nurse would say, "Yes, Mrs. Waddell, the doctor has been expecting you." The doctor would come out, "Oh, what do we have here? Come on in! Bring my boys on in here!" I would ask, "What are you going to do, Doc?" He would say, "Come on in here, I got some candy for you." You would hear them [other patients] say, "How come they get in ahead of us?" The doctor would give us a shot and tell our mother . . ., "They are getting this for diphtheria." And everything that came up, we would get a shot. He would tell her what to do. Back in those days, Dad never bought us any Easter, Fourth of July or anything. The Doc would always get that.[166]

As indicated in Chapter 4, black physicians encountered such challenges in establishing McLean County practices that only two settled in the area before 1960. Thus, African American patients were largely dependent on the good will of the local (white) medical establishment.

Black informants experienced less difficulty obtaining medical than dental care. Reginald Whitaker responded to the question, "Did you go to the dentist":

INFORMANT: That was a problem. No. Not until recent years. They wouldn't accept you. They had one black dentist here years ago, his name was Thompson, I think. I don't know how long he stayed here. He had an office uptown somewhere, downtown Bloomington, I should say. We just didn't go to the dentist. . . .

INTERVIEWER: Now, why do you suppose there was such a difference between doctors and dentists? You said the doctors didn't make any difference . . .

INFORMANT: Well, I don't know. . . . It's hard to explain prejudice. . . . Maybe a doctor is examining, putting that stethoscope on you and listening to your heart and lungs, diagnosing your problem. A dentist has got to go into your mouth with his instruments and what-have-you. I guess a black person's mouth was contaminated to them or something. I don't know.[167]

Caribel Washington also said,

I think that probably was our biggest problem for African Americans here. You could always get medical care, but it was very very hard to get dental care. . . . I can remember that people would put aspirins in their mouths around their teeth. I had very few problems, but by the time I began to have dental problems, there were dentists . . . I had a wisdom [tooth] that had to be kind of ground out, but I was married by then. I don't even remember the man who finally took me. I know I went and finally asked him. He was in the 400 block on Main Street. I went and asked him. He finally said he would. I don't know if it was real early in the morning or very late in the day, but I finally got it done. Then I didn't bother any more until we got to where it wasn't quite the problem to have a dentist.[168]

African Americans also encountered discrimination in medical institutions. For example, as we have seen, Fairview Sanitarium did not house black patients in the main building before World War II. According to Caribel Washington, "Well, of course, we were always afraid of tuberculosis. And I think probably after the sanitarium came on [1919], people had such an abhorrence to it because the African Americans couldn't stay in the sanitarium. They had a little place outside where they stayed."[169] Local hospitals varied in the ways they dealt with African Americans. According to Lucinda Brent Posey, "At Brokaw, a black patient was put in a room wherever there was an empty bed, regardless of color. This was in the early 1940s I know about. At St. Joseph's Hospital, two blacks were always put into the same room or a room by yourself. If they couldn't do this, the response was 'no beds.' Regardless of how much moving around was necessary, one never was in a room with a white person—until integration." Posey herself became Brokaw Hospital's second black employee in 1943 when she was hired as medical record administrator. The first was Elizabeth Brent Keyes who started work in the laundry in 1915.[170]

After the 1960s, in McLean County, racial discrimination in health-care provision declined. Nonwhite residents attained, at least theoretically, the same access to medical, dental, and hospital treatment as their white neighbors. However, since disproportionate numbers of African American county residents remained in poverty, economic, educational, and social class barriers continued to limit access of many black residents to a full range of services.[171]

Death

During the twentieth century, management of dying and death, like illness and childbearing, was professionalized and institutionalized. Early in the century, traditional ways of dealing with the end of life survived. The dying were cared for at home by relatives and neighbors. Bodies were prepared for burial by laypeople who learned by attending many deathbeds, sometimes as a voluntary community service, sometimes for a fee.[172] Relatives, friends, and neighbors sat up all night with the recently deceased to render respect to the bereaved family, grieve together, and care for the body. Grace Allman said, "All I remember is that people said they used to put pennies on people's eyes to keep their lids shut. Then they sat up with them all night too. I've done that. . . . Before they embalmed bodies they had to keep it as cool as they could, and they did it with cool cloths and things of that kind that they would put over their faces, you know."[173] Ralph Spencer remembered participating in wakes, which he defined as follows: "A wake is where a person is dead and two or three people sit up all night during the night. I have done that."[174] Caribel Washington also remembered,

> We always brought the dead home. That was one of the things that neighbors did. The body would go to the undertaker to be prepared and then it would come home. That time between the death and the burial, that would be a home sort of a thing . . . and people would come into our house. You'd stay up all night and have food and entertainment. Even if the dead was there, sometimes it would turn into a kind of social event. . . . the old people would call it "tarry," but we would call it the wake. But it would be the wake. We're going to tarry with them.[175]

Organizing funerals was the responsibility of family and church members.[176]

Older informants recalled that death almost always occurred at home. Martha Ferguson commented, "It was common to take care of a dying person in the home. My mother took care of my grandmother [in the 1930s]; it was just common." This is not to say that providing care was easy. Ferguson said, "I do know that she had breast cancer. . . . My mother had a lingering hard time with my grandmother going."[177]

Even the badly injured were nursed at home in the days before ambulance service and hospital emergency rooms. Marie Bostic remembered her great-grandmother's death in about 1908:

> INFORMANT: My great grandmother who lived in town here, she was the greatest thing. I can remember her just like it was yesterday. They had one of these round stoves, you know . . . of course, you'd never see her legs because they had long dresses. She used goose grease and kerosene, and she got her clothes saturated with that, you know, and was burned. . . . She lived alone. She got up and somewhere or other she turned around, and her dress tail got in that fire. It went up her back, and I guess she was really something else.
> INTERVIEWER: That's terrible!
> INFORMANT: Yes, it was. She screamed and the boys from the restaurant heard her . . . and they got burned. . . . Threw her on the ground, wrapped her up, and got her to the doctor. She burned on Tuesday. She died on Friday. She was buried on Sunday. Easter Sunday. She always went to church on Easter. She went to church, but she went in a coffin. . . .

INTERVIEWER: Was she taken to a funeral home?
INFORMANT: No. . . . It was all done at home.[178]

Despite continuation of traditional death practices until about World War I, change was under way in McLean County. It became usual, particularly in larger towns, for trained undertakers to undertake services previously performed by laypeople. Undertakers prepared bodies for burial, first in private homes, later in specially equipped funeral parlors. They offered embalming, supplied coffins, and organized funerals. While providing a welcome service, morticians and funeral directors also developed a business opportunity for which there was a steady market.

By the interwar period, informal home-based management of death was old-fashioned even in rural communities. More common was the paid undertaker who visited the homes of the recently deceased to prepare bodies for burial. Ralph Spencer's grandparents died at home within two months of each other in about 1920. He said,

> A reason why I know who the funeral personnel was was the fact that at the time it was in the spring of the year and the roads had thawed out and they had to use a horse hearse. That was the only horse hearse that was around. Mr. Otto had a horse hearse. He had a farmer out here with a big team of horses to pull that hearse. That's how I knew. Of course, knowing Otto from the time I was a little kid on, I knew he took care of my grandparents and then I knew him from then on till the time he died. You just don't forget those things either, see.[179]

Marie Bostic remembered a series of undertakers serving the village of Danvers, beginning with Mr. Lowe who looked after her grandmother.[180]

African American informants remembered some white undertakers refusing to prepare black bodies for burial. Caribel Washington recalled,

> Murray, and then Stamper, and then Kibler. Now, those were always the undertakers that would take care of us. My sister and I had a little laugh a month or so ago. Someone from Beck called and asked her if they could come and talk to her about funeral preparations. He came in, and the first thing she told him was that there was a time when you couldn't even go into the Beck establishment. . . . There was always someone, always someone who wouldn't bury us. You know. That's been a long time ago, though.[181]

After World War II, death in McLean County left homes and was managed by experts. When asked about changes since her youth, Martha Ferguson said, "I think it is nice that the body goes to the funeral home instead of the home now. It's just easier for the family to go through it than it was."[182] All aspects of the process became more costly.[183] In addition, death, like birth and illness, became increasingly remote from ordinary experience. Ferguson commented, "Nobody wears mourning. Then [in the past], they would go in black and wear it for a year or whatever. Nobody does that."[184] Grace Allman remembered a much more emotional response to death in the past. "My folks used to live across from the Presbyterian Church over there, and we've had people come out of that church and just cry until you could hear them yell clear across the street, the way that they were crying and going on. Nobody does that any more. . . . I think people have more control over their emotions than they used to. I think they shed lots of tears at home, but they try to hold up in public."[185] Perhaps as death, like illness and childbearing, moved out of homes and lay responsibility, people were less prepared for it and lost confidence about how to deal with it.

Conclusion

Lay community residents were active participants in the twentieth-century transformation of McLean County's health culture. Indeed, their faith in biomedicine facilitated the transitions from home to institutional care; from informal to formal authority and agency in health-care decisions and interventions; and from fatalist endurance of many aspects of the human condition to expectations of good health, long life, and powerful medicine.

Yet, this faith has been challenged in recent years. Racial, ethnic, and social class disparities in access to care and health outcomes persist—in McLean County as elsewhere in the United States.[186] The limitations of biomedicine to deal effectively with many health problems are increasingly apparent.[187] The reentry of laypeople into health-care negotiations and choices has positively affected childbearing and end-of-life care, to mention only two examples. As the population is overwhelmed with chronic conditions such as diabetes and heart disease, individuals are being urged to take charge of disease prevention long before expert intervention is required. Furthermore, a return to home and lay care is currently being driven by health-care costs; thus, a generation that never learned to splint a sprain, comfort a laboring mother, or pass a bedpan must, in McLean County as elsewhere, use instruments to monitor hypertension, change postsurgical drains and dressings, and care for dementia sufferers at home. At the beginning of the twenty-first century, the boundaries between lay and professional, amateur and expert, and traditional and modern are becoming increasingly porous, suggesting transition to a postbiomedical health culture.

CONCLUSION

Health Culture in Transition

The history of health, illness, and medicine is about all of us. It is about the anticipation of birth; the fear of disease; the worry over the sickbed of a beloved child; the impotence attending the decline of an aging parent; the horror and peace of dying; the finality of death. It is about where and when we live, our resources, our relationships, and our identities. It is about our dreams, nightmares, ingenuity, and mortality—those elements that are central to our humanity.

The experiences of health, illness, treatment, and care are culturally determined. They occur within communities, defined not only geographically and politically, but by social class, age, gender, race, and ethnicity. Thus, whereas national studies can document and interpret the broad outlines of change and continuity in the histories of public health and medicine, local studies both highlight the diversity of experience in the United States and remind us that research based on large cities of the East Coast or Midwest does not represent American experience in general. Furthermore, local research reveals both factors determining common experiences and the diverse experiences that occur even at the local level.

In some respects, McLean County can be viewed as a microcosm of the United States. Primarily rural with a dominant urban core, its history illustrates both the different experiences and needs of rural- and urban-dwellers and the reciprocal relationships developed across the rural-urban spectrum. McLean County is both rural and urban, depending on the observer's perspective. Remote from metropolitan centers such as Chicago and St. Louis, which have nonetheless become increasingly accessible, its twentieth-century identity has been persistently "downstate." At the same time as McLean County residents built trains and administered insurance products for regional and national markets, they have viewed themselves as small-town dwellers more familiar with ploughed fields than with skyscrapers.[1]

However, McLean County is also different from many other localities with similar populations in both the Midwest and elsewhere. Unlike many small industrial cities in the Northeast and Midwest, Bloomington has not undergone economic and population decline during the twentieth century. Its transition from a railroad and craft industry town to a financial and educational service center after World War II maintained a prosperous economic base and supported diverse commercial and human services throughout the second half of the century. And although some of the county's rural areas experienced declining populations during the mid-twentieth century—particularly a youth drain to urban centers—the late twentieth century witnessed growth of many villages, which have tended to become commuter bedroom communities to Bloomington-Normal. McLean County, along with the rest of the nation, has witnessed the decline of the family farm, but no decline in agricultural production, which since the mid-twentieth century has shifted from mixed farming to large-scale production of corn and soybeans. Although the county population is becoming increasingly diverse, with just over 10 percent of its residents reported as nonwhite in the 2000 census it is whiter than many U.S. counties. And although, like other American communities, McLean County is aging, the presence of two universities and a community college keep it younger than other downstate Illinois counties. These characteristics influence the county's health-care needs, provision, and experience.

This book has observed the transformation between 1880 and 1980 of McLean County's health culture, providing a case study of the sweeping changes in the understanding and management of health, birth, ill-health, and death that also occurred elsewhere in the United States. It has depended on the voices of diverse participants—women and men; residents of rural and urban areas; whites and blacks; doctors and nurses—to tell their own stories. This last chapter offers conclusions organized around three central themes: changes in the *place* of treatment, care, and prevention; changes in *agency and authority* regarding these matters; and changes in the *interpretations and expectations* of health experiences and management. It closes with a brief discussion of health-care needs and resources in McLean County at the end of the twentieth century.

Place

The place where birth, ill-health, death, treatment, and care happen is intimately linked to the ways people think about and deal with these matters. In 1880 McLean County residents adhered to—and did not question—the tradition common to most locations and time periods of preventing and treating illness, giving birth, managing injury and disability, and dying at home. There, health and illness coexisted; birth and death were familiar to all; and treatment and outcomes were visible. In their own homes, sufferers remained individuals whose identities were separate from their ailments. In patients' homes, physicians remained outsiders, invited to exercise their expertise at the discretion of the householder. In clients' homes, nurses served at the will of patient and doctor; failure to satisfy either patron ended in dismissal. Disease prevention was determined by family tradition and community etiquette.

Home-based care endured longer in rural than in urban McLean County— and longer in McLean County than in the urban eastern United States, but not as long as in the rural South.[2] However, in the early twentieth century, the location of treatment, care, and prevention in the county began to change. The county's hospitals, initially either homelike refuges for those few who lacked the appropriate resources for the more desirable and conventional home care or a luxurious proprietary alternative to the dwellings of the prosperous, by the interwar period were usual locations for birth, surgery, and serious illness. This transition was driven by physicians, who not only recognized the cost-efficiency of visiting and treating multiple patients in the same place, but increasingly found hospitals necessary arenas for career development. Hospitalization and medical specialization were joined at the hip, with hospitals offering facilities and equipment meeting specialists' needs, and physicians both referring within generalist-specialist networks and admitting an increasing number and range of patients to hospitals. By the 1950s McLean County's hospitals themselves had been transformed from unspecialized imitations of home-care environments to factorylike institutions with highly specialized departments designed to process interventions. These facilities generated their own business: surgically equipped delivery rooms facilitated growing numbers of caesarean sections, and pediatric wards increased the volume of tonsillectomies and child admissions.

This transformation was intimately associated with the evolution of nursing education and careers. McLean County's hospitals generated a supply of trained nurses who, as students, staffed the hospitals and, as graduate nurses, served county residents in their own homes. The county's hospital-based nursing schools institutionalized nursing from their beginning in the 1890s. Student nurses were disciplined, assigned tasks, and garbed within conventlike rules that required them to live in the hospital and subordinate their own interests and needs to those of the institution. As students, they operated within a rigid pecking order, with physicians and nursing supervisors at the top, and senior students in authority over junior students. Their workdays merged ritualized practice of traditional women's duties of housework and nurture with inculcation of shifting biomedical theories and therapies.

Yet, until the 1940s, the institutional lives of most nurses were very short; in the early twentieth century most McLean County graduate nurses did private duty in patients' homes. Thus, nurses served as a bridge between hospital and home, urban and rural, easing changes in the place, management, and interpretation of ill-health and care for the people whose bedsides they attended. After World War II, nursing education moved out of local hospitals, and graduate nurses moved in, staffing increasingly diverse and specialized services. This change created job opportunities and increased professional status for nurses; however, it also reduced the independence previously offered by nursing careers. Nurses who, in private duty accepted or refused jobs, determined their own schedules, and decided which physicians and patients to work with, in hospitals were subordinate to both physicians and increasingly powerful hospital administrators.

For sufferers, the transition to hospital care came through a combination of marketing, obedience, and fear. The advent of the germ theory and trained nursing changed the image of hospitals from smelly disorderly places staffed by uneducated servants, where poor people went to die, to sparkling clean places run by wholesome young women in starched white uniforms, where modern people went to obtain scientifically based care. Hospital buildings themselves became some of the grandest edifices in the county, exemplifying both progressive civic life and modern science. Hospitals advertised themselves as homelike in the comfort and care they offered, but better than home in providing germ-free environments equipped with the latest medical technology, and run by trained professionals. However, McLean County residents might not have responded to these marketing efforts had it not been for McLean County physicians, who ordered admission for a growing range of conditions. Once a significant number of people had experienced hospital care, that experience became "normal" and fear of hospitals became old-fashioned. That fear was replaced by another more potent one, inculcated by physicians—the fear of not taking every possible precaution, including hospitalization, against the dangers of childbirth, illness, and injury. Furthermore, consultation of physicians and use of hospitals was associated with "modern" behavior among a growing educated public for whom medical institutions represented science and progress—as well as the glamorous, newly familiar environment for many film, radio, and television dramas. Increasingly, consumers viewed hospitalization as a necessity and a right, rather than a luxury or a threat; their demand for access to hospital care and willingness to back hospital development with votes and funding aided national and local policies supporting community hospitals.

At the same time as McLean County residents were growing accustomed to hospital care, they were more frequently consulting doctors in offices, rather than expecting house calls. Although McLean County physicians had maintained offices from the days of early settlement, in the nineteenth century they spent most of their working lives visiting and treating patients in the patients' own homes. They depended on patients' families for their incomes, reputations, and career development, and competed against each other for business. In the early twentieth century, first rural, then urban doctors began to move close to each other in downtown offices. In Bloomington, several large office blocks became medical buildings, where general practitioners and specialists developed referral networks, and specialists were visible to patients. Increasingly dependent on laboratory facilities and other equipment, doctors asked patients to come to their offices. This increased the volume, efficiency, and incomes of medical practices. In the mid-twentieth century, physicians began to employ a growing range and number of nurses and clerical assistants to share routine patient care services and help manage administrative functions. By the 1980s doctors' offices had become cost centers, where a diverse range of technology and personnel supported the business of diagnosis, advice, and therapy.

Although neither as dramatic nor as obvious, the institutionalization of prevention—public health infrastructure, services, and enforcement—paralleled the institutionalization of care and treatment. In 1880 McLean County's entire official public health operation rested on the shoulders of Bloomington's voluntary health committee, a part-time health officer, and a sanitary policeman who was mainly in charge of "nuisance" (mostly garbage) abatement. Even collection and reporting of vital statistics and incidence of contagious diseases was partial and contested. Disease prevention was largely left to individuals, except during epidemics, and, like care and intervention, was done at home. Connection with new public water and sewer services was discretionary and only possible in central Bloomington.

Nudged by advocacy groups, legislation, and, ultimately, changing popular expectations regarding environment and lifestyles, by the mid-twentieth century pubic organizations such as the Bloomington and Normal Sanitary District, the McLean County Health Department, Fairview Tuberculosis Sanitarium, and the Cooperative Extension Service Home Bureau provided officially approved health information, services, and (in the case of Fairview) institutional care. The new public health infrastructure also had enforcement powers beyond those possessed by clinical medical authorities. Although dependent on local funding and power relationships, it also had the weight of science and policy behind it. Indeed, its official terminology, including words like *surveillance* and *inspection,* and its relationships with government bodies and law courts indicate linkage with a host of institutions prepared to compel individual behavior for the public good. Thus, by the second half of the twentieth century, community health culture presumed connection with public water and sewage services as preferable to private arrangements; immunization of young children against a growing number of diseases; and compliance with laws ranging from compulsory treatment for TB and use of fluoridated water to legal disposal of rubbish.

Agency and Authority

In 1880 McLean County residents' experience of disease prevention, birth, ill-health, care, and death was managed and mediated by adult laywomen—usually mothers, wives, grandmothers, or daughters of the sufferer. These women served as informal health authorities, diagnosing illness; guiding pregnancy and lying-in; composing and administering home and patent remedies; making up prescribed medications according to instructions provided by the doctor; deciding when expert help should be sought; and aiding or observing therapeutic interventions. Girls learned nursing and first aid along with other housekeeping skills; it was not uncommon for teenagers to help out when relatives and neighbors were ill or gave birth. Mothers or other women controlled access to sickrooms, chose whether and how to carry out doctors' orders, and provided most bedside care. As onerous as these tasks often were, they also comprised a component of women's special knowledge and power, both within their own homes and at the social bedsides of the community where they were the main actors in the mutual aid networks surrounding childbearing, ill-health, and death.

However, the Progressive Era in McLean County as elsewhere was a period during which formal expertise was increasingly prized. Associated with scientific progress, organized medicine was particularly successful in garnering both legal and cultural authority. That authority, which paralleled the institutionalization of care and treatment, not only supplanted, but invalidated the opinions and activities of informal health authorities. As learned and licensed medical practitioners (with a few exceptions, white men) gained a monopoly over medical information and intervention, laywomen's obligation to take charge of health care within their families and communities not only disappeared, but also became associated with ignorant destructive behavior. Without formal training or qualifications, laboring under the disadvantage of their sex during a particularly male-dominated period of professional medicine, both old wives and the tales they told were demonized. Women born after about 1920 lacked both the knowledge and skill to deal confidently with either their own or their family members' health issues. People who called the doctor for advice or treatment were regarded as responsible; obedient patients were good, whereas those who asked questions, failed to follow doctors' orders, sought multiple medical opinions, or consulted alternative practitioners were "noncompliant."

Meanwhile, other women assumed the authority of biomedicine. Trained nurses became its symbols and agents. Providing most of the bedside care to patients who, during the mid-twentieth century were often hospitalized and confined to bed for long periods of time, nurses assumed the earlier role of the home caregiver. However, they also had the might of organized medicine and hospital administrations behind them. They created, justified on the basis of science or medical need, and enforced increasingly rigid hospital rules. They served as intermediaries between patients and members of the community outside the hospital, on the one hand, and between laypeople and physicians, on the other. Their authority extended beyond the hospital walls, to doctors' offices, public health institutions, schools, and private businesses. Their advice was definitive and their decisions could make the difference in employment and educational matters: Could Miss Jones be excused from work and receive sick pay? Was Johnny ill enough to go home from school? However, the price of the nurse's authority, paradoxically, was subservience and invisibility because it was based on the doctor's power.

Among physicians, the most important change in agency and authority during the study period was associated with specialization. In the early twentieth century, virtually all local doctors were general practitioners—even those who had developed informal full- or part-time specialties. General Practitioners dominated the McLean County Medical Society and local practice until after World War II, performing most of the surgery and delivering most of the babies. However, beginning in the 1930s, the county's medical elite was comprised of board-certified specialists, and as they increased in number and coverage, the independence, authority, and incomes of GPs declined by comparison. Specialists dominated hospital staffs and determined staff membership and privileges. Specialists did the dramatic surgical procedures made possible by postwar antibiotics and new technologies—and absorbed the limelight and adulation that accompanied their new capabilities.

Agency and authority of public health institutions and officials largely resulted from popular consensus about the germ theory of disease transmission and political will to convert that consensus into laws. It also related to middle-class white convictions about the correct way to do things, ranging from infant care to trash disposal. New training and qualifications conferred authority on these new professionals—although that authority remained both less than and contested by local physicians. Armed with government powers, public health officials could compel behavior and punish disobedience. And with increasing scope, resources, and volume of regulations to enforce and programs to run, the number of McLean County's public health staff grew from two at the beginning of the twentieth century to thirty in the mid-1960s and about eighty in 1980. However, an important reason these officials succeeded in wielding authority is that county residents had internalized the worldview permeating public health regulations and services. By the second half of the twentieth century, most residents believed that it was right to drink pasteurized milk and fluoridated water, to vaccinate babies, and to investigate the sex lives of venereal disease sufferers. Public health, like modern medicine, had been incorporated into community health culture.

Interpretations and Expectations of Health, Illness, and Intervention

The transformation of McLean County's health culture changed the ways its residents prevented, identified, and managed illness. Old traditions die hard. Thus, late twentieth-century county residents still tried to keep their feet dry and put undershirts on babies to prevent illness. However, they also exercised at gyms and health clubs, and took both vitamins and an expanding range of prescription drugs to maintain health. These activities, not dictated by physical sensations but recommended by experts, were analogous to the asafetida bags worn by an older generation of county residents. They were based on faith in expert authority and the coherence of that expertise with residents' own belief systems. The definition of health changed. It became increasingly complex, beyond the competence of laypeople to identify or understand. Thus, county residents had annual medical checkups to determine the degree to which their bodies were healthy—and to identify illnesses that had not yet generated symptoms. Their bodies had become dark continents that could only be explored and interpreted by experts. Complete health became elusive—something adults associated with childhood innocence and sought, but did not expect.

By contrast, expectations of the outcomes of birth, injury, and illness rose dramatically during the twentieth century. Indeed, the professionalization and institutionalization of medicine in the interwar period raised popular expectations of intervention even before antibiotics offered the first effective treatment for infection. These expectations were reflected in hospital utilization, which mushroomed despite hard economic times.[3] After World War II, new drugs and technology-supported surgery raised popular expectations of medicine still higher. Medical scientists in white coats and surgeons in green scrubs made the covers of national magazines; medical heroes headlined broadcast news programs. Biomedicine symbolized progress and American power. During the 1950s and 1960s, expectations of medical intervention expanded beyond any possible reality. Access to formal health care became a necessity, its power an unalloyed good.

Thus, in contemporary health culture all medically managed pregnancies and deliveries are expected to result in perfect babies and robust mothers. Few illnesses are presumed to be invariably fatal; the concept of natural death has all but disappeared. Laypeople believe that physicians can cure almost any disease or repair almost any injury—that the right doctor can snatch health from the jaws of death. Their faith is encouraged by practitioners, who also have high expectations of medical intervention—if it is not limited by inadequate facilities, interference from nonpractitioners, or lack of financial resources.

As is true for other services or products, high expectations came with costs that, in turn, created a new industry. Although health insurance became available during the 1930s, and employer-based coverage was initiated during World War II, few McLean County households used insurance to pay their medical bills until the 1960s. At that point, as health-care expenses rose beyond the capacity of most wage earners to pay for them out of pocket, the third-party-payer system became part of local health culture. Very quickly, access to insurance began to influence residents' important life decisions, including family size and employment. It also influenced physicians' decisions and authority, as insurers, recognizing the feeding frenzy that was taking place in medical charges, began to set limits on what they would pay.

Rising expectations and costs of health care stimulated malpractice litigation. Because people expected to get what they paid for, they were disappointed and angry when medical intervention did not produce the projected result. In addition, because the costs of care in cases of iatrogenic disability could be astronomical, patients and their families were also forced by economic exigency to sue. Physicians and other providers, for their part, were increasingly required to insure themselves heavily and to practice increasingly defensive medicine. These developments further stimulated the rise of health-care costs. They also affected the patient-practitioner relationship. While demand for services continued to rise, consumer trust in the health-care delivery system declined, and the tendency of physicians to treat their craft as a business rather than a calling grew.

Postscript

The years after 1980 witnessed reorganization, growth, and diversification of McLean County's health-care delivery system. In 1984 Brokaw, Mennonite, and Eureka (in nearby rural Woodford County) hospitals joined to form BroMenn Healthcare, which includes hospital and medical facilities. In the late 1980s, Carle Clinic, a group practice and hospital organization based in Champaign, Illinois, forty-five miles to the east, opened a branch clinic in Bloomington-Normal. St. Joseph's Hospital's new facility on the east side, opened in the 1960s, was rapidly expanding. In addition, new stand-alone proprietary day surgery, acute care, sports medicine, and other health-care businesses now serve a regional market with McLean County at its center. Utilization, quality, and cost of services remain high.

What does this say about the health of McLean County residents? Is health a direct product of a generous supply of services? In 1999 a study of the county's resources and needs for health and human services considered this matter together with other issues.[4] *Assessment 2000,* which employed a mixture of qualitative and quantitative research methods, revealed a complex picture of community health and the extent to which its medical needs are being met. Whereas overall county mortality rates declined during the 1990s, age-adjusted rates among African Americans were higher than among other groups. Infant mortality rates rose, from 5.9 per 1,000 in 1991 to 8.1 per 1,000 in 1996. Low birth rates, often associated with infant mortality, were much higher among blacks than among whites.[5] These figures indicate a racial gap in health status similar to national trends.

Health status is also associated with income. McLean County is prosperous; yet about a quarter of its population has annual household incomes of less than $25,000.[6] Most of the 1,594 county residents participating in the *Assessment 2000* survey reported being in excellent (29 percent) or good (56 percent) health; only 15 percent were in fair or poor health.[7] However, lower-income and older respondents reported poorer health and higher-income and younger respondents reported better health. Nine percent of survey respondents indicated having a disability and 467 (31 percent) respondents said they suffer from chronic illnesses including heart and respiratory disorders (29 percent), high blood pressure (20 percent), diabetes (16 percent), and arthritis (15 percent). Over one-tenth of respondents with chronic conditions indicated that they are not receiving treatment for these ailments. In addition, a county health department study indicates that one-fifth of McLean County adults have a diagnosed mental disorder.[8]

A product of community health culture, *Assessment 2000* presumed the need for professional health care. Access to care involves factors including number and location of providers, ability of residents to see providers in a convenient and timely manner, availability of insurance, and affordability of services and insurance coverage. Access is also influenced by health-care consumers' location of residence, transportation, income, employment, health status, mobility, and insurance coverage (or lack thereof). Most primary and all specialist and hospital care in McLean County is located in Bloomington-Normal. This situation enhances access for urban residents, and limits access for rural residents.

As identified by the study, the county's major service shortages or gaps include local availability of mental health services (particularly for children and the elderly); abortion and sterilization services; geriatric and home-care services; Spanish-speaking health-care providers; and access to care generally for the un- and under-insured. Insurance governs access to services. Although 93 percent of county residents have some kind of health insurance, many lack coverage for certain types of services, including dental care (27 percent), vision care (42 percent), and prescription drugs (10 percent).[9] Because most residents are insured through their jobs, access to specific kinds of coverage depends on both employers' and residents' decisions—usually dictated by cost. According to participants in *Assessment 2000* focus groups, the number of uninsured people in the county is growing because of rising numbers of self-employed and part-time workers. Although many of these people have low incomes, an increasing number are professionals with good incomes but no job-related benefits. Furthermore, even people with coverage may lack access to care. According to study informants, there are no dentists or psychiatrists in McLean County that will accept Medicaid assignment. Some elderly people reported difficulty in finding doctors who would take new Medicare patients. Although some practitioners provide voluntary attention to the needy and there are pubic health programs and charities that serve people who would not otherwise have access to care, it is clear that in McLean County access to and quality of health care is rationed by the ability to pay.

Assessment 2000 reflects a health culture with broad consensus about health, medicine, and care. However, as is also true elsewhere in the United States, solutions to health-care challenges are elusive, in part, because proliferation of services does not eliminate ill-health but, instead, profits from it. The *Field of Dreams* adage, "If you build it, they will come," is nowhere truer than in health care, where the circle of diagnosis, referral, treatment, and payment never ends, but only expands.

Furthermore, ironically, McLean County residents are increasingly required to take responsibility for care that for at least a half-century was provided by experts. Discharged from hospitals hours after surgery and childbirth, they must apply dressings, watch for complications, and drive themselves to hospital emergency rooms if things go wrong. They are advised to inform themselves about their ailments, get multiple opinions about diagnoses and treatment options, and compare providers' charges before requesting treatment. They must increasingly care at home for physically and mentally disabled relatives as institutional care becomes unavailable or financially out of reach. These new demands reveal both the limitations of the mid-twentieth-century shift from lay and home care to professional institutional care and an educational and cultural challenge now facing Americans. We must attempt to re-create care-giving skills and confidence among laypeople in a society that can no longer depend on "natural" and nurtured female ability to care for the sick. We must also recognize the limits of intervention and emphasize prevention—not, perhaps, as glamorous or profitable an approach, but one that will be healthier for both individuals and communities.

APPENDIX

Oral History Informants

Name	Year of Birth	Residence	Occupation
Grace Allman Mrs. A1MP	1896	Stanford	Teacher
Marie Bostic Mrs. B1MP	1897	Danvers	Teacher
Loren Boon Dr. B2MP	1917	Washburn Danvers	Physician (general practitioner)
Ben Boyd Mr. B3MP	1927	Bloomington	Sanitarian
Matilda Calico B-N BHP[a]	1909 or 1910	Bloomington	Domestic service
Ruth Carpenter Mrs. C1MP	1909	Vermilion County Shirley Bloomington	Nurse
Ethel Cherry Mrs. C2MP	1911	Arrowsmith	Postmaster
Katherine Dean B-N BHP[a]	1910	Bloomington	Insurance work (State Farm Insurance)
W.L. Dillman Dr. D1MP	1920	Bloomington	Dentist
Margaret Esposito Mrs. E1MP	1923	Bloomington	Home advisor, Cooperative Extension Service
Martha Ferguson Mrs. F1MP	1916	Lexington	Factory work (General Electric)

Name	Year of Birth	Residence	Occupation
Richard Finfgeld Mr. F2MP	1906	Lexington	Newspaper work
Mary Finfgeld Mrs. F2MP	ca. 1908	Lexington	Trained teacher, homemaker
Ferne Hensley Mrs. H2MP	1894	Arrowsmith	Homemaker
Roberta Holman Mrs. H1MP	1921	Danvers	Nurse
Lavada Hunter B-N BHP[a]	1913	Bloomington	Homemaker
Marguerite Jackson B-N BHP[a]	1927	Bloomington	Caterer
Sister Judith Sr. J1MP	1922	Duseldorf, Germany Bloomington	Sister nurse
Evelyn Lantz Mrs. L1MP	1918	Danvers/ Bloomington	Nurse, homemaker
Russel Oyer Dr. O1MP	1920	Bloomington	Physician (general practitioner)
Lucinda Brent Posey B-N BHP[a]	1914	Streator/Normal	Medical record librarian
"Rebecca Rittenhouse"[b] Mrs. R1MP	1941	Eureka	Homemaker
"Betty Rueger"[b] Mrs. R2MP	1913	Cruger	Homemaker
"Linda Rohm"[b] Mrs. R3MP	1966	Eureka	Homemaker
Harriet Rust Mrs. R4MP	1919	Bloomington	Homemaker
Josephine Samuels B-N BHP[a]	1922	Normal	Domestic service, newspaper work
Harold Shinall Dr. S1MP	1909	Gibson City Bloomington	Physician (General practitioner, radiologist)
Marie Snyder Mrs. S4MP	1899	Bloomington	Hairdresser, homemaker
Alice Swift Mrs. S2MP	1927	Bloomington	Nurse

Name	Year of Birth	Residence	Occupation
Ralph Spencer Mr. S3MP	1914	Danvers	Farmer, mechanic, retail
Dorothy Jean Stewart B-N BHP[a]	1933	Bloomington	Insurance work (State Farm Insurance)
Jane Tinsley Mrs. T1MP	1924	Bloomington	Public health nurse
Paul Theobald Dr. T2MP	1922	Bloomington	Physician (general practitioner)
Sr. Theonilla Sr. T3MP	1912	Dortmund, Germany Pontiac, Illinois Bloomington	Sister nurse
Albert VanNess Dr. V1MP	1926	Bloomington	Physician (internist)
Oscar Waddell B-N BHP[a]	1917	Bloomington	Factory work (General Electric)
Ruth Waddell B-N BHP[a]	1923	Bloomington	Domestic work
Sally Wagner Mrs. W2MP	1938	Bloomington	Nurse
Caribel Washington Mrs. W1MP	1914	Bloomington	Insurance work (State Farm Insurance)
James Welch Dr. W3MP	1915	Cuba	Physician (general practitioner)
Reginald Whitaker Mr. W4MP	1925	Normal	Maintenance, telephone company (GTE)

Note: Unless indicated otherwise, informants were interviewed for the "A Matter of Life and Death: Health, Illness and Medicine in McLean County" project by project volunteers between April 1994 and September 1995. Transcripts are housed by the McLean County Historical Society, Bloomington, Illinois.

[a] Informant was interviewed in the mid-1980s for the Bloomington-Normal Black History Project. Partial transcripts and notes were used by the author with permission. Publications of the Bloomington-Normal Black History Projects were also consulted. The Bloomington-Normal Black History Project's oral history collection is housed by the McLean County Historical Society, Bloomington, Illinois.

[b] Informant was interviewed by Cynthia Baer for a class project at Illinois State University during the 1992–93 academic year. Interview transcripts were used for this project with Ms. Baer's permission.

Notes

Introduction: Matter of Life and Death

1. Pieperbeck, "A History of the Development of Nursing Education," 53.

2. *Biographical History, 1854–1954,* 83; *St. Joseph's Medical Staff Records,* 16, 34; Pieperbeck, "A History of the Development of Nursing Education," 80; "B-N hospital was order's first mission outside Peoria," *Pantagraph,* 28 August 1994, A3.

3. Porter, *Health, Civilization and the State,* 56, 149, 152; Charles E. Rosenberg, *The Cholera Years,* 17, 103, 210; Wohl, *Endangered Lives,* 84–85; Walitschek, "Historic Archaeological Investigations," 29.

4. Ingalls, "The Espy Pharmacy Records," 6–7; *The History of McLean County, Illinois,* 387.

5. Walitschek, "Historic Archaeological Investigations," 30.

6. See, e.g., Cooter, "'Framing' the End of the Social History of Medicine," 309–37; Jordanova, "The Social Construction of Medical Knowledge,"338–63; and Fissell, "Making Meaning from the Margins," 364–89.

7. See, e.g., Jordanova, "Social Construction" and Lupton, *Medicine as Culture,* 17.

8. See, e.g., Turner, *The Body and Society;* Loustaunau and Sobo, *The Cultural Context;* Lindenbaum and Lock, eds., *Knowledge, Power, and Practice;* and Augé and Herzlich, eds., *The Meaning of Illness.*

9. Loustaunau and Sobo, *Cultural Context,* 127; Oakley, *The Captured Womb;* Borst, *Catching Babies;* and Smith and Holmes, *Listen to Me Good.*

10. See, e.g., Melosh, "The Physician's Hand"; Rosenberg, *The Care of Strangers;* Porter, *Health, Civilization and the State;* and Porter, ed., *Patients and Practitioners.*

11. Lupton, *Medicine as Culture,* 17. This situation, of course, is changing, as Mary Fissel points out in "Making Meaning from the Margins."

12. See, e.g., Burnham, *How the Idea of Profession Changed,* 57–59, for discussion of the centrality of the physician as an ideal worker (rather than as a member of a professionalizing occupation) in the work of pioneering social historians of medicine.

13. For examples of research by professional scholars, see Bonner, *Medicine in Chicago, 1850–1950;* Leavitt, *The Healthiest City;* Lynaugh, *The Community Hospitals;* O'Hara, *An Emerging Profession;* Crellin, *Medical Care in Pioneer Illinois;* Numbers and Leavitt, *Wisconsin Medicine;* and Rowe, *A Representative History.* For examples of research by nonprofessionals, see *Practice and Progress;* and Livingston, *A History of the Practice of Medicine.*

14. Mahoney, "The Small City in American History," 99, 311.

15. Shaw, "Review Essay: Small Towns," 220.

16. See, e.g., Faragher, *Sugar Creek,* 87–95.

17. *Records of the McLean County Medical Society* (hereafter cited as *Records MCMS*); *St. Joseph's Hospital Accounts; St. Joseph's Hospital Admissions Records; St. Joseph's Medical Staff Records;* and "Records of Stella Bennett".

18. See, e.g., Thompson, *The Voice of the Past,* 1–21.

19. Interviews were transcribed with support from the Illinois Humanities Council. Tapes and transcripts of the twenty-nine interviews conducted for this project, together with tapes and transcripts of interviews conducted by the Bloomington-Normal Black History Project, are housed by the McLean County Museum of History.

20. Cynthia Baer took my "Oral History" course at Illinois State University in 1992. She supplied copies of her interview transcripts, which remain in my possession. Pseudonyms are used in connection with information provided by her informants.

21. This issue is discussed at length in Summerfield, *Reconstructing Women's Wartime Lives,* 17.

22. Portelli, "What Makes Oral History Different?", 71.

23. Summerfield, *Reconstructing Women's Wartime Lives,* 28–29, provides a particularly useful discussion of myth, legend, and "reality" in oral history evidence.

24. Portelli, *The Battle of Valle Giulia,* 17. See also Giles, *Women, Identity, and Private Life,* 26.

25. That work has resulted in four published papers and a forthcoming monograph: Beier, "I Used to Take Her to the Doctor's," 221–41; "Contagion, policy, class, gender," 7–24; "We Were Green as Grass," 461–80; and "Expertise and Control," 379–409. The working title of my forthcoming monograph is *For Their Own Good: The Transformation of English Working-Class Health Culture,* which has received grant support from the National Library of Medicine (G 13 LM 8353) and is scheduled for publication by the Ohio State University Press in 2008.

26. For examples of her use of oral history evidence, see Roberts, *Women and Families* and *A Woman's Place.*

27. I owe the concept of "collective responses to ill-health" to Dorothy Porter's "history of collective action in relation to the health of populations," *Health, Civilization and the State.*

Chapter 1: Living and Dying in Nineteenth-Century McLean County

1. I do not intend to give the impression that the area that would become McLean County was uninhabited when the "first settlers" arrived. Dr. E. Duis, "late professor of German in the Bloomington public schools," in his 1874 history of McLean County,

wrote that in the 1820s, "The Kickapoos ruled the country." Nonetheless, it is clear that significant Native American presence in the county was fleeting once "settlement" began, and early histories focus overwhelmingly on white experience. See Duis, *Good Old Times in McLean County*, 2–3. See also Tate, *The Way It Was*, 49–50.

2. Tate, *The Way It Was*, 67, 127; *History of McLean County, Illinois*, 337.

3. *Report on the Population of the United States*, Table 4, "Statistics of Population."

4. Wyman, "Bloomington and the Railroad," xviii–xix. See also *The McLean County Almanac 1984*, 20.

5. By the end of the twentieth century, State Farm Insurance employed more than thirteen thousand local workers.

6. Duis, *Good Old Times*, 281, 332, 334–35.

7. See Duis, *Good Old Times*, 846–54; *Biographical History, 1854–1954*, 46; Rogers, *Day Books*; and Beier. *A Matter of Life and Death*, 33–35.

8. Hasbrouck, *History of McLean County*, 189–99.

9. See, e.g., Tate, *The Way It Was*, 235.

10. Ibid., 179; Duis, *Good Old Times*, 19, 29. Jesse Fell was also involved in founding the home.

11. Teaford, *Cities of the Heartland*, 3.

12. *Dictionary of Unitarian and Universalist Biography*, "Adlai Stevenson," http://www.uua.org/uuhs/duub/articles/adlaistevenson.html.

13. Duis, *Good Old Times*, 213.

14. Mahoney, "The Small City," 316.

15. Hasbrouck, *History of McLean County*, 234–48.

16. Mahoney, "The Small City," 317, 319.

17. According to Tate, *The Way It Was*, in 1972, "There [were] 20 communities of sufficient size and virility in McLean County outside Bloomington-Normal to classify as community trading centers." (359) However, some fifty additional settlements began and disappeared in the county during the first half of the nineteenth century (363).

18. *The Illinois Fact Book*, 39–43; *Blue Book of the State of Illinois* and the McLean County Regional Planning Commission.

19. United States Census for 1880 and 1890; Geospatial and Statistical Data Center, University of Virginia Library, "County-Level Results for 1900," http://fisher.lib.virginia.edu/collections/stats/histcensus/php/county.php (accessed March 21, 2008); *County and City Data Book*; Tate, *The Way It Was*, 8.

20. Hohnenberg and Lees, *The Making of Urban Europe*, 4–5.

21. Rawlings, *The Rise and Fall of Disease*, 1:304. See Valencius, *The Health of the Country*, for a useful discussion of the ways settlers perceived the healthfulness—or otherwise—of the places to which they migrated. See also Crellin, *Medical Care in Pioneer Illinois*.

22. See, e.g., Hays, *The Burdens of Disease*, 243–50.

23. Dickens described the fever-blasted residents of Cairo, Illinois, in his *American Notes* (1842) and *Martin Chuzzlewit* (1843–44).

24. Rawlings, *The Rise and Fall*, 1:96–97, 150, 306–7, 393.

25. See, e.g., Faragher, *Sugar Creek*, 89–91; and Rawlings, *The Rise and Fall*, 1:35–43.

26. Duis, *Good Old Times*, 4.

27. Quoted in Rawlings, *The Rise and Fall*, 1:31.

28. Duis, *Good Old Times,* 353.

29. Faragher, *Sugar Creek,* 90; Duis, *Good Old Times,* 10–11; Drake, *A Systematic Treatise.*

30. Duis, *Good Old Times,* 11. See also Faragher, *Sugar Creek,* 90.

31. Rawlings, *The Rise and Fall,* 1:42, observes that the last extensive Central Illinois malaria epidemic occurred in the summer of 1872.

32. Ibid., 2:59. Ingalls, "The Espy Pharmacy Records," 6–7; *The History of McLean County,* 14, indicates one reason for prevalent resistance to vaccination: "The vaccine used was given with dried bone points that made the arm very sore and imparted dubious immunity."

33. Rawlings, *The Rise and Fall,* 2:59.

34. Ibid., 2:57.

35. Ibid., 1:311.

36. Custer, "Asiatic Cholera in Central Illinois," 6.

37. Rawlings, *The Rise and Fall,* 1:44.

38. See, e.g., Ingalls, "Espy Pharmacy," 15.

39. See, e.g., Rothman, *Living in the Shadow of Death;* and Hays, *Burdens of Disease,* 154–67.

40. "McLean County, Illinois 1860 Census." McLean County Mortality Reports for 1850 and 1860, McLean County Historical Society Museum.

41. Rawlings, *The Rise and Fall,* 1:364, 371. Since reporting of the incidence of tuberculosis was not required until 1915, these figures are certainly underestimates of tuberculosis infection in McLean County.

42. See, e.g., Abel, "A 'Terrible and Exhausting' Struggle," 478–506.

43. Leavitt, *Brought to Bed,* 24–25.

44. Although, in fact, the largest documented typhoid outbreak in Bloomington resulted in 1920 from contamination of the water supply used by Chicago and Alton Shops workers, two hundred of whom became ill, and at least twenty-four of whom died. See Rawlings, *The Rise and Fall,* 2:70; Ibid., 2:56.

45. Rawlings, *The Rise and Fall,* 1:83.

46. See, e.g., Ingalls, "Espy Pharmacy," 16–18; Rawlings, *The Rise and Fall,* 1:69–83; and Tomes, *The Gospel of Germs,* 23–27, 177.

47. Rawlings, *The Rise and Fall,* 1:55, 353–61; Ibid., 2:58–59.

48. Ibid., 1:351, 385, 391.

49. See, e.g., Whorton, *Inner Hygiene,* 29–54; and Warner, *The Therapeutic Perspective,* 91–98.

50. Rawlings, *The Rise and Fall,* 1:85.

51. Ibid., 1:394. It is noteworthy that in the early 1880s, "Birth reports were estimated to be from 40 to 50 percent incomplete and death reports from 30–40. In 1926 . . . statistics for births and deaths were complete for all practical purposes," (ibid., 1:393). In 2002 the infant mortality rate for Illinois was 7.2 per 1,000 live births. Source: Illinois Department of Public Health, *http://www.idph.state.il.us/health/infant/infmort000102.htm* (accessed March 21, 2008).

52. Rawlings, *The Rise and Fall,* 1:87. See also Viner," Abraham Jacobi," 434–63; Truax, *The Doctors Jacobi,* 171.

53. Rawlings, *The Rise and Fall,* 1:87.

54. Drake, *A Systematic Treatise,* 520–21.

55. Rawlings, *The Rise and Fall,* 1:378.

56. It would be a mistake, however, to presume a linear and inevitable increase in life expectancy at birth. As Faragher points out in *Sugar Creek,* 93, new Illinois communities experienced high mortality, with expectation of longevity at birth actually declining among settlers born after 1800 compared to those born earlier.

57. Ingalls, "Espy Pharmacy," 10.

58. Ibid.

59. Rawlings, *The Rise and Fall,* 2:57–59. Ingalls, "Espy Pharmacy," 9.

60. See Duffy, *The Sanitarians,* for a general discussion of public health history in the United States.

61. Walitschek, "Historic Archaeological Investigations," 29.

62. Ibid., 30.

63. Avery, "Privial Pursuit," 4.

64. *The History of McLean County,* 387.

65. Coal was found in Bloomington in 1868, and the Mclean County Coal Company operated from that time until the 1920s. See Hasbrouck, *History of McLean County,* 239.

66. Ibid., 388.

67. Ibid., 388.

68. Quoted in Ingalls, "Espy Pharmacy," 8.

69. Walitschek, "Historic Archaeological Investigations," 30.

70. Ibid.

71. Ingalls, "Espy Pharmacy," 6.

72. Ibid., 7.

73. Rawlings, *Rise and Fall,* 1:131 and *Biographical History, 1854–1954,* 36.

74. Armstrong, *Political Anatomy of the Body;* Rawlings, *The Rise and Fall,* 2:50.

75. *Records MCMS.*

76. Starr, *Social Transformation,* 180–97; Rosen, *Structure,* 41–43.

77. *Records MCMS.*

78. See, e.g., Abel, *Hearts of Wisdom,* 37–67; and Lawrence, "Iowa Physicians," 155–56.

79. See, e.g., Risse, Numbers, and Leavitt, eds., *Medicine Without Doctors.*

80. Hasbrouck, *History of McLean County,* 267.

81. Bateman, ed., *Historical Encyclopedia,* 2:850.

82. This issue is discussed in Rosen, *Structure,* 7–9, and Warner, *Therapeutic Perspective,* 93.

83. Orendorff, "Sketch of Major Baker."

84. Preface to Fishbein, ed., *Modern Home Medical Adviser.*

85. *The Home Cook Book of Chicago,* 267.

86. Blake, "From Buchan to Fishbein," 11–30.

87. See, e.g., *Home Care of Communicable Diseases.*

88. For a useful discussion of nineteenth-century medical sects and distinction between "regulars" (dubbed by homeopathic doctors "allopaths") and other types of practitioners, see Starr, *Social Transformation,* 93–102.

89. See, e.g., Beier, *Sufferers and Healers*, 48. See also Blake, "From Buchan to Fishbein," 20.

90. Orendorff, "Sketch of Omen and Zena Olney"; the mixture referred to was probably red precipitate or red oxide of mercury, which is both water-soluble and poisonous.

91. Faragher, *Sugar Creek*, 91.

92. Cassedy, *Medicine in America*, 60; Young, "Patent Medicines," 95–116.

93. Ibid., 98.

94. Reference to the *Pantagraph* appears in Ingalls, "Espy Pharmacy Records," 65. The names of these troops reflect both the lingering belief that cause, form, and cure of disease were geographically linked and that, consequently, Native Americans had special power to cure native ailments.

95. Wakefield had no formal medical training. He inherited his first fever remedy from his older brother, Zera, a physician who died in 1848. See Hasbrouck, *History of McLean County*, 409.

96. "An autobiography of Dr. Cyrenius Wakefield," revised by Dr. Homer Wakefield; Ingalls, "Espy Pharmacy," 126–27.

97. Duis, *Good Old Times*, 357.

98. "Plain Statement," 1891, McLean County Historical Society.

99. Armstrong, "Silas Hubbard."

100. Leavitt, *Brought to Bed*, 28–32.

101. Faragher, *Sugar Creek*, 93–95.

102. See, e.g., Bateman, *Historical Encyclopedia*, 850.

103. See,e.g., Leavitt, *Brought to Bed*, 36–38.

104. See, e.g., Blake, "From Buchan to Fishbein," 18.

105. Duis, *Good Old Times*, 541.

106. Orendorff, "Sketch of Omen and Zena Olney."

107. Espy is neither mentioned in the several catalogues of local worthies in early county histories, nor does his biography appear in the *Biographical History* published by the McLean County Medical Society in 1954, although he is named as a charter member of the society. Thus, no information about his credentials or practice history is available. However, it seems likely that he was related to John E. Espy who ran a drug store in Bloomington between 1873 and 1884 and left records used by Ingalls for "Espy Pharmacy." Orendorff, "Sketch of Major Baker."

108. Duis, *Good Old Times*, 297.

109. Rosen, *Structure*, 55–58.

110. At approximately one physician for every 635 people, the doctor-patient ratio compares favorably to the current U.S. government desirable ratio of one primary care physician per 3,500 population. It was not, however, unusually favorable for the United States at the time; in *The Structure of American Medical Practice*, 15, George Rosen writes that between 1860 and 1900, the number of physicians kept pace with growing general population at about one physician to every 575 people.

111. *Biographical History, 1854–1954*, 33, 43. Both of these physicians were charter members of the McLean County Medical Society in 1854, although Dr. Cromwell, who had tuberculosis, gave up practice in 1858 for health reasons.

112. Bateman, *Historical Encyclopedia*, 2:851.

113. Orendorff, "Sketch of Omen and Zena Olney."

114. Rogers. *Day Books.*

115. See, e.g., Warner, *Therapeutic Perspective,* 91–98.

116. Starr, *Social Transformation,* 84.

117. Hasbrouck, *History of McLean County,* 267.

118. Madison, "Preserving Individualism," 446.

119. These take the form of a reprint of the original constitution and brief biographies of early members contained in *Biographical History, 1854–1954,* cited above.

120. *Records MCMS.*

121. These figures extrapolated from the *Biographical History* entries are necessarily *under*estimates, because this source includes only allopaths who belonged to the McLean County Medical Society. It is clear from the Medical Society's records that there were many "irregular" practitioners in McLean County at the end of the nineteenth century.

Chapter 2: No Place Like Home

1. Lynaugh, "From Respectable Domesticity," 22–28.

2. *St. Joseph's Hospital Admissions Records,* 2–3.

3. Lynaugh, "From Respectable Domesticity," 22.

4. *St. Joseph's Hospital Accounts; St. Joseph's Medical Staff Records.*

5. Ibid., 17.

6. Ibid., 28.

7. Ibid., 28.

8. *St. Joseph's Hospital Accounts,* especially pages 90 and 161

9. See, e.g., Strasser, *Never Done,* 242–62. U.S. studies tend to focus on women's paid work (in and out of the home), women as consumers, and the development of home economics as an academic discipline and educational initiative. See Roberts, *A Woman's Place,* 110–68, for discussion of late nineteenth- and early twentieth-century Lancashire working-class women's roles as managers of household economies.

10. *St. Joseph's Medical Staff Records,* 16.

11. See, e.g., Strasser, *Never Done,* 162–79; and Reverby, *Ordered to Care,* 60–76.

12. *St. Joseph Hospital Accounts,* 64, 106.

13. Ibid., 26, 56, 146.

14. Ibid., 130, 132.

15. Ibid., 166, 170.

16. Another medical institution was founded in McLean County in 1892—the Willow Bark Institute, in Danvers, established by Dr. F. J. Parkhurst (d. 1916) to treat problem drinkers. Similar to the lucrative Keeley Institute established in Dwight, Illinois, in 1879, the Willow Bark Cure, offered until 1950, was based on aversion therapy. Discussion of the Willow Bark Institute is not included in this chapter because the facility served mainly patients from areas other than McLean County and was not a general hospital. For information about the Willow Bark Institute, see *Danvers, Illinois Community History;* and Ferguson, "Willow Bark Institute." For information about the Keeley Gold Cure and Keeley Institute, see Bingham, *The Snake-Oil Syndrome,* 44–45.

17. Hasbrouck, *History of McLean County,* 324. Oral history interviews with Mrs. H2MP,

5 and Mrs. R4MP, 3. (References to interview transcripts, housed in the McLean County Historical Society, are hereafter given by respondent code number and transcript page number.) *Biographical History, 1854–1934,* 59.

18. See, e.g., Rosenberg, *The Care of Strangers,* 237–52; Stevens, *In Sickness and in Wealth,* 8–11; Vogel, *The Invention of the Modern Hospital,* 1; Dowling, *City Hospitals;* and Reverby, *Ordered to Care,* 21–26.

19. That this Catholic facility should be the first general hospital opened in McLean County is not surprising, because "Illinois reported the largest cluster of Roman Catholic hospitals of any state" at the turn of the twentieth century—forty-three out of a total of 118 hospitals, according to Stevens, *In Sickness and in Wealth,* 29. Rosenberg in *Care of Strangers,* 111, explains the dramatic growth in the number of Catholic hospitals in the late nineteenth century as "a consequence not simply of the specific history and commitment of the church and its religious orders, but of the isolated and defensive character of the Catholic immigrant population in American cities."

20. Ferguson, "The McLean County Poor Farm." After hospitals were established in Bloomington, Poor Farm inmates and other county indigents received hospital care partially paid for by county funds.

21. Kelso Sanitarium brochure.

22. See, e.g., Hatty and Hatty, *The Disordered Body,* 188; and Turner, *Medical Power and Social Knowledge,* 153–66.

23. See Abel, "A 'Terrible and Exhausting' Struggle," 478–506; and Abel, *Hearts of Wisdom,* 1–176.

24. For discussion of the transition of nurses' social status from the days of untrained nurses in the mid-nineteenth century to the era of professional nursing beginning (in the United States) in the 1870s, see Reverby, *Ordered to Care,* and Melosh "The Physician's Hand." For information about Brokaw's early history, see Essig, "History of Brokaw Hospital."

25. *St. Joseph's Medical Staff Records,* 39.

26. Abel, "A 'Terrible and Exhausting' Struggle," 493.

27. Estes, *Christian Concern for Health,* 47.

28. Lynaugh, "From Respectable Domesticity," 28.

29. United States Census, 1880, Vol. 1, Table 22.

30. See, e.g., *St. Joseph's Medical Staff Records,* 34.

31. In 1916 the county was paying $1 per day to local hospitals for the care of each indigent patient. See Ferguson, "The McLean County Poor Farm."

32. *St. Joseph's Medical Staff Records,* 34.

33. Included in the category of miscellaneous illnesses are acute exyemia, anemia, brain trouble, chronic eczema, congestion of brain, general debility, granulated eyelids, jaundice, liver complaint, metritis, old age, palsy, papilonia, paralysis, shingles, hives, sore eye, spinal clinosis, tapeworms, and torpid liver. See *St. Joseph's Hospital Admissions Records.*

34. *St. Joseph's Medical Staff Records,* 55. These rooms were apparently still in use during the mid-twentieth century, according to oral history informants. See, e.g., Sr. T3MP, 67.

35. The American Academy of Otolaryngology—Head and Neck Surgery hosted an online exhibit, "Deliberate and Exquisite," which provided additional information about this

procedure. See *http.//www.entlink.net/museum/exhibits/Tonsilectomy-exhibit.cfm* (viewed March 9, 2005).

36. *St. Joseph's Hospital Admissions Records.*

37. Ibid., 246–47.

38. *St. Joseph's Hospital Accounts,* 62, 162.

39. *St. Joseph's Medical Staff Records,* 29.

40. Hasbrouck, *History of McLean County,* 1088–89.

41. See, e.g., Cassedy, *Medicine in America,* 42.

42. *Biographical History, 1854–1954,* 44; Bateman, ed., *Historical Encyclopedia of Illinois,* 2:851; Hasbrouck, *History of McLean County,* 589.

43. *Biographical History, 1854–1954,* 49.

44. *St. Joseph's Medical Staff Records,* 16, 34.

45. Ibid., 16.

46. Ibid., 12; Madison, "Preserving Individualism," 442–83.

47. *St. Joseph Medical Staff Records,* 8–9.

48. Ibid., 11, 33.

49. See, e.g., Rosenberg, *Care of Strangers,* 122, 136–41.

50. *St. Joseph Medical Staff Records,* 34.

51. Ibid., 41.

52. Ibid., 25.

53. Ibid., 24.

54. Ibid., 38.

55. Ibid., 38, 40; *St. Joseph's Hospital Accounts,* 257.

56. *St. Joseph's Medical Staff Records,* 30.

57. Ibid., 47.

58. See also, e.g., Ibid., 43.

59. Ibid., 23.

60. Ibid., 17, 19.

61. See Madison, "Preserving Individualism," for discussion of the link between medical specialization and efficiency in the early twentieth century.

62. *St. Joseph's Medical Staff Records,* 13; *St. Joseph's Hospital Admissions Records.*

63. *St. Joseph's Medical Staff Records,* 47; *St. Joseph's Hospital Admissions Records.* In the twentieth century, McLean County's mentally ill were routinely sent to the State Hospital at Bartonville.

64. It is noteworthy that the Poor Farm closed in 1954, when it was replaced by the McLean County Nursing Home, which until 1974 occupied the renovated Poor Farm residence building. See Ferguson, "The McLean County Poor Farm."

65. *St. Joseph's Medical Staff Records,* 47.

66. Essig, "History of Brokaw Hospital," 24–25. An oral history interview provided by Harriet Rust offers another example of both use of a hospital for long-term care and continuation of the home care model in the small proprietary osteopathic hospital (the Fuller Clinic) her father ran in Bloomington during the interwar period. See Mrs. R4MP.

67. The only general hospital in the county that did not have a nurse training school was the proprietary hospital started in 1921 in the small rural community, Arrowsmith, by Dr. L. M. Johnson who used the facility to treat his own patients.

68. The exact date of the opening of Deaconess/Brokaw Hospital's nursing school is hard to determine. According to Brokaw's own promotional literature, the school was established in 1902. However, Essig's 1939 "History of Brokaw Hospital," 4, mentions a graduation exercise for student nurses in 1899.

69. See, e.g., Melosh, *The Physician's Hand*, 33, 37, 168; Rosenberg, *The Care of Strangers*, 219–28; and Reverby, *Ordered to Care*, 60–76. According to Reverby, 61, in the United States, "By 1923, there were 6,830 hospitals (an increase of over 3,700 percent), and every fourth one included a nursing school."

70. Melosh, *The Physician's Hand*, 10–11; D'Antonio, "Revisiting and Rethinking," 274.

71. See, e.g., Reverby, *Ordered to Care*, 70–76.

72. The county was not alone. According to Melosh, *The Physician's Hand*, 41, "Between 1900 and 1920, the number of trained nurses rose from 11,804 to 149,128, while the population of the United States increased by less than 50 percent."

73. In this respect, also, McLean County exemplified national norms. See Melosh, *The Physician's Hand*, 77–111; and Reverby, *Ordered to Care*, 111–17.

74. A new endeavor in the late nineteenth century, hospital administration was dominated by medical superintendents (male physicians) and matrons or nursing supervisors (female graduate nurses). For information about the development of professional hospital administration, see Stevens, *In Sickness and in Wealth*, 68–75, 156–57.

75. Estes. *Christian Concern for Health*, 11, 43.

76. Ibid., 43.

77. Ibid., 43–44, 62.

78. Essig, "History of Brokaw Hospital," 12.

79. See, e.g., Lynaugh, "From Respectable Domesticity," 27.

80. Essig, "History of Brokaw Hospital," 26; Rosner, "Doing Well or Doing Good," 160.

81. Stevens, *In Sickness and in Wealth*, 172–73.

82. Kelso Sanitarium brochure, cover and 3.

83. Brokaw Hospital pamphlet, 6; Mr. F2MP, 23, 25.

84. Brokaw Hospital pamphlet, 1, 8.

85. "Medical Society Honors Dr. Rhoda Yolton," *Pantagraph*, March 8, 1938.

86. See, e.g., Stevens, *In Sickness and in Wealth*, 53–54; Rosenberg, *The Care of Strangers*, 147–50; and Howell, *Technology in the Hospital*, 30–68.

87. Brokaw Hospital pamphlet, 5. The figure of ten surgeons is actually an underestimate, since the four eye, ear, nose and throat specialists and the gynecologist also did surgery, as did the general practitioners.

88. Estes, *Christian Concern for Health*, 24, 50.

89. Ibid., 47.

90. Stevens, *In Sickness and in Wealth*, 172–73.

91. Howell, *Technology in the Hospital*, 5.

92. DeLee's, "The Prophylactic Forceps Operation," quoted in Wertz, *Lying-In*, 143. DeLee's textbook was used by students at Brokaw Hospital School for Nurses in the 1920s. See Brokaw Hospital pamphlet, 19.

93. Kelso Sanitarium brochure, 6.

94. See, e.g., Mrs. C1MP, 75.

95. Dr. W3MP, 20.

96. Dr. 01MP, 15,33.

97. Mrs. R1MP, 43. Rebecca Rittenhouse is not this informant's real name. She was interviewed by Cynthia Baer, a graduate student, for a class project in 1993. Mrs. Baer gave me permission to use this and two additional transcripts. Since these three informants did not give permission for their names to be used in my publications, I have used pseudonyms for them.

98. Ibid., 23.

99. Rosenberg, "Community and Communities," 11; Stevens, *In Sickness and in Wealth,* 52ff.

100. See, e.g., Rosenberg, "Community and Communities," 11. Expanded discussion of physicians' relationships with hospitals will be provided in Chapter 4.

101. See, e.g., Madison, "Preserving Individualism," 462.

102. Estes, *Christian Concern for Health,* 18.

103. Ibid., 58; Rosen, *The Structure of American Medical Practice,* 82.

104. See, e.g., Dr. T2MP, 31–32.

105. Ibid., 21.

106. Melosh, *The Physician's Hand,* 111; Reverby, *Ordered to Care,* 188–91.

107. Dr. V1MP, 32. According to the online *Oxford English Dictionary,* an empyema is, "A collection of pus in the cavity of the pleura, the result of pleurisy. The term has also been used to denote any chronic inflammatory effusion in the chest."

108. Mrs. T1MP, 27.

109. Melosh, *The Physician's Hand,* 59–61.

110. Mrs. E1MP, 16.

111. Mr. S3MP, 23.

112. Estes, *Christian Concern for Health,* 25; *Pantagraph,* November 28, 1943.

113. Estes, *Christian Concern for Health,* 52.

114. See, e.g., Cassedy, *Medicine in America,* 138, 143; Starr, *Social Transformation,* 348–51; and Stevens, *In Sickness and in Wealth,* 216–19.

115. Mrs. F1MP, 29.

116. Mrs. R3MP, 38. Linda Rohm is not this informant's real name (see note 97).

117. Tate, *The Way It Was,* 243–48.

Chapter 3: Nursing, Gender, and Modern Medicine

1. For information about women's healing roles in early modern England, see Beier, *Sufferers and Healers,* ch. 8, 211–41.

2. Dickens, *Martin Chuzzlewit* (1843–44).

3. See, e.g., Reverby, *Ordered to Care,* 39–59.

4. Brokaw Hospital pamphlet, 17. See also *Mennonite Hospital School of Nursing,* 18.

5. *Mennonite School Commemorative History,* 18.

6. Essig, "History of Brokaw Hospital," 12; Reverby, *Ordered to Care,* 165. Reverby compares the Goldmark Report's effect on nursing education to the Flexner Report's effect on medical education.

7. Musser, "Nursing Education at Illinois Wesleyan."

8. *Mennonite Hospital School of Nursing,* 64. During the 1970s the curriculum was augmented by both additional theoretical course work and a variety of experiential placements for students. In 1982 the Mennonite College of Nursing was established, offering a baccalaureate curriculum enhanced by partnerships with seven Illinois institutions of higher education. In 1999 the college merged with Illinois State University.

9. See., e.g., Reverby, *Ordered to Care,* 54.

10. Ibid., 61–62, 124–25.

11. This local development reflected national trends. See Melosh, *The Physician's Hand,* 44.

12. Gegel, "Formation and the First Fifty Years."

13. See, e.g., Mrs. C1MP, 57–58, 75.

14. Melosh, *The Physician's Hand,* 77–99; Reverby, *Ordered to Care,* 176–79.

15. See the "Records of Stella Bennett."

16. Sandelowski, *Devices and Desires,* 15.

17. Mrs. H1MP, 37.

18. Mrs. T1MP, 13.

19. The Sue Barton series, by Helen Dore Boylston, appeared between the 1930s and the 1960s; the Cherry Ames series, by Helen Wells, was published between the 1940s and the 1970s. See Melosh, *The Physician's Hand,* 60–61, for discussion of the image of the nurse fostered by these series.

20. Shortland, *Medicine and Film.*

21. Mrs. C1MP, 38.

22. Sr. T3MP, 1–6, 9–10.

23. Sr, J1MP, 4.

24. Mrs. L1MP, 5.

25. Ibid., 6–7.

26. Brokaw Hospital pamphlet, 17.

27. Ibid., 18.

28. Ibid., 18.

29. Mrs. C1MP, 38, 43.

30. Mrs. L1MP, 7.

31. Mrs. W2MP, 20.

32. Mrs. S2MP, 26.

33. See, e.g., Reverby, *Ordered to Care,* 63.

34. Mrs. C1MP, 39.

35. Mrs. H1MP, 38.

36. Mrs. S2MP, 21.

37. Mrs. L1MP, 3–4.

38. See, e.g., Melosh, *The Physician's Hand,* 38–39.

39. Mrs. W2MP, 17.

40. Mrs. C1MP, 40.

41. Sr. T3MP, 53–55.

42. Mrs. C1MP, 74.

43. Mrs. T1MP, 17.

44. See, e.g., Melosh, *The Physician's Hand,* 53–57

45. Melosh, *The Physician's Hand,* 49.

46. Mrs. H1MP, 30.

47. Mrs. C1MP, 49.

48. Mrs. H1MP, 30.

49. Ibid., 30.

50. Mrs. L1MP, 38.

51. Mrs. C1MP, 23.

52. Mrs. H1MP, 30.

53. Mrs. W2MP, 26.

54. Mrs. H1MP, 41, 46.

55. Sr. T3MP, 10, 21.

56. Essig, "History of Brokaw Hospital," 17.

57. Mrs. L1MP, 28.

58. Mrs. H1MP, 47.

59. Mrs. T1MP, 18.

60. Melosh, *The Physician's Hand,* 49.

61. Mrs. C1MP, 45, 52. See also, e.g., Reverby, *Ordered to Care,* 60–76.

62. Mrs. W2MP, 18.

63. Mrs. T1MP, 19.

64. Mrs. W2MP, 19.

65. See, e.g., Melosh, *The Physician's Hand,* 46–47.

66. Mrs. W2MP, 38–39.

67. Ibid., 54; See, e.g., Melosh, *The Physician's Hand,* 52.

68. Mrs. W2MP, 20.

69. Mrs. T1MP, 17. See also Mrs. L1MP, 22–24.

70. Mrs. W2MP, 27.

71. Mrs. S2MP, 19–20.

72. Mrs. L1MP, 22.

73. Mrs. H1MP, 18–19.

74. Mrs. C1MP, 44.

75. Mrs. T1MP, 18–19.

76. "BroMenn Healthcare," 4.

77. See, e.g., Mrs. T1MP, 18.

78. Estes, *Christian Concern for Health,* 56–57; *Mennonite Hospital School of Nursing,* 28.

79. Ibid., 26.

80. Ibid., 28, 37.

81. Mrs. C1MP, 61.

82. Melosh, *The Physician's Hand,* 40.

83. Mrs. L1MP, 49.

84. Mrs. S2MP, 31.

85. Sr. T3MP, 26.

86. Gegel. "6th District Illinois Nurses' Association."

87. *Brokaw Hospital Registry Rules.*

88. Brokaw Hospital directory.

89. *Historical Statistics,* 164, 167.

90. Mrs. C1MP, 57–58.

91. Ibid., 47.

92. Ibid., 48.

93. Ibid., 75–76.

94. See, e.g., Melosh, *The Physician's Hand,* 77ff.

95. Mrs. H1MP, 27.

96. See Melosh, *The Physician's Hand,* 80–85.

97. Bennett, "Receipt Book."

98. See, e.g., Melosh, *The Physician's Hand,* 93.

99. Mrs. L1MP, 50–51.

100. Ibid., 49.

101. Ibid., 49–50.

102. Bennett's work for the Union Auto Industrial Association cries out for further study, because it could be interpreted in several ways. On the one hand, her home visits and advice could be viewed as a benefit to the largely women workers, many of whom suffered from "female" problems including menstrual cramps and menopausal symptoms. On the other hand, Bennett was also investigating possible malingering, which she reported to company officials. See "Union Auto Industrial Association Notebook."

103. Bennett, "Receipt Book" and "Union Auto Industrial Association Notebook."

104. "Bloomington Woman, 66, to be Congressional Intern," *Pantagraph,* May, 4 1979.

105. BroMenn Healthcare archives, Bloomington, Illinois.

106. Mrs. C1MP, 58.

107. Estes, *Christian Concern for Health,* 56.

108. Mrs. L1MP, 33.

109. *Pantagraph,* May 5, 1946.

110. Reverby, *Ordered to Care,* 204.

111. Sandelowski, *Devices and Desires,* 1–20.

112. Sr. T3MP, 39–40.

113. Mrs. T1MP, 26.

114. Mrs. H1MP, 58.

115. Sr. T3MP, 57. See also Melosh, *The Physician's Hand,* 65–76.

116. Mrs. S2MP, 52.

117. Sr. T3MP, 40.

118. Ibid., 35.

119. Mrs. L1MP, 25.

120. Mrs. S2MP, 55–56.

121. Mrs. T1MP, 23.

122. Mrs. H1MP, 37.

123. Mrs. W2MP, 14, 27.

124. *Liquorian.* See also Hine, *Black Women in White.*

125. Mrs. L1MP, 23.

126. Mrs. T1MP, 25.

127. Mrs. H1MP, 57, 62.

128. Mrs. W1MP, 27.

129. Mrs. L1MP, 36.

130. See, e.g., Mrs. R1MP, 23; Mrs. E1MP, 16; Mr. S3MP, 23.

131. Mr. F2MP, 27.

132. Sandelowski, *Devices and Desires*, 3–4.

Chapter 4: Doctors and Organized Medicine

1. Burnham, *How the Idea of Profession Changed.*

2. O'Hara, *An Emerging Profession;* Bonner, *Medicine in Chicago;* Stowe, *Doctoring the South.*

3. See, e.g., Morantz-Sanchez, *Sympathy and Science;* Watson, *Against the Odds;* and Ward, *Black Physicians.*

4. Starr, *Social Transformation;* Rosen, *The Structure of American Medical Practice.*

5. This estimate was extrapolated from biographical sketches provided by the *Biographical History, 1854–1954,* 28–52.

6. See, e.g., Brieger, ed., *Medical America in the Nineteenth Century,* 3–4; and Starr, *Social Transformation,* 40, 63–64, 82, 89, 114.

7. Hasbrouck, *History of McLean County,* 592–93.

8. Rawlings, *The Rise and Fall of Disease,* 1:280–81. For useful information about regulation of medicine in another state, see Lawrence, "Iowa Physicians," 151–200.

9. Madison, "Preserving Individualism," 449. In 1875 the McLean County Medical Society amended its constitution to require appointment of a delegate to the Illinois State Medical Society. The revised constitution of 1904 stated, "This society shall be auxiliary to the Illinois State Medical Society, and to the American Medical Association." See *Biographical History, 1854–1954,* 18, 20.

10. *Records MCMS.*

11. See, e.g., Rosen, *Structure;* Starr, *Social Transformation;* and Madison, "Preserving Individualism."

12. In fact, McLean County allopaths had routinely advertised their services in the newspaper as recently as the 1850s, as the *Weekly National Flag,* published in Bloomington between 1856 and 1859, shows. The society's struggle against advertisement continued, as its 1898 formal protest against "the methods of illegitimate advertisement toward which some of its members have drifted" illustrates (*Records MCMS,* 85).

13. *Biographical History, 1854–1954,* 74.

14. *Ibid.,* 49.

15. *Records MCMS,* 6.

16. *Biographical History, 1854–1934,* 71.

17. *Records MCMS,* 94.

18. Ibid., 141.

19. Ibid., 264.

20. Ibid., 90.

21. See, e.g., Rosen, *Structure,* 33–36.

22. Bateman, ed., *Historical Encyclopedia of Illinois,* 852.

23. *Biographical History, 1854–1934,* 59.

24. Osteopathy was invented by rural Missouri physician Andrew Still in 1891. See e.g. Starr, *Social Transformation,* 108; Gevitz, *The D.O.s.*

25. *Records MCMS,* 69, 283.

26. The daughter of an osteopath (Dr. Fuller), Harriet Rust, was interviewed for this study. Dr. Fuller ran a small proprietary hospital in Bloomington during the 1930s.

27. Hasbrouck, *Bloomington and Normal Sanitary District,* 1089.

28. See, e.g., Reagan, *When Abortion Was a Crime.*

29. *Records MCMS,* 282. Dr. Burr appears in the 1904 list of members in the *Biographical History, 1854–1954,* 30, where it is noted that he practiced in Chicago from 1889 to 1894 and in Bloomington from 1895 to 1898. However, Burr had ongoing difficulties with the society. In June 1894, he accused members of undercharging on prescriptions, and in June 1901 he appeared at a meeting demanding to know why he was not considered a member of the society (*Records MCMS,* 33, 130). The outcome of the Board of Censors' deliberations is not clear.

30. *Biographical History, 1854–1954.* 22–23.

31. *Records MCMS,* 261.

32. Ibid., 309.

33. Muirhead, *A History of African-Americans,* 31; *Biographical History, 1854–1954,* 69.

34. Bloomington-Normal Black History Project files. Lucinda Brent Posey interviews.

35. *Records MCMS,* 67.

36. Ibid., 97.

37. Ibid., 249.

38. Starr, *Social Transformation,* 69.

39. *Records MCMS,* 70–71.

40. Ibid., 84.

41. Ibid., 240–42.

42. Ibid., 167.

43. Ibid., 64.

44. Ibid., 221.

45. See, e.g., Rogers, "Germs with Legs," 599–617; and Curry, *Modern Mothers in the Heartland,* 74–75.

46. *Records MCMS,* 271–72.

47. Ibid., 157.

48. Ibid., 240.

49. Ibid., 243. Fairview Sanitarium opened on the outskirts of Normal in August 1919.

50. See, e.g., Rosen, *Structure,* 40–43.

51. *Records MCMS,* 3.

52. Ibid., 66.

53. Ibid., 255–56.

54. Ibid., 199.

55. Ibid., 255.

56. For example, William E. Guthrie, who had a long and distinguished surgical career

in McLean County, worked at different times as county physician and surgeon for two railroad companies. See *Biographical History, 1854–1954*, 36.

57. See, e.g., Ludmerer, *Time to Heal.*

58. Starr, *Transformation*, 118.

59. Ibid., 117, 124.

60. *Biographical History, 1854–1954*, 23, 41–42; Bonner, *Medicine in Chicago*, 58–59.

61. *Biographical History, 1854–1954*, 23, 76.

62. Bonner, *Medicine in Chicago*, 108–9.

63. Ibid., 114–15.

64. Ibid., 63.

65. *Biographical History, 1854–1954*, 161.

66. Rosen, *Structure*, 54–55; Dr. V1MP, 1–6; Dr. T2MP, 11.

67. See, e.g., Livingston, *A History of the Practice of Medicine;* and Oyer, *Of Doctors and Sickness.*

68. Dr. D1MP, 7–8.

69. *Biographical History, 1854–1954*, 179.

70. Dr. W3MP, 5.

71. Dr. W3MP, 8–9.

72. Dr. B2MP, 3.

73. Dr. V1MP, 7.

74. Dr. S1MP, 8, 11.

75. Dr. O1MP, 6.

76. Dr. T2MP, 2.

77. Livingston, *History*, vii.

78. Dr. W3MP, 12–13.

79. Ibid., 4–5.

80. Dr. S1MP, 12.

81. Dr. B2MP, 2–3.

82. Dr. O1MP, 8–9.

83. Dr. W3MP, 15–17.

84. Dr. S1MP, 11.

85. Ibid., 16. Scholarships of this type are still available in Illinois. See *http://www.collegezone.com/informationzone/3392_3601.htm* (accessed March 27, 2008).

86. Dr. T2MP, 2.

87. Dr. O1MP, 4, 8.

88. Ibid., 12.

89. Dr. V1MP, 4, 6.

90. Dr. S1MP, 13.

91. Dr. V1MP, 10–11.

92. Dr. S1MP, 19, 21–22.

93. Starr, *Social Transformation*, 120–21, 354–55.

94. Dr. S1MP, 22–23.

95. Dr. O1MP, 7, 9.

96. Dr. V1MP, 12.

97. Dr. D1MP, 9–10.

98. See, e.g., Stevens, *In Sickness and in Wealth,* 10, 251–52.

99. Dr. W3MP, 21.

100. Dr. V1MP, 14.

101. Dr. S1MP, 29–30.

102. Dr. O1MP, 12–13.

103. Dr. V1MP, 20.

104. Dr. W3MP, 41, 46, 47.

105. Dr. B2MP, 2.

106. Dr. O1MP, 13–14.

107. See, e.g., Rosen, *Structure,* 85.

108. Dr. S1MP, 55, 57–58.

109. Dr. V1MP, 16.

110. Madison, "Preserving Individualism"; Dr. O1MP, 25; Dr. S1MP, 2, 66; Dr. W3MP, 48; Dr. B1MP, 8.

111. Dr. T2MP, 8.

112. Dr. V1MP, 33.

113. Dr. S1MP, 30–31.

114. Dr. B1MP, 4–5.

115. Mr. F2MP, 23–24.

116. *Biographical History, 1854–1954,* 66.

117. Mr. F2MP, 23, 24, 26.

118. According to Rosen, *Structure,* 55–56, physicians began to locate in urban centers more rapidly than the U.S. population in general during the first half of the twentieth century.

119. Dr. W3MP, 6.

120. Mr. F2MP, 24.

121. Dr. S1MP, 32.

122. Ibid., 33.

123. Dr. S1MP, 36–37.

124. Dr. W3MP, 30.

125. Dr. S1MP, 35.

126. Mr. F2MP, 24.

127. Dr. S1MP, 39.

128. Ibid., 40.

129. Dr. B2MP, 6.

130. Dr. T2MP, 8–9.

131. Ibid., 8–9, 11–12.

132. Ibid., 12.

133. Rosen, *Structure,* 25–32.

134. Dr. T2MP, 14.

135. Dr. B2MP, 5.

136. Dr. T2MP, 11, 13.

137. Sloan. *The Thyroid,* v.

138. Dr. S1MP, 66.

139. Dr. V1MP, 35.

140. Ibid., 34, 35.

141. Dr. V1MP, 36.

142. Dr. T2MP, 19.

143. Dr. O1MP, 20.

144. Dr. S1MP, 62.

145. Dr. V1MP, 37–38.

146. Dr. O1MP, 40.

147. The American College of Surgeons opposed fee splitting beginning in 1919. See Starr, *Social Transformation*, 167.

148. Livingston, *History*, 2–3.

149. Ibid., 4.

150. Dr. T2MP, 31–32.

151. Dr. B2MP, 9, 11.

152. Dr. O1MP, 15.

153. Dr. T1MP, 26–27.

154. Dr. T2MP, 19–20.

155. Sr. T3MP, 59.

156. Dr. B2MP, 11.

157. Dr. O1MP, 42.

158. Livingston, *History*, 11.

159. Dr. S1MP, 51.

160. *Historical Statistics of the United States*, 1:213.

161. Dr. O1MP, 23–24.

162. Ibid.; *Historical Statistics of the United States*, 1:169.

163. See, e.g., Rosen, *Structure*, 87.

164. Dr. V1MP, 37.

165. Ibid., 39.

166. Livingston, *History*, 14–15.

167. Dr. O1MP, 27.

168. Dr. V1MP, 40.

169. Livingston, *History*, 15.

170. Dr. T2MP, 15.

171. Starr, *Social Transformation*, 385.

172. Ibid.

173. Dr. T2MP, 32.

174. Dr. O1MP, 39.

175. Dr. T2MP, 22.

176. Dr. S1MP, 57.

177. Dr. O1MP, 37.

178. Dr. S1MP, 61–62.

179. Dr. B2MP, 14.

180. Dr. O1MP, 22–23.

181. Mrs. S2MP, 53–54.

182. Livingston, *History,* 19.

183. Dr. B2MP, 15.

184. Illich, *Medical Nemesis.*

Chapter 5: An Ounce of Prevention

1. See, e.g., Rosen, *A History of Public Health;* Sand, *The Advance to Social Medicine;* Leavitt, *Typhoid Mary;* Arnold, *Colonizing the Body;* and Jones, *Bad Blood.*

2. Porter, *Health, Civilization and the State,* 4.

3. Worboys, *Spreading Germs,* 38; Tomes, *The Gospel of Germs.*

4. Curry, *Modern Mothers in the Heartland,* 65–90.

5. See, e.g., Curry, *Modern Mothers;* and Lewis, *The Politics of Motherhood.*

6. In McLean County, mortality rates per 100,000 from tuberculosis were 139 in 1907, 101.1 in 1913, and 135.7 in 1918, the year before the county's sanitarium opened. Only influenza, with a rate of 296.4 in 1919, and pneumonia, with rates of 203.2 in 1919, and 144.8 in 1920, rivaled tuberculosis as contemporary killers (Rawlings, *The Rise and Fall of Disease,* 2:58).

7. Tomes, *Gospel of Germs,* 113–134, quotes: 118 and 123.

8. Rawlings, *The Rise and Fall of Disease,* 1:368.

9. Ibid., 1:365.

10. Ibid., 1:366.

11. *Records MCMS,* 243.

12. Hasbrouck, *History of McLean County,* 332.

13. Rawlings, *The Rise and Fall,* 1:368.

14. Hasbrouck, *History of McLean County,* 332.

15. Ibid., 333.

16. *Biographical History, 1854–1954,* 116.

17. Rawlings, *The Rise and Fall,* 2:61.

18. Ruth Carpenter worked for Fairview Sanitarium in the mid-1940s. She was paid $125 a month and given a car to use for home visits. See Mrs. C1MP, 59.

19. *Biographical History, 1854–1954,* 116; Rawlings, *The Rise and Fall,* 2:52.

20. *Biographical History, 1854–1954,* 116.

21. Mrs. T1MP, 25.

22. Mrs. C1MP, 83.

23. Leavitt, *Brought to Bed,* 68–69.

24. According to Tate, *The Way It Was,* 254, there were only four patients in Fairview Sanitarium in 1972 and a thousand empty tuberculosis beds in Illinois.

25. Mr. B3MP, 46.

26. See, e.g., Tomes, *Gospel of Germs.*

27. Ibid., 135–54.

28. Curry, *Modern Mothers,* 39–64; Tomes, *Gospel of Germs,* 185–95.

29. Curry, *Modern Mothers,* 65–98; Esposito, *Places of Pride,* 3–4; Tomes, *Gospel of Germs,* 195–204. It should be noted that the Cooperative Extension Service, funded by the Smith-Lever legislation, hired (male) agricultural advisers before funding positions for

home economists. Although the law did not specify a rural focus for the home economists, the extension's activities have been most visible and influential in rural areas.

30. Esposito, *Places of Pride.*

31. Curry, *Modern Mothers,* 81–82.

32. In Illinois, county-based extension work is funded partially by money from the United States Department of Agriculture, funneled through the University of Illinois, and partially by local taxes.

33. Esposito, *Places of Pride,* 5–6.

34. Curry, *Modern Mothers,* 85–86.

35. Ibid., 87.

36. Esposito, *Places of Pride,* 24.

37. Ibid., 14, 18.

38. Ibid., 10.

39. Ibid., 12.

40. Ibid., 20.

41. Curry, *Modern Mothers,* 75. Curry attributes this insight to medical historian Naomi Rogers.

42. Esposito, *Places of Pride,* 17.

43. Ibid., 20, 26.

44. Mrs. E1MP, 30.

45. Esposito, *Places of Pride,* 16.

46. Ibid., 26.

47. Ibid., 17.

48. Esposito's *Places of Pride* includes more than one hundred black-and-white photographs taken by Clara Brian.

49. Mrs. E1MP, 8–9.

50. Ibid., 15–16.

51. Ibid., 24.

52. Ibid., 24.

53. Ibid., 25.

54. Ibid., 26–27.

55. Ibid., 29.

56. Ibid., 30.

57. Ibid., 28.

58. Ibid., 29.

59. Ibid., 24.

60. See, e.g., Curry, *Modern Mothers,* 70–71.

61. Hasbrouck, *History of McLean County,* 143. Rawlings, *The Rise and Fall,* 2:53–56.

62. Rawlings, *The Rise and Fall,* 2:30. Quantity and quality of its well water became an ongoing issue in Bloomington. In 1929 the city dammed Money Creek, creating Lake Bloomington about fourteen miles from the city. After a water treatment plant was constructed in 1933, Bloomington abandoned its wells. The city's water supply was augmented in 1972 by the damming of the Mackinaw River to create Lake Evergreen.

63. Rawlings, *The Rise and Fall,* 2:56.

64. *Pantagraph,* July 13, 1925 and October 2, 1925. Hasbrouck, *Bloomington and Normal Sanitary District,* 5–9.

65. Rawlings, *The Rise and Fall,* 2:51–53.

66. Melosh, "The Physician's Hand," 125.

67. Mr. B3MP, 43–44.

68. Dr. D1MP, 18.

69. Ibid., 20.

70. Ibid., 21.

71. Mrs. T1MP, 14, 16.

72. Mr. B3MP, 51–52.

73. Ibid., 53.

74. Ibid., 30.

75. Ibid., 23–24.

76. Ibid., 43.

77. Ibid., 48.

78. Ibid., 56–57.

79. Ibid., 59–60.

Chapter 6: Matters of Life and Death

1. See, e.g., Porter, *The Greatest Benefit,* 3–4.

2. Mrs. A1MP, 19.

3. Mrs. B1MP, 11.

4. Mrs. C2MP, 16, 21, 22.

5. Mrs. F1MP, 33.

6. This phenomenon was also observed by public health officials. See, e.g., Rawlings, *The Rise and Fall,* 2:59.

7. Mrs. A1MP, 32.

8. Mrs. W1MP, 26.

9. Rawlings, *The Rise and Fall,* 2:59.

10. Mrs. C1MP, 29.

11. Rawlings, *The Rise and Fall,* 2:61.

12. Ibid., 2:58–59. Porter, *The Greatest Benefit,* 438–39.

13. Rawlings, *The Rise and Fall,* 2:58.

14. Ibid., 2:61.

15. *Biographical History, 1854–1954,* 88–89, 107, 116–18; Walters, "McLean County and the Influenza."

16. Rawlings, *The Rise and Fall,* 2:59.

17. This treatment, hailed by some scholars as the first true "antibiotic," involved a long course of treatment and severe side effects. See, e.g., Sutcliffe and Duin, *A History of Medicine,* 101. According to one oral history informant for this study, Mrs. L1MP, 15, in McLean County syphilis continued to be treated with mercury until penicillin became available.

18. See, e.g., Tomes, *The Gospel of Germs,* 135–56.

19. *Home Care of Communicable Diseases,* 5. It is noteworthy that this company had

a vested interest in keeping people healthy and, indeed, together with several other insurance firms, established visiting nurses services for its members. See, e.g., Buhler-Wilkerson, *No Place Like Home,* 161.

20. Ironically, it was in 1941 that the Australian, Norman McAlister Gregg, first identified a link between rubella suffered during pregnancy and the incidence of birth defects. Sutcliffe and Duin, *A History of Medicine,* 155.

21. *Home Care of Communicable Diseases,* 4.

22. Ibid., 13–14.

23. Abel, *Hearts of Wisdom.* Correspondence from Sarah Davis to David Davis for the 1860s and 1870s reveals conventional patterns of home care provision in one of McLean County's most prosperous homes. This correspondence is available through the David Davis Mansion, Bloomington, Illinois.

24. Mr. W4MP, 42–43.

25. Mrs. A1MP, 20.

26. Mrs. C1MP, 30.

27. Mrs. F1MP, 26–27.

28. Mrs. B1MP, 11.

29. Mrs. F2MP, 9.

30. Mr. S3MP, 20, 22.

31. Mrs. C1MP, 31.

32. Mr. W4MP, 26–27.

33. See, e.g., *Pantagraph,* August 27, 1931; July 21, 1935; September 22, 1940; January 20, 1943; September 8, 1944; January 21, 1946; October 29, 1946; October 30, 1949; December 18, 1949; April 15, 1951; August 21, 1952; September 13, 1952; April 2, 1954; March 31, 1955; and May 18, 1957.

34. Mrs. H1MP, 24.

35. Dr. S1MP, 36.

36. Mr. F2MP, 25.

37. See, e.g., Warner, *The Therapeutic Perspective,* 91–92.

38. Oral history transcript included in Pratt, ed., *We the People,* 18.

39. Mrs. S4MP, 17.

40. Mrs. H2MP, 4.

41. Mrs. W1MP, 10–11.

42. Mr. W4MP, 29.

43. Sutcliffe and Duin, *A History of Medicine,* 11.

44. Mrs. F2MP, 19.

45. Ibid., 20. See also Mrs. R1MP, 7. During the interwar period, fever therapy was used for several diseases. See, e.g., Humphreys, "Whose Body? Which Disease?", 53–77.

46. Mrs. W1MP, 18–21.

47. Mrs. E1MP, 22.

48. Dr. B2MP, 13.

49. See, e.g., Cooter and Luckin, eds., *Accidents in History.*

50. Mrs. S4MP, 13–14.

51. Mr. F2MP, 23.

52. Mr. S3MP, 13.

53. Ibid., 15.

54. Mrs. C1MP, 78–80.

55. Mr. S3MP, 19.

56. Mrs. C1MP, 18.

57. Mrs. F1MP, 22.

58. Pratt, *We the People*, 16; Mrs. W1MP, 12. Wearing asafetida bags to prevent disease was common among slaves in the nineteenth-century American South according to Stowe, *Doctoring the South*, 133.

59. Mr. F2MP, 31.

60. Mrs. F1MP, 21.

61. Mr. W4MP, 12.

62. See, e.g., Terrell, *This Other Kind of Doctors*.

63. Pratt, *We the People*, 16.

64. Mrs. W1MP, 12–13.

65. Mrs. A1MP, 29.

66. Mrs. C1MP, 23. See also Mrs. F1MP, 25.

67. Pratt, *We the People*, 16.

68. Mrs. C1MP, 16.

69. Pratt, *We the People*, 16.

70. Mrs. W1MP, 13; Mrs. C1MP, 15; Pratt, *We the People*, 16.

71. Mrs. W1MP, 13.

72. Mrs. C1MP, 15.

73. Mrs. C2MP, 20.

74. Mrs. C1MP, 15. See also Pratt, *We the People*, 16.

75. Mrs. F1MP, 20.

76. Mrs. E1MP, 41–42.

77. Mrs. S4MP, 21.

78. Mrs. C1MP, 16, 18.

79. Mrs. B1MP, 13.

80. Mrs. W1MP, 13–14.

81. Ibid., 28.

82. Mr. S3MP, 19.

83. Mr. W4MP, 38.

84. Mrs. C1MP, 14–15.

85. Mrs. F1MP, 22–23.

86. Mrs. C2MP, 25.

87. Abel, "A 'Terrible and Exhausting' Struggle," 493. A local example from the 1920s is provided in Chapter 4 of this volume. See also Sr. T3MP, 41.

88. Mrs. A1MP, 25–26.

89. Ibid., 28.

90. Mrs. C2MP, 19–20.

91. Mr. W4MP, 22–23.

92. Mrs. F1MP, 26, 30.

93. Mr. W4MP, 36–37, 39.

94. Mrs. A1MP, 60.

95. Mr. W4MP, 35–37.

96. Mrs. R1MP, 20–21.

97. Mrs. E1MP, 21–22.

98. Mrs. R1MP, 6.

99. Mrs. E1MP, 36.

100. Mrs. R3MP, 15–16, 26. Linda Rohm is not this informant's real name (see note 97 for Chapter 2).

101. Mrs. W1MP, 16.

102. Mrs. F1MP, 29. This example was also quoted in Chapter 2 to illustrate inflation of health-care costs between the 1930s and the 1980s.

103. Mrs. S4MP, 18–19.

104. *Historical Statistics*, 166.

105. Mr. F2 MP, 26.

106. Mrs. S4MP, 22.

107. Mrs. F1MP, 13.

108. Mrs. C1MP, 80.

109. Mrs. H1MP, 7–8.

110. Mrs. E1MP, 23

111. Dr. S1MP, 50–51.

112. Dr. T2MP, 18.

113. Mrs. R3MP, 39.

114. Oakley, *The Captured Womb*, 17.

115. Mrs. A1MP, 33.

116. See, e.g., Leavitt. *Brought to Bed.*

117. Wertz, *Lying-In*, 143; Leavitt, *Brought to Bed*, 116–41.

118. Leavitt, *Brought to Bed*, 182–85.

119. Wertz, *Lying-In*, 165.

120. See, e.g., Leavitt, *Brought to Bed*, 107.

121. Mrs. S2MP, 3.

122. Mrs. R1MP, 6.

123. Bloomington-Normal Black History Project files.

124. Mrs. R2MP, 7. Betty Rueger is not this informant's real name (see note 97 for Chapter 2). Midwives were licensed in the State of Illinois beginning in 1877, although many unlicensed, informally trained midwives continued to practice after that time. See Rawlings, *The Rise and Fall*, 1:285 and 2:348. A combination of antiabortion sentiment, which scapegoated midwives, and physicians' increasing monopoly over management of childbirth meant that midwives had disappeared from urban Illinois by the 1930s. See Reagan, *When Abortion Was a Crime*, 111.

125. Mrs. R2MP, 21.

126. Mrs. A1MP, 32.

127. Ibid., 33.

128. Mrs. C1MP, 20.

129. Ibid., 75, 76.

130. Bloomington-Normal Black History Project files.

131. Mrs. C1MP, 20.

132. Mrs. E1MP, 1.

133. Mrs. F1MP, 30.

134. Mrs. C1MP, 22.

135. Mrs. W1MP, 30.

136. Mrs. C1MP, 77.

137. Mrs. E1MP, 16–17, 19.

138. Mrs. C1MP, 61.

139. See, e.g., Mr. S3MP, 23. Also referenced in Chapter 3.

140. Mrs. E1MP, 16.

141. Mrs. R1MP, 23–24.

142. See, e.g., Leavitt, *Brought to Bed*, 214–15.

143. Mrs. W2MP, 32.

144. Mrs. R3MP, 15.

145. Mrs. B1MP, 19.

146. Mrs. C1MP, 76–77.

147. Mrs. F2MP, 18.

148. See, e.g., Reagan, *When Abortion Was a Crime*, 13, 134.

149. Mrs. R1MP, 18, 31

150. Mrs. R3MP, 12.

151. Dr. T2MP, 24.

152. Dr. 01MP, 32.

153. Dr. T2MP, 25–26.

154. Dr. O1MP, 31–32.

155. Reagan, *When Abortion Was a Crime*, 173–81, 190–91.

156. Dr. T2MP, 26.

157. Ibid., 24.

158. The Baby Fold in Normal, founded in 1903 for "homeless babies" still provides these services. See Hasbrouck, *History of McLean County*, 328–29.

159. United States Census for 1880 and 1890; Geospatial and Statistical Data Center, University of Virginia Library, "County-Level Results for 1900", http://fisher.lib.virginia .edu/collections/stats/histcensus/php/county.php (accessed March 27, 2008); *County and City Data Book, 1962;* Tate, *The Way It Was*, 8.

160. Muirhead, *A History of African-Americans*, 2–3. U.S. Censuses, 1880–1960.

161. Mrs. W4MP, 4–5; Muirhead, *A History of African-Americans*, 38–39.

162. Muirhead, *A History of African-Americans*, 39.

163. *Pantagraph*, January 7, 1996.

164. Bloomington-Normal Black History Project files, Lucinda Brent Posey interviews.

165. Mrs. W1MP, 15–16.

166. Bloomington-Normal Black History Project files, Oscar Waddell interviews.

167. Mr. W4MP, 44–45.

168. Mrs. W1MP, 35–36.

169. Ibid., 25–26.

170. Bloomington-Normal Black History Project files, Lucinda Brent Posey interviews.

171. *Assessment 2000*, 41.

172. See, e.g., Mrs. A1MP, 36.

173. Ibid., 36, 41.

174. Mr. S3MP, 32.

175. Mrs. W1MP, 36–37. See also Pratt, *We the People*, 17.

176. See, e.g., Jackson, "Death Shall Have No Dominion, 48; and Farrell, *Inventing the American Way of Death*, 146–48.

177. Mrs. F1MP, 35–36.

178. Mrs. B1MP, 8–9.

179. Mr. S3MP, 29–30.

180. Mr. B1MP, 9.

181. Mrs. W1MP, 38–39.

182. Mrs. F1MP, 39.

183. Mitford, *The American Way of Death*.

184. Mrs. F1MP, 39.

185. Mrs. A1MP, 46.

186. See, e.g., *McLean County Illinois Project* and *Assessment 2000*.

187. See, e.g., Fox, *Power and Illness*.

Conclusion: Health Culture in Transition

1. See, e.g., Seabrook, *The Myth of the Market*. Chapter 12, "The Apotheosis of the Market Economy" (134–55) argues that Bloomington-Normal represents "the kind of community in which the majority of Americans live" (134).

2. See, e.g., Smith and Holmes, *Listen to Me Good*.

3. Estes, *Christian Concern for Health*, 25, 52; *Pantagraph*, November 28, 1943.

4. *Assessment 2000*. The author of the present volume, Lucinda McCray Beier was the director of this project, which also included contributions from Sharon Mills and other Applied Social Research Unit staff members. The final report and appendices containing "Household Survey" results may be accessed at http://www.asru.ilstu.edu. Most information reported in this section comes from pages 63–69 of that report.

5. *McLean County Illinois Project*, 13.

6. *Assessment 2000*, 41.

7. Of the six thousand McLean County households sent a randomized survey, 5,699 household proved eligible to participate and 1,594 responded. The 28 percent response rate is acceptable for a mail survey.

8. *McLean County Illinois Project*, Appendix C, Appendix E.

9. *Assessment 2000*, "Household Survey."

Bibliography

Primary Sources

Assessment 2000: Health and Human Services in McLean County. Normal, Illinois: Applied Social Research Unit, Illinois State University, 2000.

An Autobiography of Dr. Cyrenius Wakefield. Revised by Dr. Homer Wakefield. Unpublished ms., Bloomington, IL: McLean County Historical Society, 1889?

Bennett, Stella Reiner. "Receipt Book," Reiner-Bennett Collection, 95–10–27, McLean County Historical Society.

Bevier, Isabel. *Home Economics in Education.* Philadelphia: J. B. Lippincott, 1924.

Biographical History of the Members of the McLean County Medical Society, 1854–1904, Bloomington, Ill.: McLean County Medical Society, 1904.

Biographical History of the Members of the McLean County Medical Society, 1854–1934. Bloomington, Ill.: McLean County Medical Society, 1934.

Biographical History of the Members of the McLean County Medical Society, 1854–1954. Bloomington, Ill.: McLean County Medical Society, 1954.

Bloomington-Normal Black History Project files. Lucinda Brent Posey interviews. Bloomington, Illinois: McLean County Historical Society.

Blue Book of the State of Illinois. Springfield, Ill.: Office of the Secretary of State, 1910–1960.

Brokaw Hospital directory (graduate nurses card with schedule of prices). September 6, 1920.

Brokaw Hospital pamplet. Bloomington, Ill.: McLean County Historical Society, 1921.

Brokaw Hospital Registry Rules, ca. 1920.

County and City Data Book. Washington, D.C., U.S. Department of Commerce, 1962.

Drake, Daniel. *A Systematic Treatise Historical, Etiological, and Practical on the Principal Diseases of the Interior Valley of North America,* vol. 2. 1854. Reprint, New York: Burt Franklin, 1971.

Fishbein, Morris, ed. *Modern Home Medical Adviser.* New York: Doubleday, 1935.

Hasbrouck, J. L. *Bloomington and Normal Sanitary District, 1919–1936.* Bloomington, Ill.: privately published, 1936.

Home Care of Communicable Diseases. Boston, Mass: John Hancock Mutual Life Insurance Company, 1942.

The Home Cook Book of Chicago. Chicago: J. Fred. Waggoner, 1874.

Kelso Sanitarium brochure. Bloomington, Ill.: McLean County Historical Society, 1916.

Liquorian 57, no. 6 (1969)

Livingston, Edward A. *A History of the Practice of Medicine in McLean County, Illinois, 1930–1980,* self-published, 1989.

The McLean County Almanac 1984. Bloomington, Ill.: Pantagraph Books, 1983.

"McLean County, Illinois 1860 Census and Mortality Schedule." Lexington, Ill.: Lexington Genealogical and Historical Society, 1985.

McLean County Illinois Project for Local Assessment of Need (IPLAN): Community Health Plan and Needs Assessment. Bloomington, Ill.: McLean County Health Department, 1999.

Orendorff, J. B. *Sketch of Omen and Zena Olney, Sketch of Major Baker,* unpublished ms., Bloomington, Ill.: McLean County Historical Society, 1897.

The Pantagraph, Bloomington, Ill.: 1879–1995.

"Plain Statement," McLean County Historical Society, 1891.

Rogers, Thomas P. *Day Books, 1839–1854,* unpublished ms., Bloomington, Ill. .: McLean County Historical Society.

"Records of Stella Bennett," Reiner-Bennett Collection, 95–10–27. Bloomington, Ill.: McLean County Historical Society.

Records of the McLean County Medical Society, 1891–1910, unpublished ms., Bloomington, Ill.: McLean County Historical Society.

Sloan, E. P. *The Thyroid: Surgery, Syndromes, Treatment.* Springfield, Ill.: Charles C. Thomas, 1936.

St. Joseph's Hospital Accounts, 1880–97, Peoria, Ill.: Archives of The Sisters of the Third Order of St. Francis.

St. Joseph's Hospital Admissions Records, 1880–1906. Peoria, Ill.: Archives of The Sisters of the Third Order of St. Francis.

St. Joseph's Medical Staff Records, 1885–1902. Peoria, Ill.: Archives of The Sisters of the Third Order of St. Francis.

United States Censuses of Population, 1880–1980.

Wakefield, Homer. "An Autobiography of Dr. Cyrenius Wakefield," unpublished ms., Bloomington, Ill.: McLean County Historical Society, [1889?]

Weekly National Flag. Bloomington, Ill.: 1856–59.

Secondary Sources

Abel, Emily K. *Hearts of Wisdom: American Women Caring for Kin.* Cambridge, Mass.: Harvard University Press, 2000.

———. "A 'Terrible and Exhausting' Struggle: Family Caregiving during the Transformation of Medicine." *The Journal of the History of Medicine and Allied Sciences* 50, no. 3 (1995): 478–506.

Armstrong, Beatrice. "Silas Hubbard, Early Physician of McLean County," unpublished ms., Bloomington, Ill.: McLean County Historical Society, [1970?].

Armstrong, David. *Political Anatomy of the Body: Medical Knowledge in Britain in the Twentieth Century.* Cambridge: Cambridge University Press, 1983.

Arnold, David. *Colonizing the Body: State Medicine and Epidemic Disease in 19th-Century India.* Berkeley: University of California Press, 1993.

Augé, Marc, and Claudine Herzlich, eds. *The Meaning of Illness: Anthropology, History and Sociology.* Luxembourg: Harwood Academic Publishers, 1995.

Avery, Kevin W., "Privial Pursuit: A Research Paper on Outhouses," unpublished paper, McLean County Historical Society, 1985.

Bateman, Newton, ed. *Historical Encyclopedia of Illinois and History of McLean County,* vol. 2. Chicago: Munsell, 1908.

Beier, Lucinda McCray, "Contagion, Policy, Class, Gender, and Mid-20th-Century Lancashire Working-Class Health Culture," *Hygiea Internationalis: An Interdisciplinary Journal for the History of Public Health,* 2, no. 1 (2001): 7–24.

———. "Expertise and Control: Childbearing in Three Twentieth-Century Working-Class Lancashire Communities," *Bulletin of the History of Medicine* 78, no. 2 (2004): 379–409.

———. *For Their Own Good: The Transformation of English Working-Class Health Culture.* Columbus: Ohio State University Press, forthcoming.

———. "I Used to Take Her to the Doctor's and Get the *Proper* Thing": Twentieth-Century Health Care Choices in Lancashire Working-Class Communities. " In *Splendidly Victorian,* edited by Michael Shirley and Todd Larson, 221–41. Aldershot, Hants: Ashgate Press, 2001.

———. *A Matter of Life and Death: Health, Illness and Medicine in McLean County, 1830–1995.* Bloomington, Ill.: McLean County Historical Society, 1996.

———. *Sufferers and Healers: The Experience of Illness in Seventeenth-Century England.* London: Routledge, 1986.

———. "We Were Green as Grass: Learning about Sex and Reproduction in Three Working-Class Lancashire Communities, 1900–70," *Social History of Medicine* 16, no. 3 (2003): 461–80.

Bingham, Walker. *The Snake-Oil Syndrome: Patent Medicine Advertising.* Hanover, Mass.: Christopher Publishing House, 1994.

Blake, John B. "From Buchan to Fishbein: The Literature of Domestic Medicine." In *Medicine Without Doctors: Home Health Care in American History,* edited by Guenter B. Risse, Ronald L. Numbers, and Judith Walzer Leavitt, 11–30. New York: Science History Publications, 1977.

Bonner, Thomas Neville. *Medicine in Chicago, 1850–1950: A Chapter in the Social and Scientific Development of a City,* 2d ed. Urbana, Ill.: University of Illinois Press, 1991.

Borst, Charlotte G. *Catching Babies: The Professionalization of Childbirth, 1870–1920.* Cambridge, Mass.: Harvard University Press, 1995.

Brieger, Gert H., ed. *Medical America in the Nineteenth Century: Readings from the Literature.* Baltimore: Johns Hopkins University Press, 1972.

Buhler-Wilkerson, Karen. *No Place Like Home: A History of Nursing and Home Care in the United States.* Baltimore: Johns Hopkins University Press, 2001.

Burnham, John C. *How the Idea of Profession Changed the Writing of Medical History.* London: Wellcome Institute for the History of Medicine, 1998.

Cassedy, James. *Medicine in America: A Short History.* Baltimore: Johns Hopkins University Press, 1991.

Cooter, Roger. "'Framing' the End of the Social History of Medicine." In *Locating Medical History: The Stories and their Meanings,* edited by Frank Huisman and John Harley Warner, 309–37. Baltimore: Johns Hopkins University Press, 2004.

Cooter, Roger, and Bill Luckin, eds. *Accidents in History,* Clio Medica 41. Amsterdam: Rodopi, 1997.

Crellin, John K. *Medical Care in Pioneer Illinois.* Springfield, Ill.: Pearson Museum, Southern Illinois University School of Medicine, 1982.

Curry, Lynne. *Modern Mothers in the Heartland: Gender, Health, and Progress in Illinois, 1900–1930.* Columbus: Ohio State University Press, 1999.

Custer, Milo. "Asiatic Cholera in Central Illinois, 1834–1873," *Journal of Illinois State Historical Society* 23, no. 1. (April 1930): 1–50.

D'Antonio, Patricia. "Revisiting and Rethinking the Rewriting of Nursing History," *Bulletin of the History of Medicine* 73, no. 2 (1999): 274.

Danvers, Illinois Community History. Danvers, Ill.: Danvers Historical Society, Inc., 1987.

Dictionary of Unitarian and Universalist Biography, "Adlai Stevenson," http://www.uua.org/uuhs/duub/articles/adlaistevenson.html (accessed March 21, 2008).

Dowling, Harry. *City Hospitals: The Undercare of the Underprivileged.* Cambridge, Mass.: Harvard University Press, 1982.

Duffy, John. *The Sanitarians: A History of American Public Health.* Urbana, Ill.: University of Illinois Press, 1990.

Duis, E. *Good Old Times in McLean County.* Bloomington, Ill.: Leader Publishing and Printing House, 1874.

Esposito, Margaret. *Places of Pride: The Work and Photography of Clara R. Brian.* Bloomington, Ill.: McLean County Historical Society, 1989.

Essig, Maude F. "History of Brokaw Hospital," unpublished essay, Normal, Ill.: Mennonite College of Nursing Library, 1939.

Estes, Steven R. *Christian Concern for Health: The Sixtieth Anniversary History of the Mennonite Hospital Association.* Bloomington, Ill.: The Association, 1979.

Faragher, John Mack. *Sugar Creek: Life on the Illinois Prairie.* New Haven: Yale University Press, 1986.

Farrell, James J. *Inventing the American Way of Death, 1830–1920.* Philadelphia: Temple University Press, 1980.

Ferguson, Corlin R., "The McLean County Poor Farm," unpublished ms., Bloomington, Ill.: McLean County Historical Society, 1995.

———. "Willow Bark Institute," unpublished ms., Bloomington, Illinois: McLean County Historical Society, 1995.

Fissell, Mary E. "Making Meaning from the Margins: The New Cultural History of Medicine." In *Locating Medical History: The Stories and their Meanings,* edited by Frank Huisman and John Harley Warner, 364–89. Baltimore: The Johns Hopkins University Press, 2004.

Fox, Daniel. *Power and Illness: The Failure and Future of American Health Policy.* Berkeley: University of California Press, 1993.

Gegel, Brian T. "Formation and the First Fifty Years of the 6th District Illinois Nurses' Association," unpublished paper, Bloomington, Ill.: Illinois Wesleyan University, 1992.

Gevitz, Norman. *The D.O.s: Osteopathic Medicine in America.* Baltimore: Johns Hopkins University Press, 1982.

Giles, Judy. *Women, Identity, and Private Life in Britain, 1900–50.* New York: St. Martin's Press, 1995.

Hasbrouck, Jacob L. *History of McLean County Illinois,* vol. 1. Topeka: Historical Publishing Company, 1924.

Hatty, Suzanne E., and James Hatty. *The Disordered Body: Epidemic Disease and Cultural Transformation.* Albany: State University of New York Press, 1999.

Hays, J. N. *The Burdens of Disease: Epidemics and Human Response in Western History.* New Brunswick, N.J.: Rutgers University Press, 1998.

Hine, Darlene Clark. *Black Women in White: Racial Conflict and Cooperation in the Nursing Profession, 1890–1950.* Bloomington: Indiana University Press, 1989.

Historical Statistics of the United States, Colonial Times to 1970, Part 1. Bureau of the Census, 1975.

The History of McLean County, Illinois. Chicago: Wm. LeBaron, 1879.

Hohnenberg, Paul M., and Lynn Hollen Lees, *The Making of Urban Europe 1000–1950.* Cambridge, Mass.: Harvard University Press, 1985

Howell, Joel D. *Technology in the Hospital: Transforming Patient Care in the Early Twentieth Century.* Baltimore: Johns Hopkins University Press, 1995.

Humphreys, Margaret. "Whose Body? Which Disease? Studying Malaria while Treating Neurosyphilis." In *Useful Bodies: Humans in the Service of Medical Science in the Twentieth Century,* edited by Jordan Goodman, Anthony McElligott, and Lara Marks, 53–77. Baltimore: Johns Hopkins University Press, 2003.

Illich, Ivan. *Medical Nemesis.* New York: Pantheon, 1976.

The Illinois Fact Book and Historical Almanac 1673–1968. Carbondale, Ill.: Southern Illinois University Press, 1970.

Ingalls, Marlin Ray. "The Espy Pharmacy Records." Master's thesis, Illinois State University, 1986.

Jackson, Charles O. "Death Shall Have No Dominion: The Passing of the World of the Dead in America." In *Death and Dying: Views From Many Cultures,* edited by Richard A. Kalish, 47–55. New York: Baywood Publishing, 1980.

Jones, James Howard. *Bad Blood: The Tuskegee Syphilis Experiment.* New York: Free Press,1993.

Jordanova, Ludmilla. "The Social Construction of Medical Knowledge." In *Locating Medical History: The Stories and their Meanings,* edited by Frank Husman and John Harley Warner, 338–63. Baltimore: The Johns Hopkins University Press, 2004.

Lawrence, Susan C. "Iowa Physicians: Legitimacy, Institutions, and the Practice of Medicine. Part One: Establishing a Professional Identity, 1833–1886," *The Annals of Iowa,* 62 (Spring 2003): 151–200.

Leavitt, Judith Walzer. *Brought to Bed: Childbearing in America, 1750–1950.* New York: Oxford University Press, 1986.

————. *The Healthiest City: Milwaukee and the Politics of Health Reform.* Princeton: Princeton University Press, 1982.

————. *Typhoid Mary: Captive to the Public's Health.* Boston: Beacon Press, 1996.

Lewis, Jane. *The Politics of Motherhood: Child and Maternal Welfare in England, 1900–1930.* London: Croom Helm, 1980.

Lindenbaum, Shirley, and Margaret Lock, eds. *Knowledge, Power, and Practice: The Anthropology of Medicine and Everyday Life.* Berkeley: University of California Press, 1993.

Livingston, A. Edward. *A History of the Practice of Medicine in McLean County Illinois, 1930–1980.* Bloomington, Ill.: Privately published, 1989.

Loustaunau, Martha O., and Elisa J. Sobo. *The Cultural Context of Health, Illness, and Medicine.* Westport, Conn.: Bergin and Garvey, 1997.

Ludmerer, Kenneth M. *Time to Heal: American Medical Education from the Turn of the Century to the Era of Managed Care.* New York: Oxford University Press, 1999.

Lupton, Deborah. *Medicine as Culture: Illness, Disease and the Body in Western Societies.* Thousand Oaks, Calif.: Sage, 1994.

Lynaugh, Joan E. *The Community Hospitals of Kansas City, Missouri, 1870–1915.* New York: Garland, 1989.

————. "From Respectable Domesticity to Medical Efficiency: The Changing Kansas City Hospital, 1875–1920." In *The American General Hospital: Communities and Social Contexts,* edited by Diana Elizabeth Long and Janet Golden, 22–39. Ithaca: Cornell University Press, 1989.

Madison, Donald L. "Preserving Individualism in the Organizational Society: 'Cooperation' and American Medical Practice, 1900–1920." *Bulletin of the History of Medicine,* 70, no. 3 (1996): 442–83.

Mahoney, Timothy R., "The Small City in American History," *Indiana Magazine of History* 99 (2003): 311–30.

Matejka, Michael G., and Greg Koos, eds. *Bloomington's C&A Shops: Our Lives Remembered.* Bloomington, Ill.: McLean County Historical Society, 1987.

McKeown, Thomas. *The Modern Rise of Population.* London: Edward Arnold, 1976.

Melosh, Barbara. *The Physician's Hand: Work Culture and Conflict in American Nursing.* Philadelphia: Temple University Press, 1982.

Mennonite Hospital School of Nursing: The Passing of the Flame, a Commemorative History, 1919–1985. Bloomington, Ill.: Mennonite College of Nursing, 1985.

Mitford, Jessica. *The American Way of Death.* New York: Fawcett World Library, Crest Books, 1963.

Morantz-Sanchez, Regina Markell. *Sympathy and Science: Women Physicians in American Medicine.* New York: Oxford University Press, 1985.

Muirhead, John W. *A History of African-Americans in McLean County, Illinois, 1835–1975.* Bloomington, Ill.: The Bloomington-Normal Black History Project, 1998.

Musser, Lori Ann, "Nursing Education at Illinois Wesleyan University: 1923 to 1976," unpublished paper, Bloomington, Ill.: Illinois Wesleyan University, [1976?].

Numbers, Ronald L., and Judith Walzer Leavitt. *Wisconsin Medicine: Historical Perspectives.* Madison: University of Wisconsin Press, 1981.

Oakley, Ann. *The Captured Womb: A History of the Medical Care of Pregnant Women.* Oxford: Basil Blackwell,1986.

O'Hara, Leo J. *An Emerging Profession: Philadelphia Doctors, 1860–1900.* New York: Garland Publishing, 1989.

Ott, Katherine. *Fevered Lives: Tuberculosis in American Culture since 1870.* Cambridge, Mass.: Harvard University Press, 1996.

Oyer, R. L. *Of Doctors and Sickness in Chenoa: A Historical Perspective.* Chenoa, Ill.: Chenoa Historical Society, June 1992.

Pieperbeck, Sister Mary Ludgera. "A History of the Development of Nursing Education in the Community of the Sisters of the Third Order of Saint Francis, Peoria, Illinois." Ph.D. diss., Loyola University of Chicago, 1990.

Portelli, Alessandro. *The Battle of Valle Giulia: Oral History and the Art of Dialogue.* Madison: University of Wisconsin Press, 1997.

———. "What Makes Oral History Different?" In *The Oral History Reader,* edited by Robert Perks and Alistair Thomson, 63–74. London: Routledge, 1998.

Porter, Dorothy. *Health, Civilization and the State: A History of Public Health from Ancient to Modern Times.* London: Routledge, 1999.

Porter, Roy. *The Greatest Benefit to Mankind: A Medical History of Humanity.* New York: Norton,1997.

———, ed. *Patients and Practitioners: Lay Perceptions of Medicine in Pre-industrial Society.* Cambridge: Cambridge University Press, 1985.

Practice and Progress: Medical Care in Central Illinois at the Turn of the Century. Springfield, Ill.: The Pearson Museum, Department of Medical Humanities, Southern Illinois School of Medicine, 1994.

Pratt, Mildred, ed. *We the People Tell Our Story.* Normal, Ill.: Bloomington-Normal Black History Project, Illinois State University, no date.

Rawlings, Isaac D. *The Rise and Fall of Disease in Illinois.* 2 vols. Springfield, Ill.: The State Department of Public Health, 1927.

Reagan, Leslie. *When Abortion Was a Crime: Women, Medicine, and the Law in the United States, 1867–1973.* Berkeley: University of California Press, 1997.

Reverby, Susan M. *Ordered to Care: The Dilemma of American Nursing, 1850–1945.* Cambridge: Cambridge University Press, 1987.

Risse, Guenter B., Ronald L. Numbers, and Judith Walzer Leavitt, eds. *Medicine without Doctors: Home Health Care in American History.* New York: Science History Publications, 1977.

Roberts, Elizabeth. *A Woman's Place: An Oral History of Working-Class Women, 1890–1940.* Oxford: Blackwell, 1984.

———. *Women and Families: An Oral History, 1940–1970.* Oxford: Blackwell, 1995.

Rogers, Naomi. "Germs with Legs: Flies, Disease, and the New Public Health," *Bulletin of the History of Medicine,* 63 (1989): 599–617.

Rosen, George. *A History of Public Health.* New York: MD Publications, 1958.

———. *The Structure of American Medical Practice 1875–1941.* Philadelphia, Pennsylvania: University of Pennsylvania Press, 1983.

Rosenberg, Charles E. *The Care of Strangers: The Rise of America's Hospital System.* New York: Basic Books, 1987.

———. *The Cholera Years: The United States in 1832, 1849 and 1866.* Chicago: University of Chicago Press, 1962.

———. "Community and Communities: The Evolution of the American Hospital." In *The American General Hospital: Communities and Social Contexts,* edited by Diana Elizabeth Long and Janet Golden, 3–17. Ithaca: Cornell University Press, 1989.

Rosner, David. "Doing Well or Doing Good: The Ambivalent Focus of Hospital Administration." In *The American General Hospital: Communities and Social Contexts,* edited by Diana Elizabeth Long and Janet Golden, 157–69. Ithaca: Cornell University Press, 1989.

Rothman, Sheila M. *Living in the Shadow of Death: Tuberculosis and the Social Experience of Illness in American History.* New York: Basic Books, 1994.

Rowe, Beverly J. *A Representative History of Local Hospital Development, Wadley Hospital, Texarkana.* Lewiston, N.Y.: Edwin Mellen Press, 2002.

Sand, René. *The Advance to Social Medicine.* London: Staples Press, 1952.

Sandelowski, Margarete. *Devices and Desires: Gender, Technology and American Nursing.* Chapel Hill: University of North Carolina Press, 2000.

Seabrook, Jeremy. "The Apotheosis of the Market Economy: McLean County" Chap. 12 in *The Myth of the Market: Promises and Illusions.* Hartland Bideford, Devon: Green Books, 1990.

Shaw, Diane. "Review Essay: Small Towns and Nineteenth-Century Urbanization," *Journal of Urban History,* 28, no. 2 (2002): 220–30.

Shortland, Michael. *Medicine and Film: A Checklist, Survey and Research Resource.* Oxford: Wellcome Unit for the History of Medicine, 1989.

Smith, Margaret Charles, and Linda Janet Holmes, *Listen to Me Good: The Life Story of an Alabama Midwife.* Columbus: Ohio State University Press, 1996.

Starr, Paul. *The Social Transformation of American Medicine.* New York: Basic Books, 1982.

Stevens, Rosemary. *In Sickness and in Wealth: American Hospitals in the Twentieth Century.* New York: Basic Books, 1989.

Stowe, Steven M. *Doctoring the South: Southern Physicians and Everyday Medicine in the Mid-Nineteenth Century.* Chapel Hill: University of North Carolina Press, 2004.

Strasser, Susan. *Never Done: A History of American Housework.* New York: Pantheon Books, 1982.

Summerfield, Penny. *Reconstructing Women's Wartime Lives: Discourse and Subjectivity in Oral Histories of the Second World War.* Manchester: Manchester University Press, 1998.

Sutcliffe, Jenny, and Nancy Duin. *A History of Medicine.* New York: Barnes and Noble, 1992.

Tate, H. Clay. *The Way It Was in McLean County 1972–1822.* Bloomington, Ill.: McLean County History '72 Association, 1972.

Teaford, Jon. C. *Cities of the Heartland: The Rise and Fall of the Industrial Midwest.* Bloomington: Indiana University Press, 1993.

Terrell, Suzanne J. *This Other Kind of Doctors: Traditional Medical Systems in Black Neighborhoods in Austin Texas.* New York: AMS Press, 1990.

Thompson, Paul. *The Voice of the Past: Oral History,* 2d ed. New York: Oxford University Press, 1988.

Tomes, Nancy. *The Gospel of Germs: Men, Women, and the Microbe in American Life.* Cambridge, Mass.: Harvard University Press, 1998.

Truax, Rhoda. *The Doctors Jacobi.* Boston: Little, Brown, 1954.

Turner, Bryan S. *Medical Power and Social Knowledge,* 2d ed. London: Sage, 1995.

Turner, Bryan S. *The Body and Society.* Oxford: Basil Blackwell, 1984.

Valencius, Conevery Bolton. *The Health of the Country: How American Settlers Understood Themselves and Their Land.* New York: Basic Books, 2002.

Viner, Russell. "Abraham Jacobi and German Medical Radicalism in Antebellum New York," *Bulletin of the History of Medicine* 72, no. 3 (1998): 434–63.

Vogel, Morris J. *The Invention of the Modern Hospital.* Chicago: University of Chicago Press, 1979.

Walitschek, David A. "Historic Archaeological Investigations at the Reuben Benjamin House." Master's thesis, Illinois State University, 1988.

Walters, Karen A. "McLean County and the Influenza Epidemic of 1918–1919," (unpublished paper, Illinois State University, 1980).

Ward, Thomas J. *Black Physicians in the Jim Crow South.* Fayetteville: University of Arkansas Press, 2003.

Warner, John Harley. *The Therapeutic Perspective: Medical Practice, Knowledge, and Identity in America, 1820–1885,* 2d ed. Princeton, N.J.: Princeton University Press, 1997.

Watson, Wilbur H. *Against the Odds: Blacks in the Profession of Medicine in the United States.* New Brunswick: Transaction Publishers, 1999.

Wertz, R. W., and D. C. Wertz. *Lying-In: A History of Childbirth in America.* New York: The Free Press, 1977.

Whorton, James C. *Inner Hygiene: Constipation and the Pursuit of Health in Modern Society.* Oxford: Oxford University Press, 2000.

Wohl, Anthony S. *Endangered Lives: Public Health in Victorian Britain.* London: J. M. Dent, 1983.

Worboys, Michael. *Spreading Germs: Disease Theories and Medical Practice in Britain, 1865–1900.* Cambridge: Cambridge University Press, 2000.

Young, James Harvey. "Patent Medicines and the Self-Help Syndrome." In *Medicine Without Doctors: Home Health Care in American History,* edited by Guenter B. Risse, Ronald L. Numbers, and Judith Walzer Leavitt, 95–116. New York: Science History Publications, 1977.

Index

Abel, Emily, 26; *Hearts of Wisdom,* x–xi
abortion, 78, 121, 159, 170–71, 189
adoption, 171, 220n158
African Americans: as doctors, 82, 172–73;
health care for, 95, 151, 171–74, 188; health
outcomes among, 188; home remedies/
informal health authorities among, 151;
as hospital patients, 27; in the McLean
County Medical Society, 78–79; mortality
rates among, 188; as nurses, 70–71, 172;
perspectives on ill health and medical
care, 144–45, 150; population of, 3, 171–72;
poverty among, 174; racial discrimination
against/segregation of, 121, 172, 174; white
undertakers' discrimination against, 176
Agatha, Sr., 24
ague, 4–5
AIDS, 125
Allin, James, 2–3
Allman, Grace, 191; on childbirth, 162, 165;
on death practices, 174–75, 177; healthy
childhood of, 137–38; on home remedies,
151; on influenza deaths in husband's
family, 141; relationship with her doctor,
155–56
allopaths. *See* doctors
alternative medical practitioners. *See* irregular medical practitioners
Alton and Sangamon. *See* Chicago and Alton Railroad Company
AMA (American Medical Association), 75,
82, 209n9

American College of Surgeons, 107, 213n147
American Medical Association (AMA), 75,
82, 209n9
Ames, Cherry (fictional nurse), 48, 206n19
Anderson, Dr., 20
Anderson, S. T., 76
antibiotics, 41, 85, 100, 186, 216n17
appendectomy, 54, 79
Armstrong, David, 10–11
Arrowsmith community hospital (Illinois),
24, 203n67
asafetida, 150, 186, 218n58
Assessment 2000, 188–89
Augustina, Sr., ix–x, 22, 30

Baby Fold (Normal), 220n158
Baker, Mrs. Charles, 20
Baker, Seth, 12
Barnes, A. T., 31
Barton, Sue (fictional nurse), 48, 206n19
Bath, T. W., 79
Beier, Lucinda McCray: *A Matter of Life and
Death,* xii
Bennett, Stella Reiner, 65, 208n102
Bennett Medical College of Eclectic Medi-
cine and Surgery, 83
Bevier, Isabel, 122
Bigelow's Kickapoo Indian Shows, 14,
200n94
biomedicine: critique of, 116; as a cultural
product, x–xi; expectations of, 186–87; lay
health culture pervaded by, 159–60, 177,

186; limitations of, 177, 190; as unalloyed good, xi

birth. *See* childbirth

birth control/family planning, 108, 169–70

birth defects, 217n20

Bismarck, Otto von, ix

blacks. *See* African Americans

Bloomington (Illinois): African American population of, 171; as a central place, 3–4; coal in, 9, 199n65; economy of, 180; incorporation of, 1; livestock ordinance in, ix; paving in, ix, 8, 128; population growth/distribution in, 3, 3 (table); public health initiatives in, 128; public works built in, 10–11; sewage system and water supply in, ix, 8–10, 21, 128–29, 183, 215n62; wells in, 9, 80, 215n62

Bloomington and Normal Sanitary District, 128

Bloomington Health Committee/Department, 10–11, 81, 129, 183

Bloomington-Normal Black History Project, xiv, 136

Boon, Loren: anesthesia training of, 104; career choice of, 87; general practice of, 108–9; on house calls, 102; on malpractice suits, 114–15, 191; medical training of, 89; on need for hospital care, 147–48; professional relationships of, 98; rural practice of, 84, 85 (table); as a specialist, 96

Bostic, Marie, 138, 142, 153, 169, 175–76, 191

Boyd, Ben, 118, 121, 130–34, 191

Boyle, Dr., 77

Boylston, Helen Dore, 206n19

Brett, Mrs., 120

Brian, Clara R., 123–27, 215n48

Brokaw Hospital (*formerly* Deaconess Hospital; Bloomington): African American patients/employees at, 174; charity mission of, 24; doctors associated with, 30; fees collected by, 25; founding of, 24; home care model in, 33, 203n66; home for life offered by, 33; management of, 36; merger with Mennonite Hospital, 43 (*see also* BroMenn Healthcare); School for Nurses, 34, 36, 44–45, 50, 52, 59–61, 204n68; surgeons/surgery at, 37–38, 204n87

BroMenn Healthcare (*formerly* Brokaw, Mennonite and Eureka Hospitals; Bloomington), 43, 188

brucellosis (undulant fever), 145–46

Bull, E. Martha, 98–99

Burnham, John, 73

burns, 148, 175

Burr, L. A., 78, 210n29

Calico, Matilda, 191

cancer, 22, 28–29, 31, 147, 157–58, 175

Carle Clinic, 188

Carpenter, Ruth, 191; background/oral history of, 46, 47 (table); car accident suffered by, 149–50, 161; on disinfection, 142; on family planning, 169; on father's aversion to doctors, 154; on fear of infectious diseases, 141; on home births, 165; on home remedies, 151–52; on maternal deaths after childbirth, 166; on newborns, 167; nurse training of, 50, 52–55, 57, 59–61; nursing career of, 63, 66, 121, 214n18; on patent medicines, 153; pregnancy/childbirth of, 166; on purging, 150; on vaccinations, 138

Catholic hospitals, 24–25, 35, 202n19. *See also individual hospitals*

charitable hospitals, 24–25, 29–30, 34–35

Cherry, Ethel, 138, 152, 155, 191

Chicago and Alton Railroad Company (*formerly* Alton and Sangamon; McLean County), 1–2, 82, 198n44, 210–11n56

Chicago Tuberculosis Institute, 119

childbirth: with anesthetics, 94, 163, 165–68; by caesarian section, 163, 166–67, 181; changing expectations/management of, 94, 155, 163–64, 168, 187, 219n124; as dangerous/pathological, 38–39, 166, 182; with episiotomy, 38, 163, 167; with forceps, 38, 163, 204n92; at home, 15–16, 38, 42, 88, 94–95, 102, 160, 162–65, 180–81; in hospitals, 38–39, 42, 94–95, 102, 160, 162–63, 166–67, 204n92; husbands present during, 41, 167–68; lying-in period after, 16, 166–67; maternal death after, 16, 155, 166; midwives for, 15–16, 164, 219n124; natural, 168; newborns kept with mother, 167; patient fees for, 42–44, 162–63; stillbirth, 16, 166

chiropractors, 77

cholera, 5

Christian Science, 77

Christmas Seals, 119–21

Clover Lawn (McLean County), 10

coal, 9, 199n65

Coleman, J. W., 7

Comstock Law, 169
condoms, 169
consumption. *See* tuberculosis
contagious diseases. *See* infectious/contagious diseases *and specific diseases*
contraceptives. *See* birth control/family planning
cookbooks, home remedies in, 12–13
Cooperative Extension Service Home Bureau, xviii, 118, 122–28, 214–15n29, 215n32
cough-syrup recipes, 15, 151, 153
Country Life movement, 122
Covington, E. G., 78–79
Cromwell, William, 18, 200n111
Curry, Bernice, 120
Curry, Lynne, 118, 124, 215n41

Daily Pantagraph, 143
Davis, David, 2, 10
Davis, Sarah, 10, 217n23
Dawson, Aunt Ann, 12
Deaconess Hospital. *See* Brokaw Hospital
Dean, Katherine, 191
death: after childbirth, 16, 155, 166; from disease, 5–7, 21, 119, 121, 139, 141, 144, 174–77, 198n41, 198n44, 214n6; at home, 175–76; infant mortality, 7, 21, 117, 188, 198n51; mortality rate at hospitals, 31; preventable vs. inevitable, 31
DeLee, Joseph, 38, 204n92
Deneen, Frank, 83
dentists, 86, 93, 130–31, 173–74, 189
diarrheal diseases, 5–7
Dickens, Charles, 4
diet, 127, 150
Dillman, W. L., 85 (table), 86, 93, 118, 130–31, 191
diphtheria, 5–6, 81, 87, 139–41
diseases. *See* infectious/contagious diseases *and specific diseases*
doctors, 73–116; advertising by, 75, 100, 209n12; African American, 78, 82, 172–73; age of, 17–18, 89, 107, 110, 112–13; authority of, 82, 84, 99, 113, 115–16, 156–57, 159–60, 168, 184–85; birth control information from, 169–70; career choices of, 85–88, 112; changing roles/reputations/expectations of, 17–18, 73, 115–16, 157–58, 185–87; competence of, 110; contract practice, 82, 210–11n56; critique of, 116; doctor-nurse relationship, 58, 63, 69–70, 108–9; doctor-patient relationship, 74, 82, 86–87, 89, 94,

113–16, 133, 153–60, 168, 183, 185, 187; education/training of, 18, 30, 82–83, 87–97; before 1880, 16–21; fees charged by, 19–20, 42–43, 75, 78, 82, 107, 110–12, 160–62, 187; fee splitting by, 107, 213n147; female, 78, 82, 92, 98–99; focus on, xi; general practitioners vs. specialists, xviii, 34, 40, 74, 85, 96–97, 102, 104–9, 111, 113–14, 156–57, 185; going into practice, 97–104; and hospitals, 29–34, 39–40, 93–94, 102, 181; house calls by, 18–20, 62, 83–84, 88, 99–103, 112, 183; income/status of, xviii, 39, 85, 89, 107–8, 110–13; internships for, 95–96; Jewish, 82; licensing of, 74–75, 82; malpractice litigation against, xviii, 74, 79, 81, 85, 114–15, 168, 187; media representation of, 116, 182, 187; military, 157–58; military service by, 96; number of, 18, 21, 99–100; office practice, xviii, 19, 74, 84, 87, 97, 99–104, 183; oral histories of, 84–85, 85 (table); and organized medicine (*see* McLean County Medical Society); paperwork for, 68–69, 81; professionalization of, 73–74; professional relationships of, 97–98, 100, 103–10, 183; and public health, 11, 75, 79–81, 132–34, 141, 155, 186; ratio to patients, 99–100, 200n110; rural, 84, 98–102; specialists, 37, 39–40, 84, 104–5, 111, 183, 185 (*see also individual specialties*); substance abuse by, 110; therapeutic approaches of, 19–20, 84, 144; urban, 111, 183, 212n118; work environment of, 20, 74, 83–84, 86, 99. *See also under* McLean County, nineteenth-century; surgery/surgeons
Dolan, Jim and Archie, 29
domestic science. *See* home economics
Douglas, Stephen, 2
Duff, John, 141
Duis, E., 196–97n1
dysentery, 7

Ebo, Betty, 70–71
Elder, William, 30–31
empyema, 41, 205n107
Erlich, Paul, 139
erysipelas, 5, 63
Esposito, Margaret, 191; childbirth of, 166–67; on grandmother's nursing care, 147; as home bureau adviser, 118, 127–28; on home remedies, 152–53; husband's lung cancer, 157–58, 161; husband's presence during childbirth of, 41, 167–68;

on maternal deaths after childbirth, 166; *Places of Pride*, 126, 215n48

Espy, Dr., 17, 19, 200n107

Espy, John E., 200n107

Essig, Maude F., 36, 56–57, 66, 204n68

Eureka Hospital. *See* BroMenn Healthcare

Ewing, Mrs. Spencer, 122

Fairview Tuberculosis Sanitarium (Normal), xviii, 120–21, 125, 139, 145, 174, 210n49, 214n18, 214n24

Faragher, John Mack, 15, 199n56

Fell, Jesse, 2

Fell, Kersey H., 2

Ferguson, Martha, 42, 138, 141–42, 150, 152, 154–55, 160–61, 166, 176–77, 191

fevers/fever therapy, 4–5, 145–46, 217n45

Finfgeld, Mary, 142, 145–46, 169, 192

Finfgeld, Ray, 143–44

Finfgeld, Richard, 192; on brother's infection, 143–44; on family planning, 169; on female doctors, 98–99; on Lexington doctors, 101; on medical bills, 160–61; on nurses, 72; treated for broken leg, 37, 148

Flanagan, Rosie, 22

Flexner Report, 82, 89

flies, 80, 124

flu. *See* influenza

fluoridated drinking water, 130–31, 184, 186

4-H Clubs, 124–25

Fox, A. L., 76

Frances, Reverend Mother, ix–x, 30

Fuller, Dr., 24, 210n26

funerals, 175–76

Gailey, Watson, 37

General Electric, 161

German Measles (rubella), 140, 217n20

germ theory of disease, x, 7–8, 31, 80, 117–18, 122, 134–35, 182, 185

G.I. Bill, 90–92

Girls' Industrial Home (Bloomington), 125

Glackin Act, 120

Godfrey, F. H., 82

Goffman, Erving, 57

goiter, 104

Goldmark Report, 45

gonorrhea, 133–34, 139

The Gospel of Germs (Tomes), x–xi

Gray, Elias W., 10

Greenwood, Hiram, 10–11

Gregg, Norman McAlister, 217n20

Guthrie, William E., 84, 210–11n56

Haines, Dr., 20

Hasbrouck, Jacob, 77

Hatcher, W. B., 78–79

Hawks, Joseph P., 84

Healey's Kickapoo Indian Shows, 14, 200n94

health culture, 21, 179–80, 186–87; definition of, x; and doctors, xii, 74, 89, 114–16, 157, 184; and hospitalization, 36, 42–43, 111, 182; and ideas about cause of disease, 7; and lay people, 12, 115, 136–37, 149–51, 157, 159, 167–68, 177; and nurses, 72, 182; and oral history evidence, xv; and public health, 128–29, 134–35; and women, 12, 89, 184

hearing testing, 129

Hearts of Wisdom (Abel), x–xi

Hendrix, Aunt Jane, 12

Hensley, Ferne, 144, 192

herb lore, 11, 14, 150

Hill, William, 74, 76, 81

Hill-Burton legislation, 42–43

Hinkle Pill, 153

Holman, Roberta, 192; background/oral history of, 47 (table); on the doctor-nurse relationship, 70; husband's TB, 143, 161; nurse training of, 52, 54–55, 59; nursing career of, 48, 64, 68, 71

home care, 11–12, 21, 122, 147, 181; and childbearing, 15–16; and doctors, 19, 154; and hospitals, 25, 37, 149–50; and infectious diseases, 139, 142, 144–45; and injuries, 148; and remedies, 13–15, 150; and women, 11–12, 153, 184, 190

Home Care of Communicable Diseases (John Hancock Mutual Life Insurance Company), 140

The Home Cook Book of Chicago, 12–13

home economics, 122–28, 214–15n29

Home Improvement Association (McLean County), 122–23

home medical reference books, 12–13

homeopaths, 24, 29, 76–77, 119

home remedies, 11–15, 150–53, 200n90, 218n58

Hoover, Noble and Esther, 35–36

hospitals, xvii, 22–43; admissions to, 26–29, 38, 106, 111, 146, 149, 182; anxiety about

using, 25, 182; and care for African Americans, 174; childbirth in, 26, 29, 38, 41, 204n92; doctors' relationship with, 29–34, 39–40, 102, 181; economy benefited by, 43; growth of, 41–42; home care model of, 22–26, 29, 32–34, 40–42, 203n66; vs. home treatment, 37; length of stay at, 29, 40–41, 111, 185; management of, 23, 30, 35–36, 40, 204n74; medical staff privileges at, 29–34, 39–40, 79, 84, 97, 101, 105, 107, 181; nurse training at (*see under* nursing); patient fees at, 25, 27, 28 (table); rivalries among, 106; rules at, 41, 49, 71, 167–68, 185; sanitary conditions/inspectors at, 31–32; scientific efficiency at, 36–43, 182; serious illnesses treated at, 146–48; serious injuries treated at, 149–50. *See also individual hospitals*
Howell, Joel D., 38
Hubbard, Silas, 14
humoral theory of disease causation, 6–7, 150
Hunter, Lavada, 144, 192
Huth, Agnes, 123
Hyndman, Eliza, 78, 80

Illich, Ivan: *Medical Nemesis,* 116
Illinois Central railroad, 1–2
Illinois Eye and Ear Infirmary (Chicago), 156–57
Illinois Graduate Nurse's Association, 45
Illinois Homeopathic Medical Association, 119
Illinois State Board of Health, 10, 119
Illinois State Medical Society, 10, 75, 119, 209n9
Illinois State Normal University (ISNU)/ Illinois State University (ISU), 2, 45, 172, 206n8
Illinois Wesleyan University, 45, 52
immigrants, 24–25, 27, 202n19
immunizations, 5, 130, 133, 135, 138, 146, 173, 186
Indianapolis General Hospital, 40–41
Indiana University, 93
infant mortality, 7, 21, 117, 188, 198n51
infectious/contagious diseases: deaths from, 5–7, 21, 81, 117, 119, 121, 139, 141, 198n41, 198n44, 214n6; disinfection following, 139, 142; families/communities affected by, 141–46; fear of, 141–42; incidence/ virulence of, 138–39; isolation for, 5, 8,
10–11, 117, 140; management of, 80–81, 140–41; prevention of, 117, 127, 138 (*see also* immunizations); quarantine for, 25, 139–42; sickroom precautions for, 140–41; spread of, 5–6, 80; tests for, 129. *See also specific diseases*
influenza, 86, 125, 139, 141–42, 144, 152, 214n6
informants, xiv–xvii, 136–37, 137 (table), 191–93. *See also individual informants*
injuries, 28, 31, 148–50, 152, 175
insurance, health, 85, 111–12, 161, 187, 189
insurance, malpractice, 114, 187
interviews. *See* informants
irregular medical practitioners, 21, 75–77, 80, 201n121
I.U.D.s, 169

Jackson, Marguerite, 192
Jacobi, Abraham, 7
Jenner, Edward, 5
John Hancock Mutual Life Insurance Company, 140, 216–17n19
Johnson, L. M., 24, 203n67
Joseph, Sr., 24
Judith, Sr., 47 (table), 48–49, 192
Justis, Lula, 36

Keeley Institute and Cure (Dwight, Ill.), 76, 201n16
Kelso, George and Annie, 24, 29, 77
Kelso Home Sanitarium (Bloomington): founding of, 24, 77; homelike atmosphere of, 36–37; on hospital vs. home births, 38; middle-/upper-class clientele of, 25–26, 29; nurse training at, 30, 34, 44; patient fees at, 25, 29; physician/nursing care at, 29–30; scientific efficiency at, 37
Kennedy, Beulah, 172
Keyes, Elizabeth Brent, 174
Kickapoo Indian Shows, 14, 200n94
Kickapoo tribe, 196–97n1
Knox College, 89
Koch, Robert, 5–6, 119

Lake Bloomington, 215n62
Lake Evergreen, 215n62
Lamaze classes, 168
Lampe, John L., 33
Lantz, Evelyn, 47, 47 (table), 49–52, 55–56, 59, 64–67, 69–71, 192

Larned, Ezra R., 80
laudanum, 153
laxatives, 7, 152
Lexington, 99, 101
life and death in the twentieth century,
136–77; abortion, 170–71; adoption, 171,
220n158; birth control/family planning,
169–70; childbearing, 39, 162–69, 219n124;
death/burial, 144, 174–77; doctor-patient
relationship, 113–15, 153–60; doctors' fees,
160–62, 187; health care and race, 171–74;
infections/people before World War II,
137–48, 216n17, 217n20, 217n45; informants' backgrounds, 136–37, 137 (table);
mutual aid, 144, 164, 175, 184. *See also
under* home care
life expectancy, 7, 117, 199n56
Lincoln, Abraham, 2
Little, Jehu, 80
livestock, xi, 9
Livingston, A. Edward, 88, 110, 112, 115
Loyola University, 83
Luce, A. H., 30
Ludovica, Sr., 22–23
Lupton, Deborah, xi
Lynaugh, Joan, 22, 26

Mahoney, Timothy, 3
Major, John M., 17–18
malaria, 4–5, 7
malpractice litigation, xviii, 79, 81, 85,
114–15, 168, 187
Mammen, Ernest, 79–80, 83–84
A Matter of Life and Death (Beier), xii
A Matter of Life and Death museum exhibit
(McLean County Historical Society), xii,
xiv
McCormick, Dr., 61
McHugh, Anne, 29
McLean County: agriculture in, 180; health-
culture research, ix–x, xii–xviii, 179–90;
health levels in, 188; household incomes
in, 188; population distribution in, xiii; as
representative, 179–80, 221n1
McLean County, nineteenth-century, xvii,
1–21; agriculture in, 1; doctors consulted
in, 16–18, 200n107; doctors/doctoring
before 1880 in, 18–21, 200n111, 201n121;
employment in, 2, 197n5; geography of,
1; health/illness in, 4–7, 198n32, 198n41,
198n44, 198n51, 199n56; home care in,
11–16, 180–81, 200n90; Native Americans

in, 196–97n1; political/business leaders
in, 2–3; population of, 2–3, 3 (table), 18;
public health/services in, 7–11, 117–35;
rural history of, xiii, 3, 24, 37–38, 84, 118,
123–24, 128, 179–80, 214n29; settlement/
industries of, 1–3, 196–97n1, 197n17; urban
history of, xiii, 1–4, 9, 118, 128, 179–80;
water sources in, 9
McLean County Anti-tuberculosis Society,
120–21
McLean County Coal Company, 199n65
McLean County Health Department: establishment of, 127, 130; funding for, 130;
size of, 132; testing/services by, 130–33;
venereal disease enforcement activities of,
133–34, 186
McLean County Historical Society, xii–xiv
McLean County Medical Society, 20–21,
74–84; on abortion, 78; admission of applicants to, 75–76; on advertising by doctors, 209n12; African American members
of, 78–79; and the AMA, 209n9; benefits
to members of, 79, 109; *Biographical History*, 76–77; and the Bloomington Health
Committee/Department, 11, 81; charter/
early members of, 20, 74; code of conduct
for members of, 75, 109; Committee on
Law, 76; competition fought by, 76–77;
and contract practice, 82; educational/
social activities at, 109; ethical image of,
78; female members of, 78; founding of,
2, 74; goals of, 75; and the Illinois State
Medical Society, 75, 209n9; on infectious-
disease management, 80–81; lectures at,
79–80; on malpractice cases, 81; medical
fees regulated by, 75, 82; osteopathy opposed by, 77; presidents of, 82–83; referral networks fostered by, 109; scientific/
technological innovations introduced at,
80; on tuberculosis, 81, 119–20; on water
supplies, 80
McLean County Nursing Home, 203n64
McLean County Poor Farm, 25, 33, 202n20,
203n64
measles, 6, 138, 142
Medicaid, 111–12, 189
medical fees. *See* doctors, fees charged by
Medical Nemesis (Illich), 116
Medical Practice Act, 10
medical schools: African Americans at, 82,
91; curriculum at, 89, 92–93; educational
requirements before attending, 89; Jews

at, 82; scholarships to, 90, 211n85; tuition
at, 89–90; urban locations of, 93–94;
women at, 82, 92
Medicare, 111–12, 131–32, 189
medicine shows, 14, 153, 200n94
Melosh, Barbara, 34, 54, 57, 204n72
Mennonite College of Nursing (Illinois State
University), 71, 206n8
Mennonite Hospital (Kelso Home Sanitarium; Bloomington): admissions increase at, 42; doctors associated with, 40;
founding of, 24; management of, 35–36;
merger with Brokaw Hospital, 43 (*see
also* BroMenn Healthcare); Nurses' Cadet
Corps, 66; nurse training at, 34, 44–45,
206n8; School of Nursing, 60, 71, 87; surgeries at, 38
mental/emotional illnesses, 19, 33, 188,
203n63
mercury, 13–14, 200n90, 216n17
Methodist Illinois Wesleyan University, 2
miasma theory of disease causation, 4–5, 8,
31, 117, 140
midwives, 15–16, 162, 164–65, 219n124
Miller, Jennie, 60
Minnick, Dr., 63
Moore, Dwight O., 11
mourning, 177
mustard plasters, 55, 144

narrators, xv
Noble, Harrison, 18, 200n111
Noble, Joseph Price, 83
Noble, R. A., 79
Normal (Illinois): African American population of, 171–72; incorporation of, 2;
paving in, 128; population growth/distri-
bution in, 3, 3 (table); sewage system and
water supply in, 128
Northwestern University Medical School, 83
nostrum, 14
nuns, ix–x, 22–25, 30, 32, 35, 44, 48–49, 56,
71, 109
Nurses' Cadet Program, 66–67
nursing, xvii–xviii, 44–72; African American nurses, 70–71, 172; after World War
II, 67–71; authority of nurses, 41, 49, 64,
71–72, 182; careers in, 44, 47–49, 61–68;
and the community, 71–72, 129–30; degree programs, 45, 49, 52–53, 57–58, 68,
206n8; demographic makeup of nurses,
34, 44–45, 70–71; diploma programs, 45,

52–53, 57–58, 61, 206n8; doctor-nurse
relationship, xvi, 58, 63, 69–70; in doctors'
offices, 101, 103; and gender, 44, 68, 70–71,
182; home, 15, 21, 165; hospital training of
nurses, 23, 30, 34–35, 40, 44–45, 50–61,
181–82, 203–4nn67–69, 204n72; idealized
images of, 48, 206n19; instructors in, 52,
57–59, 66; licensed nurses, 62; male nurses, 71; and marriage, 46, 59, 67; by nuns,
22–25, 32; oral histories of, 46–47, 47
(table), 50–51; paperwork in, 68–69; private duty, 35, 45–46, 61–65, 182; registered
nurses, 45–46, 61–63; school rules, 59–61;
schools for, 44, 48–61, 51 (table), 65,
204n69; social status of, 35, 44, 46, 48–49,
64, 182; specialization in, 69; staff nurses,
46, 63, 65–66, 182; stipends for students,
45, 56–57, 66; technology's effects on,
67–68; training/careers in McLean
County, 44–46, 206n8; uniforms/caps, 48,
50–52, 60, 64, 87; unqualified, 44; visiting
nurses, 120, 122; wages for nurses, 46, 56,
62–64, 66–67, 214n18

obstetricians, 38–39, 41, 105, 108, 159, 163,
166–67
Olney, Catherine, 13
Olney, Omen, 13, 19
Olney, Simon, 16–17
opiates, 20, 153
oral history, xiv–xvi, 46
Orendorff, John Berry, 12, 16–17, 19
organized medicine. *See* American Medical
Association; Illinois State Medical Society; McLean County Medical Society
Orth, James, 24
osteopathy, 24, 77, 210n24, 210n26
Our Bodies, Ourselves (Boston Women's
Health Book Collective), 116
outhouses (privies), 8–10, 129
Oyer, Russell, 192; on abortion, 170; career
choice of, 87; funding for education,
90–91; general practice of, 39, 108–9; in-
come/status of, 110–13; medical training
of, 89, 92–93, 95; on pregnancies out of
wedlock, 170; professional relationships
of, 105–6; on relationship with patients,
113–14; rural practice of, 84, 85 (table);
specialization considered by, 96

Parke, Charles Ross, 18, 30, 32–33
Parke, Dr., 23

Parkhurst, F. J., 201n16
Parsons, Dr., 17–18
pasteurization, 146, 186
patent medicines, 11–12, 14, 19–20, 75–76, 152–53
patients. *See* life and death in the twentieth century
penicillin, 54, 71, 140, 161–62, 216n17
Pennsylvania Society for the Prevention of Tuberculosis, 119
Pettit, J. W., 119–20
Philadelphia's public waterworks, 8–9
physicians. *See* doctors
Places of Pride (Esposito), 126, 215n48
pleurisy, 205n107
pneumonia, 40, 53, 55, 139, 153, 214n6
polio, 138–41, 143
poor people, 24–25, 27, 93–95, 112, 119, 128, 161, 188, 202n20, 202n31
Porter, Dorothy, 117, 196n27
Posey, Lucinda Brent, 79, 150–52, 174, 192
poultices, 15, 55, 144, 148, 151–52
pregnancy, 159–60, 162–63, 169–70, 187. *See also* childbirth
prevention. *See* public health services, infrastructure/services/enforcement
privies (outhouses), 8–10, 129
Progressive Era, 36, 75, 118, 122, 184
public health, 117–35; Cooperative Extension Service Home Bureau, 118, 122–28, 214–15n29, 215n32; Home Improvement Association, 122–23; infrastructure/services/enforcement, 127–34, 183–86, 215n62; issues, ix, 7, 10; overview of, xviii, 117–19; tuberculosis control, 119–22, 184
puerperal fever, 5
purging, 150

quacks. *See* irregular medical practitioners
"Quilts for Infants with AIDS" project, 125
quinine, 5, 20, 153

Raber, Daniel, 83
race and health care, 171–74
railroads, 1–3
Randolph, Mrs. Gardner, 12
rats, 124
Red Cross, 125
red precipitate (red oxide of mercury), 13, 200n90
Reverby, Susan M., 45, 67, 204n69

Richardson, James, 156
Rigby, Della, 77
Rittenhouse, Rebecca, 39, 157–58, 168–69, 192
Roberts, Elizabeth, xvi–xvii
Rockwell Salts, 20
Rogers, Naomi, 215n41
Rogers, Thomas P., 2, 19–20
Rohm, Linda, 42–43, 159–60, 162, 168–69, 192
Rosen, George, 73–74, 200n110
Rosenberg, Charles, 39
Rosner, David, 36
Rothmann, Mr., 22–23
rubella (German Measles), 140, 217n20
Rueger, Betty (*pseud.*), 164, 192
Rush Medical College, 83
Rust, Harriet, 192, 203n66

Salvarsan, 139, 216n17
Samuels, Josephine, 192
Sandelowski, Margarete, 46, 67, 72
sanitation. *See* Bloomington; public health
scarlet fever, 5–6, 71, 138–42, 155
Seabrook, Jeremy, 221n1
Shinall, Harold, 192; career choice of, 87; on health insurance, 161; medical training of, 89–92, 95; on number of patients with infections, 143; professional relationships of, 98, 106; relationship with patients, 100, 113–14; rural practice of, 84, 85 (table), 101–2; as a specialist, 96–97; specialization by, 104
Shultz, Gordon, 149
6th District of the Illinois State Association of Graduate Nurses, 45, 62
Sloan, Edwin Palmer, 37, 39–40, 84, 104
smallpox, 5, 8, 101, 138, 140–41, 198n32
Smith, Lee, 30, 79
Smith-Lever Act, 122, 214–15n29
Snyder, Marie, 144, 148, 153, 160–61, 192
Soldiers' Orphans' Home, 2, 30
Spencer, Ralph, 142, 148–50, 153–54, 175–76, 193
St. Joseph's Hospital (McLean County, Ill.): and abortion, 171; admissions records for, 26–27; African American patients at, 174; alcoholics admitted to, 27–28, 202n.34; charity mission of, 24, 27; discharges from, 29; doctor-nurse relationship at, 109; doctors associated with, 23–25, 30–

31; early capacity/growth of, 22–23; early patient demographics at, 26–27; farming/livestock at, 23; finances of, 23–24; first patient at, 22; founding of, ix, 30; home for life offered by, 27, 29, 33; homelike atmosphere of, 22–23, 32–33; length of stay at, 29; management of, 23, 30, 32, 35; mental/emotional illnesses treated at, 28, 33, 203n63; mortality rate at, 31; nuns' activities at, 23–25, 32; nurse training at, 44–45; Nursing School, 70–71; operating room built at, 32; outpatient treatment at, 146–47; patient fees at, 23, 25, 27, 28 (table); patients, 22–23, 25–29; polio treatment at, 139; reasons for admission to, 27–29, 28 (table), 202n33; student nurses at, 23

St. Mary's Infirmary (St. Louis), 71
Starr, Paul, 73–74, 112, 116
State Board of Health Act, 10
State Farm Insurance, 2, 197n5
Stevens, Rosemary, 38–39
Stevenson, Adlai, I, 2
Stevenson, Adlai, II, 2
Stevenson, Ed, 64, 98, 103
Stewart, Dorothy Jean, 165–66, 193
Still, Andrew, 210n24
Stowe, Steven M., 218n58
streptomycin, 145
suffering, contemporary experience of. *See* life and death in the twentieth century
sulfonamides, 139
surgery/surgeons, 12, 16, 26, 28–30, 32, 37–38, 54, 204n87; among pioneers, 12, 16, 92; in hospitals, 26, 28–30, 32, 84, 204n87; and medical specialization, 37–38, 107–8, 185; and Medicare, 111; and nurses, 54, 65–66, 69; and professional controversies, 79–80, 107; and surgical nurses, 65–66, 69
Sweeney, John, 30
Swift, Alice, 47, 47 (table), 49, 51–52, 59, 61, 68, 163–64, 192
syphilis, 139, 216n17

Tate, H. Clay, 197n17, 214n24
Taylor, Dr., 80
Taylor, James Branch, 75–76
TB. *See* tuberculosis
tetanus, 139
Theda, Reverend Mother, 24
Theobald, Paul, 193; on abortion, 170–71;

on adoption, 171; on birth control/family planning services, 169–70; on cost of penicillin, 161–62; on doctors' relationship with hospitals, 40; general practice of, 107–9; income/status of, 112–13; medical training of, 88, 90, 97; oral history of, 85 (table); practice established by, 102–4; professional relationships of, 105
Theonilla, Sr., 46–48, 47 (table), 53, 56, 61, 67–69, 109, 193
Theresa, Sr., 24
Third Order of the Sisters of St. Francis, ix, 34
Tillson, Mrs., 4
Tinsley, Jane, 193; background/oral history of, 47 (table); on the doctor-nurse relationship, 70; nurse training of, 41, 53–54, 56–58, 60; nursing career of, 48, 68, 71, 118, 131; on TB, 121
toilets, flush, 10, 129, 134
Tomes, Nancy: *The Gospel of Germs*, x–xi
tonsillectomies, 28–29, 38, 129–30, 181
tuberculosis: bacillus discovered, 5–6, 119, 144; control of, 81, 119–22, 144–45, 184, 210n49; deaths from, 5–6, 28, 31, 119, 121, 198n41, 214n6; decline in, 117, 121; employment affected by, 121, 143; as incurable, 16; lifestyes/decisions affected by, 91, 143–45; marriage affected by, 121; media attention on, 143; nurses for, 120–24; sanatoria for, 119–21, 145 (*see also* Fairview Tuberculosis Sanitarium); spread of, 5; tax support for sufferers, 121–22; therapies for, 5–6, 120–21, 145
typhoid, 5–6, 10, 80, 139–41, 198n44

undertakers, 176
undulant fever (brucellosis), 145–46
Union Auto Industrial Association, 65, 208n102
United States Department of Agriculture, 215n32
University of Illinois, 89–90, 92, 95, 122–23, 215n32
Unzicker, Kenneth, 71

vaccinations. *See* immunizations
Vandervort, Franklin, 80
Van Ness, Albert, 40–41, 85 (table), 87, 91–93, 95–98, 104–6, 111–12, 193
venereal disease enforcement, 133–34, 185
Veterans Administration, 161

Vinzent, Sr., 24
vision testing, 129

Waddell, Oscar, 172–73, 193
Waddell, Ruth, 193
Wagner, Sally, 46, 47 (table), 51, 53, 55, 57–58, 70, 168, 193
Wakefield, Cyrenius, 14, 76, 200n95
Wakefield, Homer, 75–76
Wakefield, Zera, 200n95
Walburga, Sr., 24
Washington, Caribel, 71, 144–47, 150–53, 160, 166, 172–75, 193
waste (animal and human) disposal, 8–10, 129, 184
water supplies, ix, 8–9, 80, 127–29, 183, 215n62
Weaver, Fanny, 26
Weismuller, Kath, 29
Welch, James, 39, 84, 85 (table), 86–89, 94, 96–97, 100–101, 193
Wellmerling, Herman, 37
wells, 8–9, 129, 215n62
Wells, Helen, 206n19
Whitaker, Oliver, 172
Whitaker, Reginald, 141, 143, 145, 150, 154–57, 172–73, 193

White, John L., 79
whooping cough, 6, 133, 138–39
Willow Bark Institute (Danvers, Ill.), 201n16
women: as consumers and household managers, 23, 201n9; as doctors, 82, 92, 98–99; home economics education for, 122–28, 214–15n29; as managers and home nurses, 11–13, 25, 44, 122, 141, 153–54, 184–85, 190; in the McLean County Medical Society, 78; pregnancy rate/fertility of, 15; as volunteers, 122–23, 125–26
Women's and Children's Hospital (Chicago), 92
World War I, 122
World War II, 66–71, 89–92, 95–96, 102, 104
Worrell, T. F., 30
Wunderlich, R., 30

X-rays, 36, 80, 97, 120–21

Yolton, Rhoda Galloway, 37, 78–79
Young, William M., 83
Young Women's Christian Association (YWCA), 125

LUCINDA McCRAY BEIER is a professor of history at Illinois State University. She is the author of *A Matter of Life and Death: Health, Illness, and Medicine in McLean County, 1830–1995*, *Sufferers and Healers: The Experience of Illness in Seventeenth-Century England*, and *For Their Own Good: The Transformation of English Working-Class Health Cultures, 1880–1970*.

The University of Illinois Press
is a founding member of the
Association of American University Presses.

———————————————————

Composed in 10.5/13 Adobe Minion Pro
by Jim Proefrock
at the University of Illinois Press
Manufactured by Cushing-Malloy, Inc.

University of Illinois Press
1325 South Oak Street
Champaign, IL 61820-6903
www.press.uillinois.edu